CONTENTS

Preface

The prediction in the preface to the first edition of this book published 7 years ago, that CT scans would probably never be available in small communities, has turned out to be very wrong. In fact, advances in computerized medical technology have been revolutionary. In most communities now, CT scans are not only readily available, but also considered routine in the evaluation of neurologic disorders. At the present time, magnetic resonance imaging (MRI) with its superb resolution of detail is the leading technological innovation for evaluating nervous system structural integrity, but is only available at the larger medical centers. However, considering the fate of our prediction regarding CT scans, it is possible that in half a dozen more years MRI scans will also be readily available throughout the country.

Also since the last edition, two diseases — Alzheimer's disease and the acquired immunodeficiency syndrome (AIDS) — have moved to the forefront of the health concerns of the general public. With our increasingly aged population, more and more cases of the progressive dementing disorder Alzheimer's disease are being recognized. With the greater public awareness of this devastating and untreatable condition, it is imperative that physicians not only recognize the clinical symptoms and provide patient counseling, but also identify treatable conditions with similar symptomatology. On the other hand, AIDS provides a much more difficult problem, since the causative viral agent is highly neurotropic and can produce a wide variety of symptoms related to this infection. In many respects this infection deserves the appellation once applied to syphilis infections — "the great imitator."

In this edition, we bid farewell to Dr Lee A Christoferson who was a valued collaborator in the first edition. Fortunately, his place has been amply filled by Dr Vasudeva Iyer as a new coauthor. We would also like to acknowledge the helpful comments of Mr Larry Burd and Drs Philip Becker, Jack Kerbeshian, and Ed Harder concerning several of the chapters.

Preface to the First Edition

This book was written to assist the primary care physician in diagnosing and managing the common, the treatable, and the emergency neurologic problems. No attempt was made in this text to write an exhaustive treatise of neurologic disease, to present neurologic pathophysiology, or to detail the diagnosis of rare, untreatable neurologic disorders. We believe that this book will enable primary care physicians to take a neurologic symptom and arrive at a neurologic diagnosis; this in turn will improve patient service and reduce referrals to tertiary care centers.

The content and philosophy of this manual was based on a paper by Dr T. J. Murray (Concepts in undergraduate teaching. *Clin Neurol Neurosurg* 1976; 79[4]:237-284) which addressed the issue of common neurologic complaints presenting to family physicians in Canada. Although 10% of all patients seen in family practice had neurologic complaints, only 2% received a "neurologic diagnosis." For example, the diagnosis of a patient whose major presenting problem is diabetic neuropathy instead of fluctuating blood sugar levels is still diabetes rather than peripheral neuropathy.

Dr Murray's list of primary care complaints is based on frequency of the problem, potential seriousness of the disease, and the effect of intervention on the outcome. Headache is included because it is a frequent complaint, although intervention is rarely a life-or-death matter. Infections of the nervous system are also included because, although they are relatively rare, they require immediate diagnosis and treatment. Our chapter headings closely follow Dr Murray's list.

Primary care physicians are forced by circumstances to see a large number of outpatients per day. There is often insufficient time to evaluate each patient's problem in depth. While it is an easy approach for the specialist in neurodiagnosis to advise the primary care physician to do a "complete history and neurologic examination," such advice is unrealistic. Therefore, we have prepared a symptom-oriented, problem-oriented manual, which falls short of complete neurologic diagnosis and treatment, but which should improve present patient care. The "minimum histories" and "minimum examinations" suggested in the text certainly do not define every patient's problem but have been developed to encourage a uniform, reasoned approach, which is more efficient and increases the probability of a correct diagnosis in the majority of cases. Specific diagnosis will assist in making appropriate referrals for special tests and treatment. Once a diagnosis is established, the primary care practitioner may refer to any one of a number of fine neurologic textbooks for a more detailed description of the disorder. In addition, selected references are listed at the end of each chapter.

A major problem in writing a text of this sort is a lack of uniformity of diagnostic resources available to the primary care physician. For example, the authors believe that most stroke victims need four-vessel cerebral angiography and computed tomographic (CT) scans for optimal care, but (1) angiography has its risks and should be undertaken only by a radiologist with considerable experience; and (2) it is unlikely that CT scans will be available in every community in this country. Therefore the use of these diagnostic procedures in establishing the diagnosis may be unrealistic in a particular community. A similar statement may be applied to other neurodiagnostic tests such as electromyography, electroencephalography, myelography, etc. Although we have no solutions, we have considerable empathy with the primary care physician faced with limited resources. In such situations we believe that this text will help the primary care physician to make an accurate diagnosis and to confidently make a clinical judgment regarding the need for further tests and appropriate treatment.

I

THE NEUROLOGIC EXAMINATION

Contrary to popular opinion, there is no "standard" neurologic examination. When we are requested to teach the neurologic examination, our response is "The neurologic examination of what? The ambulatory adult? The infant? The comatose patient?" A neurologic examination should be *problem-oriented*, and in reality there are different examinations for different clinical situations. Therefore we have included many of our suggestions for the neurologic examination under specific chapter headings. In most circumstances we suggest that common sense should prevail. For example, testing smell is of little help in the diagnosis of a primary muscle disease, and testing the anal wink is of little value in diagnosing the average patient with a headache. In essence, the neurologic examination is a process of gathering objective data for the hypotheses formed during the process of history taking.

THIS CHAPTER IS INTENDED TO PROVIDE HINTS ON THE MORE COMMONLY USED (AND ABUSED) PORTIONS OF THE NEURO-LOGIC EXAMINATION. IT IS NOT A COMPLETE GUIDE TO THE ENTIRE PROCEDURE.

Screening of Neurologic Abnormalities — Station and Gait

Table 1.1 outlines the procedure for station and gait testing, and Figure 1.1 illustrates the procedure. It usually can be performed in less than a minute. Table 1.2 emphasizes that virtually every aspect of the central and peripheral nervous system is tested. A patient with a normal station and gait is unlikely to have any serious structural neurologic abnormality. Twenty feet of straight walking space is desirable, and the patient should be barefooted and clothed only in underwear or a gown.

1

TABLE 1.1
Procedure for Station and Gait Testing

INSTRUCTIONS	THINGS TO NOTE
1. Walk the distance normally	Asymmetric arm swing, abnormal arm and hand postures, and instability of the trunk
2. Rapidly turn around and walk on tiptoes	Extra steps while turning around and inability to rise completely on the tips of the toes
3. Rapidly turn and walk on heels	Foot drop
4. Turn and walk with heels touching toes (tandem walk)	Instability characteristic of midline cerebellar lesions
5. Turn and "walk on outsides of feet like a bowlegged cowboy does" (walking on lateral aspects of feet)	This maneuver specifically brings out hemiplegic posturing of an arm from subtle or old upper motor neuron damage
6. Do a deep knee bend (preferably with hands on hips; if there is an obvious balance problem, patient may hold onto an object, such as a chair)	Loss of balance indicates cerebellar difficulties; inability to rise indicates proximal weakness
7. Stand with feet together, eyes closed, arms outstretched with palms facing ceiling and fingers spread apart	Increased swaying with eyes closed indicates either posterior column disease or a peripheral neuropathy; with subtle hemiparesis affected arm will pronate, while in more obvious hemiparesis the arm will pronate and then drift downward and outward.

By observing the station and gait, a skillful examiner can obtain in one minute a glimpse of mental status (how well the patient comprehends and follows instructions), upper motor neuron function (posturing of arms and gait), lower motor neuron function (muscle atrophy and weakness), muscle disease (proximal weakness), basal ganglia function (abnormal posture and movement), cerebellar function (balance and tandem walk), and the sensory system (poor

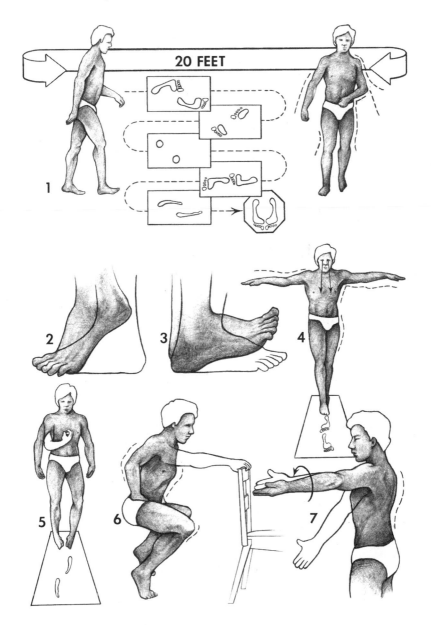

Figure 1.1 Testing of station and gait. Pay particular attention to arm swing, arm posture, body posture, instability while turning around, tendency to look at floor. See text for additional information.

TABLE 1.2
Possible Abnormalities of Station and Gait

Abnormal mentation: Patient follows directions poorly, slowly; needs examiner to demonstrate instructions; tendency to continue doing same task (perseveration)

Hemiplegia: Decreased arm swing on affected side, circumduction of leg, pronation of arms when held outstretched with palms up, flexion of arm when walking on sides of feet

Cerebellum: Unsteadiness when turning around, in tandem walking, and in deep knee bending

Sensation: Increased swaying when eyes are closed (positive Romberg test)

Muscle disease: Difficulty with deep knee bend, waddling gait

Basal ganglia: Abnormal postures and movement (eg, Parkinson's syndrome, Huntington's disease)

Lumbar disc: Inability to walk on heels or toes on one side; spinal list

Peripheral neuropathy: Bilateral foot drop; cannot walk on heels

---

balance with eyes closed — the Romberg test). A patient who can perform all the maneuvers normally will rarely have a significant neurologic abnormality. Abnormalities noted can be more specifically tested in the remainder of the neurologic examination. For example, if station and gait testing suggests a cerebellar abnormality, more specific cerebellar tests should be performed.

Deep Tendon Reflexes

The most difficult part of the neurologic examination to perform correctly (and one that medical students think is easiest) is the evaluation of deep tendon reflexes (Figures 1.2 — 1.5). If at all possible, have the patient undressed and sitting with legs dangling freely over the edge of the table. The reflex elicited will depend on:

1. Whether or not the tendon is struck
2. How hard the tendon is struck
3. How quickly the tendon is struck

To avoid striking an improper area, the tendon should first be palpated. The lightest tap that will still elicit the response should be given. A hammer with a relatively soft rubber end and a flexible handle will best allow the rapid, light tap. The examiner will most often find asymmetry of reflexes rather than gross hyperactivity or absence of reflexes. Reflexes may be normal, hyperactive or hypoactive, clonic or absent, or symmetric or asymmetric and should be recorded as such. Recording pluses, minuses, or whatever, unless carefully defined, do little to convey accurate information in the chart.

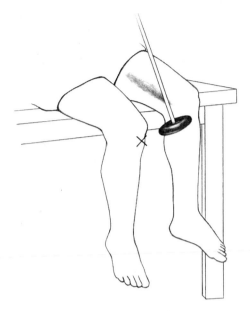

Figure 1.2 The patellar reflex: Note that legs do not touch the floor. The type of hammer illustrated was developed in England and is especially effective. Look not only for reflex contraction of the quadriceps but also contralateral contraction of the adductor muscle and the number of swings the leg makes. *Remember*: Dysfunction of either the afferent or efferent nerves may diminish the reflex.

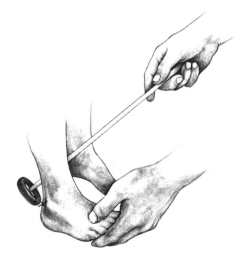

Figure 1.3 Achilles reflex: While striking the tendon, have the patient apply *light* pressure with the sole of his foot to the palm of the examiner.

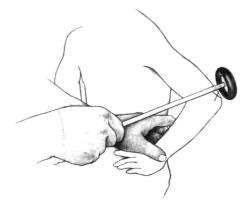

Figure 1.4 Triceps reflex: This reflex is most easily elicited when the patient rests his arms on his hips.

The Babinski Reflex

The Babinski reflex (Figure 1.6) is the eponym given to the plantar response, which may be present depending on:

1. Type of stimulation used
2. Rapidity with which the stimulus is delivered
3. The position of the patient

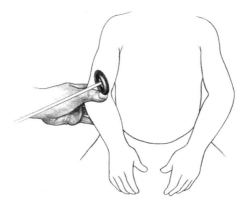

Figure 1.5 Biceps reflex: It is very important to have the arms symmetrically flexed and relaxed as illustrated.

A sharp object (safety pins or the sharpened ends of some hammers) will produce little more than a withdrawal response, while too light a touch will produce no response. We find a key to be the most readily available, appropriate stimulus. The key is used to stimulate the *lateral* aspect of the plantar surface of the foot, beginning at the heel and moving up to the ball of the foot but staying lateral to the great toe. Examples of some responses to plantar stimulation are shown in Table 1.3.

Because the abnormal response is such an important sign of nervous system disease, the best approach to recording the results, if in doubt, is to record exactly the observed movements. It is totally inadequate simply to say "Babinski absent." Of course he is — he died a half century ago.

Examination of the Optic Fundus

Examination of the optic fundus with the ophthalmoscope is the only opportunity the physician has to look directly at the brain, and it is imperative to do so on *every* patient with neurologic symptoms. This should be done even in difficult cases, such as a crying, hyperactive 4-year-old child. Mentally make a list of those parts of the fundus which must be seen to confirm the hypotheses formed during the history; for example, in the patient with suspected multiple sclerosis, look particularly for temporal pallor of the optic disc. Adjust the size of the beam to match the size of the pupil (too large a beam causes light to reflect from the iris). Using too bright a beam may cause excessive pupillary constriction. In general, use the brightest light possible that still allows visualization of the retina. Darkening the room may be helpful in certain difficult patients. Pupillary dilating agents are usually not necessary.

The Pharyngeal Reflex

The pharyngeal reflex (see Figure 1.7) should be tested on each side by stimulating the pharyngeal pillars with a cotton swab on an applicator. After observing the motor response (elevation of the palate), ask the patient if the sensation was the same on both sides of the pharynx. (Simply jamming a tongue depressor down the patient's throat not only gives very little neurologic information but is downright ungentlemanly.) Response is significant only if it is asymmetric; the normal gamut of responses runs from hyperactive to hypoactive.

Sensory Examination

The sensory examination under most clinical conditions does not produce objective, "hard" data because it involves subjective judgments by both the patient and the examiner. Beginning medical students are often fascinated by

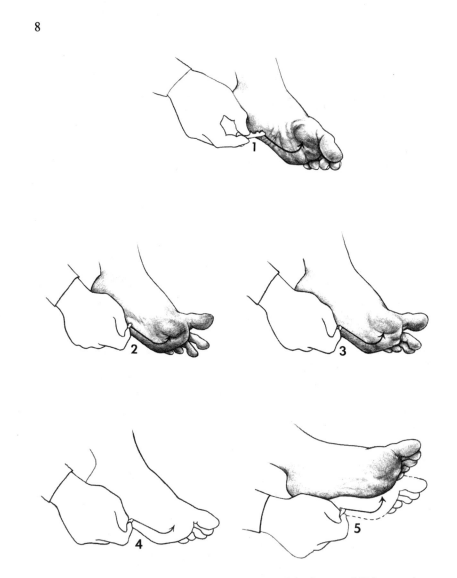

Figure 1.6 Plantar stimulation: Note that only two of the five possibilities constitute a ''positive Babinski.'' See text for additional information.

the sensory examination and spend an inordinate amount of time performing it. If pinprick, vibration, light touch, and position sensation are present in the feet and if the patient can recognize numbers written on the palms of the hands with eyes closed, a major sensory deficit in unlikely. On the other hand an intelligent, cooperative patient with a circumscribed sensory deficit, given a pin and a marking pencil, can often outline the deficit accurately. Likewise, when looking for a sensory level, have the patient run his or her own finger

TABLE 1.3
Responses to Plantar Stimulation

NAME	OBSERVATION	INTERPRETATION
1. Normal response (flexor plantar response)	First movement of great toe is flexion	Normal
2. Classic Babinski reflex (classic extensor plantar response)	Extension of great toe with extension and fanning of other toes	Most often seen in upper motor neuron lesions (above the L-5 spinal segment)
3. Babinski reflex (extensor plantar response)	First movement of great toe is extension (there may be subsequent flexion of great toes); other toes either show no movement or flexion	Seen in all types of upper motor neuron lesions (above the L-5 spinal segment)
4. Mute plantar response	Nothing happens	Severe sensory loss or paralysis of foot
5. Withdrawal	Patient pulls foot back	Often seen in metabolic neuropathies or if examiner uses excessively sharp object
6. Asymmetric response	Mute plantar response on one side and flexor plantar response on other side	Indication of need to look for other signs of neurologic disease

up the body until sensation changes. When a peripheral neuropathy is suspected, ask the patient to compare a single pinprick proximally (such as on the chest) with a single pinprick distally (such as on the foot). Use a hat pin and allow the shaft to slide through the finger in order to deliver a relatively quantitative response (see Figure 1.8). Simply comparing sharp and dull on the foot is inadequate. The examiner should attempt to quantitate any difference between the proximal and distal stimulation sites. For example, say, "If this [chest] pinprick is worth $100, how much is this [foot] pinprick worth?" and consider a response less than $75 as significant. A useful, objective sign

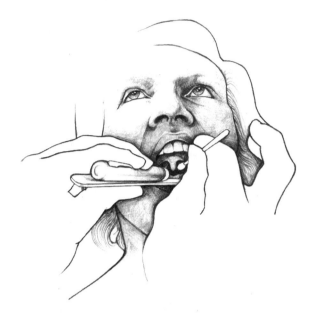

Figure 1.7 Pharyngeal reflex: Touch both sides of the posterior pharynx and watch for elevation of the palate. Ask the patient if the sensation on both sides is the same. In some patients, it may be necessary, as illustrated, to press down on the tongue by holding the tongue blade and flashlight in one hand.

of sensory loss is *summation*; that is, repeated quick pinpricks of the same intensity will suddenly become very painful and will result in the patient withdrawing the extremity and grimacing. Ordinarily, repeated pricking will not become more painful. This phenomenon is most frequently present in toxic metabolic peripheral neuropathies such as diabetic polyneuropathy.

Only when the examination basics — mental status, cranial nerves, reflexes, motor system, sensory system — have been thoroughly mastered are the "curiosities" and "toys" utilized. These include the Hoffmann reflex, optokinetic drums, etc. In specialized situations these may be useful but need not be routinely employed by the student or the time-pressed physician.

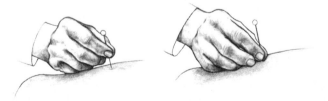

Figure 1.8 Testing sensation of pain: Grasp pin shaft and allow the pin to slide through the fingers until the pin makes contact with the skin. *Compare* a normal area (eg, chest) with a suspected area of involvement (eg, foot).

BIBLIOGRAPHY

Barrows H: *Neurologic Examination*. Division of Marketing Services, American Medical Association, 535 North Dearborn St, Chicago IL 60616, 1981 (videotape).

DeJong R: *The Neurologic Examination*. New York, Hoeber Medical Division, Harper & Row, 1967.

DeMyer W: *Technique of the Neurologic Examination, A Programmed Text*. New York, McGraw-Hill Book Co, 1980.

Goldberg S: Principles of neurologic localization. *Am Fam Physician* 1981; 23:131-141.

Mayo Clinic Foundation: *Clinical Examinations in Neurology*. Philadelphia, WB Saunders, 1981.

Van Allen M: *Pictorial Manual of Neurologic Tests*. Chicago, Year Book Medical Publishers, 1980.

II

NEURODIAGNOSTIC PROCEDURES

A well-elicited history and an adequate neurologic examination should enable the physician to form a provisional diagnosis. Such a diagnosis will include the probable site of the lesion and the probable type or etiology of the neurologic disorder. There will be a number of differential diagnoses, particularly with regard to the type of lesion and these can often be settled only by suitable investigative procedures. It is essential for the physician to have a clear idea regarding the indications as well as the specificity and sensitivity of the various procedures. The goal would be to put the patient through minimum discomfort (choosing the least invasive investigations) and obtain the most specific information that will point to the correct diagnosis. The neurodiagnostic procedures may not only be diagnostic but sometimes serve as prognostic indicators as well. In this chapter, brief descriptions of the common neurologic procedures will be given, along with their indications and side effects.

Lumbar Puncture

Lumbar puncture (LP) is perhaps the commonest neurodiagnostic procedure that a physician will be called upon to perform in person.

Indications

1. Suspected CNS infection (meningitis or encephalitis): CSF study should be done *without delay* when meningitis or encephalitis is suspected. *Caution*: If there are focal findings, such as a hemiplegia, or if there is papilledema, a CT scan is strongly recommended prior to the LP.

2. When subarachnoid hemorrhage is suspected: Most cases of subarachnoid hemorrhage can be diagnosed by CT scan alone. Lumbar puncture

is indicated more specifically in those patients in whom the CT is negative and a hemorrhage is still suspected on clinical grounds.

3. A lumbar puncture may be done in those patients in whom alterations in CSF biochemistry can be of diagnostic value: eg, Guillain-Barré syndrome (albuminocytologic dissociation), multiple sclerosis (oligoclonal bands and myelin basic protein, elevated gamma-globulin).

4. To determine CNS involvement in cases of leukemia and lymphoma (cytology).

5. When CNS syphilis is suspected.

6. To introduce contrast media or drugs into the spinal fluid.

7. Measurement of CSF pressure for the diagnosis and management of pseudotumor cerebri.

8. Repeated CSF removal is used for the management of increased intracranial pressure following neonatal intraventricular hemorrhage.

Contraindications

1. Local infection at the site of puncture (if CSF sample must be obtained in such a patient, a cisternal puncture or lateral cervical puncture can be done).

2. When a cerebral mass lesion is suspected as evidenced by signs of increased intracranial pressure such as papilledema: A sudden decrease in intraspinal CSF pressure can potentially lead to herniation of either the tonsils of the cerebellum through the foramen magnum or portions of the temporal lobe through the tentorium cerebelli; such a complication if not detected and treated promptly will be fatal. This underscores the importance of examining the ocular fundi and doing a CT scan before doing a lumbar puncture. There are two situations where LP may still have to be done despite the presence of papilledema: (1) when there is a high index of suspicion of meningitis, and (2) when pseudotumor cerebri is strongly suspected. In either case, a neurologic or neurosurgical consultation needs to be made before lumbar puncture is done.

Note: When future diagnostic studies, such as myelography, are contemplated, postpone the LP since a sample of CSF can be obtained at the time of performing the radiologic procedure.

Technique

1. Explain the procedure thoroughly to the patient and be sure to ask for a history of allergy to local anesthetics and iodine.

2. Site of puncture: The lumbar puncture is carried out usually at the L3 - L4 or L4 - L5 (same level as the highest point of the iliac crest) interspinous space.

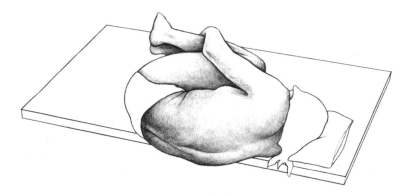

Figure 2.1 Positioning for a lumbar puncture. Note that the patient is placed on a firm surface so that the spinal column is relatively straight. Once the subarachnoid space is entered, the legs should be gently extended in order to relax the patient and relieve pressure on the abdomen.

3. Position of patient: Have the patient lie on a hard surface on his side with the knees pulled up toward the chest with the head flexed ("fetal position") (see Figures 2.1-2.5). Make sure that the spine is straight and not curved (bent) sideways. Alternatively, the patient may be made

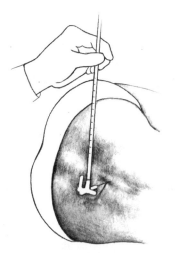

Figure 2.2 Once the subarachnoid space is entered, place stopcock in upright position and record pressure. If a moderately high pressure is recorded (eg, 250 mm of water), this is most often secondary to patient anxiety. Wait a few minutes and the pressure will frequently return to normal (<200 mm of water).

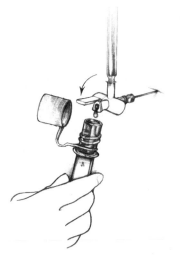

Figure 2.3 After pressure measurement is taken, turn stopcock as illustrated and obtain appropriate amount of fluid.

to sit up; this makes it easier to locate the correct space for puncture. For patients who are agitated or delirious, restraint may be necessary; if sufficient personnel are not available, the patient may be trussed (see Figure 2.4).

4. Prepare the skin surface for puncture with povidone-iodine (Betadine) or another equally effective anti-infective topical solution with vigorous rubbing. Sterile technique including gloves and drapes is very important. Commercially available sterile disposable LP trays and disposable (rather than reusable) spinal needles are preferred. Always use a spinal needle with a stylet.

5. Using local anesthetic, make a skin wheal and then infiltrate more deeply, particularly around the bone. Insert the needle with the bevel parallel to the long axis of the body so that it separates rather than cuts through the fibers of the ligamentum flavum (see Figure 2.5). When the needle enters the subarachnoid space (a pop will be felt as it passes through the posterior spinal ligament and dura), withdraw the stylet, allowing only 1 drop of CSF to escape, to verify that the needle is indeed in the subarachnoid space. Reinsert the stylet immediately and tell the patient to relax; have the assistant extend the patient's head and legs. Attach the manometer and record the opening pressure. Normal CSF pressure is less than 200 mm of water.

6. The needle must be strictly parallel to the bed and the tip is to be pointed toward the patient's umbilicus. If the needle encounters bone, withdraw

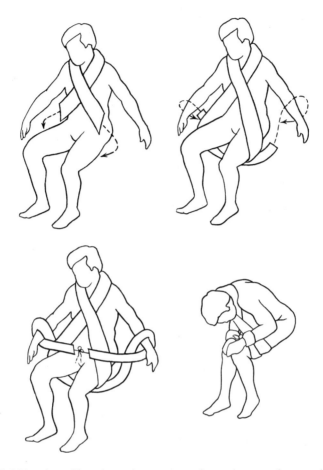

Figure 2.4 Trussing with a sheet: An uncooperative patient may be restrained with a sheet as illustrated.

the needle up to the subcutaneous tissue and then reintroduce it at a different angle. If the needle does not enter the subarachnoid space on the second attempt, it is better to try the procedure in the sitting position which enables one to gauge the midline better. Do not make repeated, unsuccessful attempts to perform an LP, but let someone else try.

7. After measuring the opening pressure, CSF is removed for laboratory study. Know how much CSF is required before attempting the lumbar puncture. About 5 mL of CSF is required for biochemical studies for determination of glucose (0.5 mL), protein (1 mL), and protein electrophoresis (4 mL). Microbiologic studies require about 8 mL of CSF for a routine culture (1 mL), acid-fast and fungal cultures (2-3 mL), syphilis serology (1 mL), cryptococcal antigen and antibody, Gram stain,

and India ink preparation. Cell count requires 0.5 mL. It is always a good idea to have an extra 2 mL of CSF labeled and frozen, in case the quantity originally sent to the laboratory was not sufficient for the tests ordered, or if confirmation is desired. In general, the first collected tube should go for routine culture and the second tube for protein and other biochemical studies.

Caveat: At the completion of the fluid collection and needle removal there is a hole through the dura into the subcutaneous paravertebral tissue. The continuously produced CSF (at the rate of about 20 mL/hr) may leak through this hole until normal repair processes obliterate the hole. With normal technique the leakage occurs for only a short period, but nonetheless may amount to 30 mL or more. Continuing leakage can result in greater fluid loss and may cause post-LP headache. The fluid removed for the study constitutes only a small proportion of the extra fluid that can be lost with leakage. Therefore one should always be certain to collect adequate amounts for laboratory study and not be concerned about "taking too much." The leakage may be minimized by

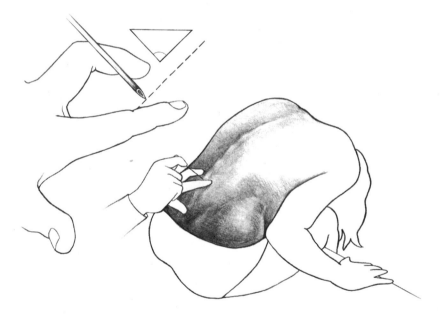

Figure 2.5 In performing a difficult lumbar puncture, it may be necessary for the patient to be in a sitting position, which often makes the landmarks clearer. Increased hydrostatic pressure in the lumbar area tenses the dura, making needle penetration easier. Note that the needle must be inserted with the bevel parallel to the long axis of the spine. Once the needle has entered the subarachnoid space (and with the stylet in place), the patient should be assisted to the lying position; appropriate pressure measurements may then be taken.

18

keeping the bevel of the needle parallel to the long axis of the spine to avoid a dural and posterior ligament tear.

8. If the CSF appears bloody, spin it down *immediately* and compare that tube in the sunlight with an identical tube containing water, looking down from the tops of the tubes (see Figure 2.6). If the lumbar puncture was traumatic, the CSF should appear clear; if the patient has had a sub-arachnoid hemorrhage, the CSF should appear xanthochromic (yellow). Elevated CSF protein (over 100 mg/dL) or peripheral bilirubin may also result in xanthochromic fluid.

9. A cell count should be done *immediately*, preferably by the physician, since white blood cells lyse quickly at room temperature. There is a 50% loss of cells in the first half-hour at room temperature. If red blood cells are present, they can be lysed with acetic acid. This is done by drawing acetic acid up the capillary hematocrit tube (or white cell pipette) and then blowing it out; the capillary tube is then introduced into the CSF solution and the CSF drawn up into the capillary tube. The red cells are lysed leaving only the white blood cells to be visualized.

It will be easier to see the cells if they are stained; crystal violet may be used (mix 0.1 g of crystal violet, 1 mL of glacial acetic acid, 50 mL of distilled water, and 2 drops of phenol). The solution is drawn up into the capillary hematocrit tube (or white cell pipette) and then blown out.

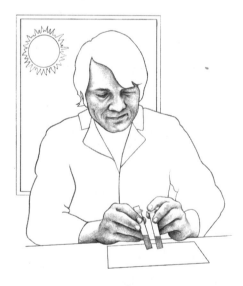

Figure 2.6 Xanthochromia may best be appreciated by comparing CSF with water in sunlight against a white sheet of paper as illustrated.

The capillary tube is then introduced into the CSF solution. The CSF is drawn up into the capillary tube and after mixing well the CSF is placed into the counting chamber. Under these conditions red cells appear green and white cells appear purple.

Normal CSF contains less than five lymphocytes and no polymorpho-nuclear leukocytes per microliter (cubic millimeter). In addition to look-ing for WBCs and doing a differential count, cytology may be done for the presence of malignant cells. When meningitis or encephalitis is sus-pected, Gram stain and acid-fast stain (on centrifuged sediment) need to be done. An India ink preparation to identify *Cryptococcus* is done when fungal meningitis is suspected.

Protein is less than 40 mg/dL in the lumbar subarachnoid fluid and much lower (10-20 mg/dL) in the ventricles. Marked increase (750-1000 mg/dL) in protein may be seen in spinal block (Froin's syndrome), while mild to moderate elevation may be seen in Guillain-Barré syndrome, meningitis, diabetes, polyneuropathy, and certain types of brain tumors. In multiple sclerosis (MS) the elevation is seldom above 80 to 100 mg/dL.

An elevated CSF gamma globulin percentage (normal is less than 13%) by CSF protein electrophoresis indicates the possibility of MS, tuber-culosis, myeloma, or other inflammatory or immunologic disorders. An IgG index is a sensitive test of excessive IgG synthesis in the CNS; it is calculated by the formula:

$$\frac{CSF\ IgG/serum\ IgG}{CSF\ albumin/serum\ albumin} \qquad [normal < 0.7]$$

Demonstration of oligoclonal (IgG) bands and myelin basic protein (> 1.0 ng/mL) in the CSF are highly useful in the diagnosis of MS. If meningitis is suspected in a diabetic patient or a patient receiving intravenous (IV) glucose, it may be advantageous to compare the blood sugar and the CSF sugar. The blood should be drawn at least one hour prior to the lumbar puncture for such comparison. The CSF glucose level normally is about two-thirds of that in blood.

CSF sugar is decreased in bacterial and fungal meningitis, while it tends to be normal in viral meningoencephalitis. It may also be low in carcinomatous and granulomatous meningeal infiltration.

Complications of Lumbar Puncture

1. Post-LP headache occurs in about 10% to 20% of patients. The diag-nostic feature is marked exacerbation of pain on sitting up and dramatic relief on lying down. Onset is within 1 to 3 days after LP and lasts for

days to weeks. Bed rest and liberal fluid intake are useful but in persistent post-LP headache autologous epidural blood patch is useful.

2. Iatrogenic meningitis: This complication should not occur if adequate sterile precautions are taken.

3. Herniation: A CT scan easily identifies mass lesions which increase the probability of herniation.

> Caveat: Millions of lumbar punctures were done safely before the invention of the CT scanner; lack of a CT scan should never delay a lumbar puncture when infection is suspected.

NEURORADIOLOGIC PROCEDURES

Computed Tomographic (CT) Scan

Computed tomographic scans give adequate information about the brain anatomy, even though they do not demonstrate most blood vessels. Since its inception, this procedure has totally revolutionized the practice of neurology. The study involves small-dose x-ray penetration of the head in multiple directions with quantification of the absorption of the x-rays by various structures. Using computer analysis, an entire cross section of the brain can be mapped out with clear differentiation of the densities of all areas. Such tomographic "slices" can be visualized as a picture on a cathode ray tube (television screen) in which the shading of each picture point is proportional to its density. Intravenous injection of iodinated contrast material ("IVP dye") may be used to enhance the density of the vascular structures, and areas where the blood-brain barrier is disrupted as in tumors, abscess, etc. The CT scan is an easy, safe procedure (noninvasive if done without contrast injection) that gives a picture of the brain resembling the brain slices ordinarily only available for neuropathologic analysis.

Newer whole body scanners permit visualization of similar "slices" of the spinal cord. Injection of a water-soluble iodinated contrast material into the subarachnoid space permits improved visualization of the spinal and intracranial contents on these slices.

A CT scan is indicated in patients presenting with focal neurologic deficits, altered mental status, head trauma, new-onset seizures, increased intracranial pressure, and suspected mass lesions or subarachnoid hemorrhage. A CT scan done after injection of contrast will improve diagnostic yield in the case of intracranial tumor, abscess, chronic subdural hematoma, infarct, and vascular malformation.

While a CT scan is highly sensitive and somewhat specific in documenting many types of intracranial pathology, its limitations include an inability to show very small lesions and those lesions that are isodense with brain tissue. Thus small plaques of multiple sclerosis may not be visible on CT scans, whereas they are easily visualized by MRI. Similarly an infarct in the first 24 to 48 hours may not be seen on CT scan. Subdurals that are bilateral and isodense may be totally missed by CT scan.

Caveat: A normal CT scan does not rule out intracranial pathology. Also, a CT scan may show lesions that may not be relevant to the patient's current illness (eg, agenesis of corpus callosum, old infarcts in a patient presenting with unrelated new symptoms). Remember that you are treating the patient and not the CT scan.

Magnetic Resonance Imaging

Magnetic resonance imaging (MRI) affords visualization of the anatomy of the brain and spinal cord with clarity that is unmatched by any other test. Sagittal, coronal, and horizontal views can be obtained. The patient is placed in a powerful magnetic field which tends to make the atoms of the tissues align themselves in the orientation of the magnetic field. A specific radiofrequency pulse is introduced into the magnetic field which makes the protons resonate; subsequently they return to their original positions when the radiofrequency pulse is discontinued. By computer analysis of the radiofrequency energy emitted by the protons, an image of the tissue is created. While MRI has proved to be superior to the CT scan in the diagnosis of neurologic disorders, the cost and limited availability of the test mandates careful selection of those patients most likely to benefit. This technique has maximum value in diagnosing multiple sclerosis, posterior fossa lesions (no artifact due to the bone as in CT), and spinal cord lesions like syringomyelia.

Myelography

Myelography is indicated when external pressure on the spinal dura and its contents or when a mass within the spinal subarachnoid space is suspected. Radiopaque material is injected into the subarachnoid space through a spinal (lumbar or lateral cervical) puncture or cisternal puncture. Contrast media such as Pantopaque is heavier than spinal fluid, and by tilting the patient it can be made to travel up and down the subarachnoid space. It will outline anything deforming the subarachnoid space. Since Pantopaque may cause delayed arachnoiditis if left in the subarachnoid space, water-soluble media are currently used. Metrizamide and iohexal are the two commonly used agents. The major complication is the occurrence of seizures and encephalopathy, if a significant amount of the material escapes into the cranial subarachnoid space. It is often advisable to discontinue drugs like phenothiazines and antidepressants before metrizamide myelography to reduce the chance of seizures. The technique is commonly used to demonstrate a herniated intervertebral disc, extrinsic tumors compressing the spinal cord, intramedullary lesions, etc. More information can be obtained if CT scanning is combined with myelography using water-soluble contrast media. Since the advent of CT scanning and MRI, the number of myelograms performed has markedly decreased.

Cerebral Angiography (Arteriography)

The most important indication for cerebral angiography is suspicion of an abnormality of the blood vessels of the brain; these abnormalities are not usually seen on CT scan. The most common indications are suspected aneurysm or arteriovenous malformation, evaluation of extracranial and intracranial portions of cerebral blood vessels in patients with a transient ischemic attack (TIA) prior to surgical treatment, arteritis involving intracranial vessels, and in tumors like meningioma to assess vascularity. The preferred technique is catheter study. This method of cerebral angiography is much safer than direct puncture of the carotid or vertebral arteries. The catheter is inserted into the femoral artery and threaded up the aorta. At the aortic arch the carotid and vertebral arteries are individually catheterized. A series of x-rays is then taken during injection of a radiopaque contrast material. Fine detail of cerebral circulation can be seen as well as the larger arteries in the chest and neck. It is usually the best method for demonstrating aneurysms, arteriovenous malformations, vascular tumors, occlusive vascular diseases, subdural and intracerebral hematomas, and abnormal vascular shunts (the subclavian steal phenomenon).

Spinal X-Ray Films

Spinal x-ray films are often taken for any complaint referable to the spine or the spinal cord. Films of the spine are only as useful as the technical competence of the x-ray technician in obtaining correctly positioned views and the ability of the radiologist to interpret the films. Especially important in cervical spine films are views of all seven vertebrae. In cervical and lumbar spine films, good oblique views are important. Remember when ordering the films that the segmental spinal cord levels are higher than the vertebral spine levels (in adults, the cord ends at approximately L-2). Pathologic conditions producing changes seen on spinal films include congenital lesions (eg, fusion, anomalies, syringomyelia), tuberculosis, trauma, spondylolisthesis, tumors, metabolic bone disease, and degenerative disc disease.

Skull X-Ray Films

Skull films are most useful in assessing abnormalities in cranial bones, pituitary fossa, abnormal calcifications, and shifts of normal calcified structures. They are occasionally useful in picking up abnormalities in facial bones, vertebrae, and pericranial structures. Skull films are only as useful as the technical competence of the x-ray technician. Pathologic conditions that produce abnormalities that can be seen on skull films include changes in bone structure (single or multiple areas of destruction as in metastases and multiple myeloma), fractures, intracranial calcifications (normal, eg, pineal, choroid plexus; or abnormal, eg, tuberous sclerosis, Sturge-Weber syndrome, certain tumors), increased intracranial pressure, craniostenosis, cerebellopontine angle tumor, enlarged sella from pituitary masses, sinus changes, and congenital or acquired disorders of the skull base. If the odontoid process is not seen on spine films, it should be included in the skull series. There is controversy about the need for routine skull films for minor head injuries, since the yield of therapeutically useful information is very low.

Digital Vascular (Subtraction) Imaging (DVI)

In this technique x-ray images are taken and recorded digitally before and after injection of contrast material; by computer subtraction an enhanced image of the blood vessels is obtained. This procedure is less invasive than arteriography, since the contrast can be injected intravenously rather than intra-arterially. Visualization is acceptable in the carotid and vertebral arteries in their extracranial course. Intracranial vasculature is not properly visualized by this procedure. Many surgeons may still want an arteriogram before carotid endarterectomy.

Isotope Cisternography

Isotope cisternography, formerly called radioiodinated serum albumin (RISA) scan, consists of the injection of a radioactive nuclide into the lumbar subarachnoid space. The substance usually employed is technetium-99m. It may be useful in the investigation of normal pressure hydrocephalus (NPH), CSF leakage, and the patency of ventricular shunts.

NEUROPHYSIOLOGIC TESTS

Electroencephalography

Electroencephalography records the spontaneous electrical activity of the brain. Electrodes are placed on the scalp in a specific pattern, and the electrical voltage fluctuations between any pair of these electrodes is amplified and recorded permanently on moving paper. Indications include: (1) finding the origin and type of electrical discharge associated with clinical seizures and more often in detecting epileptiform abnormalities in between seizures (interictal tracing), (2) localizing and assessing changes resulting from trauma, neoplasm, infection, or vascular disease, (3) assisting in the diagnosis of coma and dementia, and (4) assisting in the diagnosis of cerebral death. It is particularly useful in the diagnosis of *Herpes simplex* encephalitis and Jakob's disease where diagnostic patterns may be seen. This technique is only as good as the skills of the technician recording the tracing and the physician (electroencephalographer) interpreting the tracing. In addition, during the short time of the recording, an intermittent abnormality (eg, epileptiform abnormality) may or may not occur.

Caveat: A normal EEG does not rule out a true seizure disorder.

In order to increase the chances of recording epileptiform abnormalities in the interictal EEG, it is recommended to sleep-deprive the patient on the previous night and to make sure that waking and sleep tracings are obtained. Other measures include use of special electrodes such as nasopharyngeal and sphenoidal electrodes, long-term ambulatory cassette EEG monitoring, or in hospital video EEG with or without telemetry.

Electromyography

Electromyography (EMG) refers to the recording of the electrical activity of muscle fibers through a needle electrode inserted into the muscle belly. Abnormal spontaneous electrical activity in the form of fasciculations, fibrillations, or positive sharp waves may be recorded. Fasciculations are seen most often in chronic anterior horn cell disorders like amyotrophic lateral sclerosis (ALS). Fibrillations and positive sharp waves are detected 3 to 6 weeks after the motor nerve is injured. Reinnervation of denervated muscle fibers may be documented by detecting polyphasic motor units on volitional contraction. Changes in the morphology of units are helpful in the detection of myopathies and neurogenic disorders. Certain EMG abnormalities are diagnostic, such as myotonia (myotonia congenita, myotonic dystrophy). By delineating the distribution of denervation changes among different muscles, the site of the lesion (nerve, plexus, nerve root, anterior horn cell) can be accurately localized. For instance, in doubtful cases, objective evidence for a nerve root compression can be obtained by documenting denervation changes limited to those muscles supplied by that particular nerve root. Recovery from a nerve injury can also be predicted or confirmed on the basis of serial EMG studies.

Nerve Conduction Study

A nerve conduction study consists of stimulation of a nerve (motor or sensory) at different points and calculating the velocity of conduction of the propagated impulse. The measured velocity is that of the fastest conducting fibers (large myelinated nerve fibers) and will be normal if the myelin sheath is intact. Demyelination leads to a decrease in conduction velocity. However, there may be no slowing if the conduction measurement is not through the area of myelin destruction. Thus, initially, a conduction study distal to the site of pressure injury to the nerve may be normal. In Guillain-Barré syndrome where the nerve roots are involved early, distal conduction may be normal, while the proximal conduction (measured as F wave latency and/or H reflex latency) tend to be abnormal.

Nerve conduction studies are useful in the diagnosis of:

1. Entrapment neuropathies: ie, median nerve at the wrist (carpal tunnel syndrome), tibial nerve at the ankle (tarsal tunnel syndrome), ulnar nerve at the elbow, etc

2. Confirming the presence of peripheral neuropathies and distinguishing predominantly demyelinating from predominantly axonal polyneuropathies (see Chapter 15)
3. Localization of site of injury and follow-up of recovery in nerve trauma

> *Remember*: Normal nerve conduction velocity does not rule out the existence of polyneuropathy; it only excludes a demyelinating neuropathy involving the larger, thickly myelinated fibers. Small fiber neuropathies (thinly myelinated or unmyelinated) and predominantly axonal neuropathies may not cause significant slowing of nerve conduction.

Evoked Potentials

Evoked potentials are a recording of the electrical activity in the CNS produced by stimulation of peripheral sensory receptors. Signals are recorded by placing electrodes over the scalp (as in an EEG) or over the spine and are analyzed by a computer that averages and amplifies the signal. Auditory stimuli are delivered by clicks through earphones and visual stimuli by stroboscopic flash or more reliably by a changing checkerboard pattern on a television screen (pattern shift visual-evoked potential). For somatosensory evoked potentials, electric stimuli are delivered to the peripheral nerves, such as the median, peroneal, and tibial.

Neurosonography

Diagnostic ultrasound was originally used to detect shift of midline structures or hydrocephalus (A-mode echoencephalography). With the advent of the CT scan the method was abandoned. Recently, high-resolution, portable, real-time ultrasound scanners have become available which are highly useful in detecting intracranial hemorrhage in premature infants (ultrasound is passed through the fontanels).

Duplex scan: B-mode ultrasound with pulsed Doppler ultrasound has become a frequently used investigation of the extracranial carotid arteries. The technique gives a graphic image of the arterial wall and analyzes the velocity pattern of the blood flow. This noninvasive technique detects stenosis and plaques.

Muscle and Nerve Biopsy

Muscle and nerve biopsy specimens are very fragile, and special care must be taken in obtaining and processing the tissue. Muscle biopsies should only be done where the specimen can be quick-frozen and histochemistry performed. Nerve biopsy should only be done where facilities are available for in vitro physiologic studies, electron microscopy, and teased fiber preparation of the specimen.

Note: Muscle and nerve biopsies should be done under local anesthetic, since general anesthesia in susceptible patients may precipitate malignant hyperthermia (see Chapter 15).

Muscle biopsy may be of value in:

1. Evaluation of congenital weakness, proximal or distal weakness, or muscle wasting without sensory loss
2. Diagnosis of lipid and glycogen storage diseases, sarcoidosis, vasculitis, and polymyositis
3. Searching for microscopic changes seen in myotonic disorders, endocrine myopathies, and congenital myopathies

Nerve biopsy may be of value in:

1. Differentiating between axonal and demyelinating neuropathies
2. Showing infiltration of peripheral nerves as in myeloma, carcinoma, sarcoidosis, amyloidosis, vasculitis, and leprosy
3. Characterizing congenital hypertrophic neuropathies

Urine Neurometabolic Screening Tests

Urine Ferric Chloride Test

Reaction of the urine specimen with a ferric chloride solution can be used at the bedside for rapid evaluation of the presence of various drugs or toxic substances in the body. This test is of particular value in patients who are comatose because of possible drug ingestion and in infants and children with developmental disorders suspected of having an inborn metabolic error. The test can be performed either with ferric chloride solution or with impregnated dipsticks (Phenistix).

1. The ferric chloride test solution consists of:

Ferric chloride ($FeCl_3$)	1.0 g
Ferrous ammonium sulfate	1.0 g
0.02 mol/L hydrochloric acid	100 mL

   Procedure: Place 1.0 mL $FeCl_3$ test solution in a clean test tube. Add 10 drops (0.5 mL) of urine and mix well. Observe color immediately. Normally there will be no change in color.
2. Phenistix (impregnated cellulose strips manufactured by Ames Division of Miles Laboratories, Elkhart, IN).

   Procedure: Dip the test end in fresh urine; wait 30 seconds to read color.
3. *Results* (see Table 2.1).

Dinitrophenylhydrazine Test (DNPH Test)

Reaction of the urine with dinitrophenylhydrazine solution can be used to detect excessive excretion of ∝-keto acids as found in phenylketonuria, maple

TABLE 2.1
Results of Urine Ferric Chloride Test

Substance	10% FeCl$_3$	Phenistix
Phosphates	Brown to white precipitate (may obscure other colors)	-------
Bilirubin	Green (stable)	-------
Salicylates	Purple (stable; negative if urine is strongly acid)	Purple
p-Aminosalicylic acid	Red-brown	Red-brown
Isoniazid	Gray	--------
Phenothiazine	Blue-purple	Purple
Lysol	Green (stable)	--------
Acetaminophen or antipyrine	Cherry red	--------
Phenols	Red-brown-mauve	--------
Levodopa metabolites	Green	--------
Acetoacetic acid	Purple-red (negative if urine is heated)	--------
$\propto$-ketobutyric acid	Purple fading to red-brown	Green-brown
Pyruvic acid	Yellow	Yellow
Lactic acid	Gray	Gray
Melanin	Gray precipitate turning black	--------
5-Hydroxyindolacetic acid	Blue-green	--------
Phenylpyruvic acid	Green (fades over a few hours)	Gray-green
p-Hydroxyphenyl-pyruvic acid	Green (fades in seconds)	Green
Imidazolpyruvic acid	Dark green	--------
Branched-chain ketoacids	Blue-green	Blue-green
Homogentisic acid	Blue-green (fades in seconds)	--------

syrup urine disease, tyrosinosis, pyruvic acidemia, hypermethioninemia, or histidinemia. Ketone bodies (such as found in the fasting state or with diabetes or lactic acidosis) may also react positively in the DNPH test. To differentiate ∝-keto acids from ketone bodies, Acetest tablets (Ames Division of Miles Laboratories, Elkhart, IN) are used; urine containing ∝-keto acids is negative with Acetest tablets, while ketone bodies react positively with Acetest tablets.

1. The dinitrophenylhydrazine test solution consists of:

2,4-dinitrophenylhydrazine	0.7 g
2.0 mol/L hydrochloric acid	250 mL

(store the filtered clear yellow solution in dark bottle)

Procedure: Filter urine. Place 1.0 mL filtered urine in clean test tube. Add 1.0 mL of DNPH test solution. Observe reaction.

2. *Results*: A yellow to yellow-white opalescent turbidity or precipitate will form within three to four minutes in a positive urine.

Nitroprusside Test

The nitroprusside test may be used as a screening test for detecting cystinuria, homocystinuria, and β-mercaptolactate-cysteine disulfiduria. Since homocystinuria is associated with a high incidence of arterial thrombosis, children or adolescents with a stroke syndrome or undergoing angiography should be screened with the nitroprusside test.

1. Reagents necessary for the reaction are:
   Ammonium hydroxide, concentrated
   5% sodium cyanide solution (sodium cyanide 5.0 g in 100 mL distilled water)
   5% sodium nitroprusside (sodium nitroferricyanide 5.0 g in 100 mL distilled water)

   Procedure: Place 5.0 mL urine in clean test tube. Add 5 drops of concentrated ammonium hydroxide. Add 2.0 mL of 5% sodium cyanide and mix well. Allow to stand for 10 minutes, then add 5 drops of 5% sodium nitroprusside. Mix well and observe color immediately.

   Caution: Never add sodium cyanide to an acid solution, since it will result in the production of poisonous cyanide gas.

2. *Results*: A deep purple color that fades gradually is positive.

Cetyltrimethylammonium Bromide Turbidity Test (CTAB Test)

The CTAB test is used to detect mucopolysaccharides in the urine as found in patients with mucopolysaccharidosis.

1. The CTAB test solution consists of:

Hexadecyltrimethylammonium bromide	5.0 g
1.0 mol/L citrate buffer pH 6.0	100 mL

(Citrate buffer made from citric acid monohydrate 105 g in
250 mL water plus 19 mol/L sodium hydroxide 75 mL)
Procedure: Place 5.0 mL of *room-temperature* fresh urine in a clean test
tube. Add 1.0 mL CTAB test solution. Allow to stand at room temperature for 30 minutes, then observe for turbidity.

2. *Results*: A cloudy precipitate constitutes a positive test.
   Caution: Cold urine will give a false-positive test.

Benedict's Test

Benedict's test is used to detect the increased urinary excretion of various reducing substances (sugars) such as those found in diabetes mellitus, Fanconi
syndrome, galactosemia, or fructose intolerance.

1. Clinitest tablets (Ames Division of Miles Laboratories, Elkhart, IN).
   Procedure: Place 5 drops of urine in a clear test tube. Add 10 drops
   of water. Add one Clinitest tablet. After reaction bubbling has ceased,
   wait 15 seconds and then shake tube. Compare color with chart provided with tablets.

2. *Results*: Positive test indicates the presence of a reducing substance in
   urine. To differentiate glucose from other reducing substances, use glucose oxidase urine dipstick (Diastix by Ames Division of Miles Laboratories, Elkhart, IN), which will be positive only in the presence of
   glucose.

BIBLIOGRAPHY

Aminoff MJ: Electrophysiologic evaluation of patients with multiple sclerosis. *Neurol Clin* 1985;3:663-674.

Chiappa KH: *Evoked Potentials in Clinical Medicine*. New York, Raven Press, 1983.

Davis KR, Kistler JP, Buonanno SF: Clinical neuroimaging approaches to cerebro-vascular diseases. *Neurol Clin* 1984;2:655-665.

Grant EG, White EM: Pediatric neurosonography. *J Child Neurol* 1986; 1:319-337.

Jablecki CK: Electromyography in infants and children. *J Child Neurol* 1986; 1:297-318.

Kovanen J, Sulkava R: Duration of postural headache after lumbar puncture. *Headache* 1986;26:224-226.

Mayo Clinic and Mayo Foundation. Neurologic procedures, in *Clinical Examinations in Neurology*. Philadelphia, WB Saunders Co, 1981, pp 259-277.

Sato S, Rose DF: The electroencephalogram in the evaluation of the patient with epilepsy. *Neurol Clin* 1986;4:509-529.

Strokes HD, O'Hara CM, Buchanan RD, et al: An improved method for examination of cerebrospinal fluid cells. *Neurology* 1975;25:901-906.

Taveras JM, Wood EH: *Diagnostic Neuroradiology*. Baltimore, Williams & Wilkins Co, 1976.

Thomas GH, Howell RR: *Selected Screening Tests for Genetic Metabolic Diseases*. Chicago, Year Book Medical Publishers, 1973.

Weissberg L, Nice C, Katz M: *Cerebral Computed Tomography*. Philadelphia, WB Saunders Co, 1984.

III

HEADACHE

Headache is one of the commonest conditions for which patients seek medical treatment. It has been estimated that 5% to 20% of the population may suffer from migraine and that it is the fifth commonest reason for outpatient visits. Remember that headache is *a symptom, not a disease*, and successful therapy depends on correct diagnosis. The physician who simply prescribes an analgesic or tranquilizer does the patient no service and runs the risk of causing an iatrogenic drug dependency problem. *NEVER* treat chronic or recurrent headaches with narcotics. A minimum of one half-hour should be scheduled and spent with each patient complaining of headache. The primary aim is to differentiate serious or life-threatening conditions that present with headache (eg, brain tumor, subarachnoid hemorrhage, meningitis) from relatively benign conditions (eg, migraine, tension headache), and develop appropriate strategies for treatment.

History and Examination of the Patient with Headache

The determination of etiology of headache is most often made from the history. During the course of the interview, the following information should be obtained (avoid leading questions):

1. Location of pain
    a. Frontal, temporal, occipital, or vertex
    b. Unilateral, bilateral, or shifting
2. Type of pain
    a. Constant or throbbing.
    b. Mixed (constant and throbbing; which is first?)

30

3. Duration and timing of pain
   a. Worse in morning or evening
   b. Worse with a Valsalva maneuver (bowel movement, coughing, sneezing)
   c. Consistent associations (premenstrual, weekends, emotional stress, alcohol intake, seasonal, specific foods)
4. Severity of pain: Pain severe enough to wake up the patient from sleep may be seen with increased intracranial pressure, cluster headache, and intracranial bleeding. On the other hand, the patient may find it difficult to go to sleep with any form of severe headache.
5. Associated symptoms preceding, accompanying, or following the headache (visual changes, dizziness or other sensations may precede classic migraine).
6. Family history (migraine, epilepsy, psychiatric illness).
7. Past medical history (hypertension, infection, allergy, head trauma, recent lumbar puncture).
8. Medication history (vasodilators, oral contraceptives, alcohol, or street drugs).

   Caution: Sudden onset of a severe headache without past history should be considered ominous and warrants immediate exclusion of potentially life-threatening conditions such as subarachnoid hemorrhage or meningitis.

On examination, particular attention should be given to the following signs:
1. Blood pressure, pulse rate, temperature
2. Sharpness of optic discs, intact venous pulsations, presence of hemorrhages
3. Tenderness of temporal arteries
4. Presence of spasm in cervical muscles
5. Cranial bruits
6. Tenderness to percussion over sinuses
7. "Trigger" areas for pain as in trigeminal neuralgia
8. Asymmetry of reflexes or other focal neurologic signs

Headache of Increased Intracranial Pressure
1. *The most important diagnostic clue is a* bilateral, nonthrobbing headache that is worse in the morning.
2. Initially mild and intermittent, increasing in severity to steady, nonthrobbing pain.
3. May awaken the patient at night.

4. Worse with Valsalva maneuver.

5. When severe, associated with vomiting.

6. Often associated with signs of early papilledema (see Chapter 13).

7. Often associated with focal neurologic signs (asymmetric reflexes, palsy of extraocular muscles, pupillary asymmetry).

Treatment: Immediate hospitalization and additional diagnostic studies such as a CT scan are necessary. Treat the underlying cause.

Migraine Headache

Migraine is a periodic or cyclic disorder in which recurrent headaches occur often associated with photophobia and autonomic disturbances such as nausea and vomiting. It is considered to be a disorder of vascular regulation and is characterized by an initial phase of intracranial vasoconstriction followed by a phase of extracranial vasodilation. There are four usual varieties: classic migraine, common migraine, complicated migraine, and cluster headache.

1. Classic Migraine

   a. *The most important diagnostic clue* is an aura followed by the sudden onset of a unilateral throbbing headache.

   b. Aura may consist of transient visual (scotoma, monocular blindness, or hemianopsia), sensory, or motor (paraesthesia, weakness) phenomena or simply an indescribable feeling; prodromal symptoms include changes in mood and/or appetite.

   c. Typically throbbing, but occasionally may evolve to a dull, aching, nonthrobbing discomfort.

   d. Although unilateral, often shifts sides with different attacks, commonly temporal, orbital, frontal, or (rarely) occipital.

   e. Occurs at any time of day.

   f. Often associated with nausea, vomiting, and photophobia (or other gastrointestinal or autonomic symptoms).

   g. May last minutes to days; may be relieved by sleep.

   h. Onset is often in the teens; frequency and severity may diminish after the age of 50 years.

   i. Commonly premenstrual in females; usually less frequent during pregnancy.

   j. May be precipitated by certain foods or chemicals (especially monosodium glutamate, chocolate, cheddar cheese, red wine, or sodium nitrite as in hot dogs) or with fasting.

   k. Onset or exacerbation often follows administration of oral contraceptives or reserpine-containing drugs.

l. Family history of headaches is common.

m. Past history of motion sickness or cyclic vomiting as a child.

n. Neurologic examination normal; if abnormal, the patient should have further studies such as an EEG and CT scan to exclude a structural lesion.

Caution: If the headache is always on the same side, if seizures and headache occur together, if the neurologic examination is abnormal, or if a cranial bruit is heard, consider the possibility of an arteriovenous malformation. Refer for further study including cerebral angiography.

Treatment:

1. General measures
    a. Migraine victims often are intelligent, obsessive-compulsive individuals; a thorough explanation of the pathophysiology of the headache is an important part of therapy.
    b. Discontinue oral contraceptives and look for other triggering factors such as alcohol, specific foods, etc, taking appropriate measures to reduce exposure.

2. Specific management
    Patients with migraine fall into two categories: (A) those who have frequent attacks (one or more per week), or attacks of such severity as to interfere with their life style or work, and (B) those who have infrequent or sporadic attacks. Category A patients need regular prophylactic or interval therapy to prevent recurrence of the attacks, while category B patients need only abortive treatment at the onset of headache.
    a. Abortive treatment: Treatment should be given at the earliest warning of an impending attack, in order to be effective. The following are the usually recommended measures:
        i. In children and in those in whom the attacks are seldom severe, prompt administration of analgesics such as aspirin or acetaminophen should be tried as the initial measure. In some patients, sleep alone may abort the attack. If nausea or vomiting is a prominent feature, combine this with metoclopromide hydrochloride (Reglan) 10 mg orally or intramuscularly (IM).
        ii. Ergotamine is the mainstay in the abortive treatment of migraine. Ergot is an α-adrenergic blocking agent with direct stimulating effect on vascular smooth muscle. It may also produce depression of central vasomotor centers and have antiserotonin effects. To be

effective, ergot should be administered at the very beginning of an attack. It is available in oral, sublingual, suppository, inhalant, and injectable forms (see Table 3.1).

Caution: Ergot can induce nausea and vomiting and may lead to ergotism (loss of peripheral pulses with weakness, muscle pain, paresthesia of extremities, precordial distress, and pain) if consumed in large quantities. Use with great care or avoid in organic heart disease, peripheral vascular disease, hypertension, pregnancy, hepatic disease, and septic states.

iii. If simple measures (as outlined above) fail to stop an attack and the pain persists continuously for more than 72 hours, hospitalization and more vigorous measures become necessary:

Table 3.1.
Commonly Used Ergot Preparations

Form	Brand Name	Constitutents	Dosage
Oral	Cafergot Wigraine	Ergotamine tartrate 1 mg and caffeine 100 mg	2 tablets at onset followed by 1 tablet every half-hour to maximum of 6 tablets per attack
Suppository	Cafergot Wigraine	Ergotamine tartrate 2 mg and caffeine 100 mg	1 at onset followed by 1 every half-hour up to maximum of 3 suppositories per attack
Sublingual	Ergostat	Ergotamine tartrate 2 mg	1 tablet at first warning of impending attack followed by 1 tablet every half-hour if needed to maximum 3 tablets per attack or 5 tablets/wk
Aerosol	Medihaler-Ergotamine	Ergotamine tartrate 9 mg/mL (0.39 mg per measured dose)	1 measured dose at first warning of attack followed by 1 measured dose every 5 minutes as needed up to a maximum of 6 doses per attack or 15 doses/wk
Parenteral	DHE-45	Dihydroergotamine mesylate 1 mg/mL	1.0 mL IM at first warning of attack followed by 1.0 mL every hour to maximum of 3.0 mL per attack or 6.0 mL/wk; for more rapid effect initial dose may be given IV

Dihydroergotamine mesylate (DHE-45) 0.75 mg IV after prochlorperazine maleate (Compazine) 5 mg may be effective in stopping the attack.

Narcotic treatment should only be a last and desperate measure due to its potential for addiction. If pain is severe enough to require narcotics, meperidine hydrochloride (Demerol) 50 to 100 mg IM may be given.

An occasional patient who is resistant to these measures and goes into "status migrainus" may respond to high-dose, short-term corticosteroid therapy (dexamethasone 8 mg daily for five days).

Caution: Keep in mind that a patient known to have migraine can develop other conditions which cause severe headache and hence if there is any question about the diagnosis, further studies such as a CT scan may be necessary.

b. Interval and prophylactic treatment

For patients with one or more attacks per week or those in whom the attacks are of such severity as to interfere with life style and work, prophylactic treatment should be instituted.

i. Propranolol hydrochloride (Inderal), a nonselective β-adrenergic blocking agent may be started at a dose of 40 mg orally twice a day or 80 mg of the long-acting preparation (Inderal LA). The dose may be increased to 160 mg or more gradually or until the headaches are abolished. Maintain therapeutic doses for 6 months and then gradually reduce over a 2 month period. If headaches recur restart the drug. The aim is to achieve a sustained remission from headache. Common side effects include fatigue, general weakness, insomnia, and mental depression. Contraindications include bradycardia, postural hypotension, bronchial asthma, and congestive heart failure. Use with great caution in diabetic patients since propranolol may mask the warning symptoms of hypoglycemia. Patients prone to depression should not be given propranolol since it may worsen this condition. Other β-adrenergic blockers reported to be useful in migraine are atenolol (component of Tenormin), metoprolol tartrate (Lopressor), and timolol maleate (Blocadren).

ii. Patients who have both depression and migraine benefit from amitriptyline hydrochloride (Elavil, Endep) at an initial dose of 25 mg at bedtime; gradually increase to maximum effectiveness (usually 100 mg at bedtime). Use with caution in patients prone to cardiac arrhythmias.

iii. In patients with disabling headaches, methysergide maleate (Sansert), 4 to 8 mg total daily dose with meals is effective. Efficacy should be established in 3 weeks. It should be taken for 8-week intervals with 4 weeks off to avoid retroperitoneal fibrosis or other serious side effects. Cyproheptadine hydrochloride (Periactin) is another antiserotonin agent which has been found to be effective in some patients. Side effects include weight gain and somnolence.

c. Recent studies have shown that calcium channel blocking agents may also be used as prophylactic treatment. Currently available drugs include nifedipine (Procardia), diltiazem hydrochloride (Cardizem), and verapamil hydrochloride (Isoptin); flunarizine hydrochloride is not yet available in the United States.

d. Biofeedback: Thermal biofeedback techniques designed to prevent the vasodilatory phase of migraine may be helpful as a prophylactic measure in some patients with migraine, but have not been uniformly successful.

e. Patient and physician information about migraine can be obtained from the National Headache Foundation, 5252 North Western Ave. Chicago, IL 60625 (telephone: 312-878-7715).

2. Common Migraine

Common migraine is similar to classic migraine, but the essential difference is the lack of visual and other neurologic symptoms. As the name indicates, this is the commonest form of migraine headache; features of migraine may coexist with those of muscle contraction headache, thus giving rise to a combination of throbbing and constant headaches. Although drug therapy is similar for both classic and common migraine, the disorders differ in that cerebral blood flow changes typically occur only in the classic migraine.

Treatment:

Treatment is the same as for classic migraine.

3. Complicated Migraine

In complicated migraine significant neurologic complications (such as hemiplegia presumably secondary to ischemia from the intracranial vascular constriction) occur and may outlast the headache phase. In complicated migraine the headache phase may be relatively minor. Very rarely there may be permanent neurologic sequelae. Before making a diagnosis of complicated migraine it may be necessary to rule out an underlying arteriovenous malformation (especially if the deficit always occurs in the same location). The common types of complicated migraine are:

   a. *Hemiplegic migraine*: The hemiplegia often shifts from side to side during different attacks.

   b. *Ophthalmoplegic migraine*: Oculomotor paralysis occurs on the same side as the headache; recurrent painful oculomotor palsy in a child strongly suggests complicated migraine.

   c. *Basilar artery migraine* occurs mostly in children and adolescents; vertigo, tinnitus, diplopia, and ataxia accompany occipital throbbing headache.

   d. *Acute confusional migraine* occurs in adolescents, manifested as recurrent episodes of confusion and disorientation along with headache.

Treatment:

Prophylactic (interval) treatment, as in classic migraine, is strongly recommended even when the attacks are infrequent.

4. Cluster Headache (Horton's headache, histamine cephalgia, migrainous neuralgia)

   a. *The most important diagnostic clue* is the sudden onset of severe unilateral retro-orbital lancinating pain that tends to occur repeatedly.

   b. Frequently associated with tearing or unilateral nasal discharge on the side of the headache; other features include partial ptosis and smaller pupil (Horner's syndrome) on the side of the headache.

   c. May last from 30 minutes to several hours.

   d. Often awakens patient at night.

   e. Tends to occur in a series followed by remission for months or even years (hence the name cluster headache).

   f. Often precipitated by a small amount of alcohol.

   g. May be familial.

Treatment

Patients with cluster headache need two forms of therapy: (1) abortive treatment for an attack and (2) prophylactic treatment to stop future attacks.

1. Abortive treatment: Ergotamine preparations are often effective if the attacks occur at a predictable time (see classic migraine treatment). Oxygen inhalation (100% oxygen through mask) for ten to fifteen minutes has been found to be effective in some patients.

2. Prophylactic treatment
   a. Propranolol may be tried first (see section on classic migraine for dosage). If this fails, methysergide is effective in many patients.
   b. For patients that are resistant to these prophylactic agents, corticosteroid therapy may be useful; prednisone 60 mg daily for three days with the dose reduced progressively to the minimum that is effective in stopping the attacks from recurring; continue for the duration of the bout.
   c. This type of headache may occur in chronic form on an almost daily basis; lithium carbonate treatment has been reported to be an effective therapy (300 mg 2 to 3 times a day to provide a blood level of 0.7-1.2 mEq/L).
      Note: Lithium carbonate has a number of side effects and caution is necessary.
   d. In one variety of cluster headache, chronic paroxysmal hemicrania (CPH), in which the clusters are strictly unilateral (does not shift from side to side), indomethacin (Indocin) has been found to be highly effective (dose may vary from 25 to 100 mg/day).

Tension Headache (Muscle Contraction Headache)

1. *The most important diagnostic clue* is a bilateral, nonthrobbing constant headache that begins in the occipital area and spreads to the frontal area.
2. Although the initial pain is viselike, it may eventually assume a vascular quality.
3. Not affected by a Valsalva maneuver.
4. Worse in the evening.
5. May last for days.
6. Occurs in situations of tension, such as family problems and job stress; verify by history.
7. Neurologic examination is normal except for possible palpable spasm of cervical muscles.

Note: Cervical spine disease can produce pain in the neck and occipital area either from paraspinal spasm or compression of nerve roots. Cervical spine x-ray films are necessary in such patients.

Treatment

1. Muscle relaxants may be of little value. A brief course of minor tranquilizers such as diazepam (Valium) may be useful symptomatically, but may be addictive, and relief in most instances is only temporary. Nonnarcotic analgesics may also be of benefit.
2. If cervical spine disorder is detected appropriate treatment will be necessary (see Chapter 18).
3. Biofeedback with EMG may train the patient to voluntarily relax contracted cervical musculature and alleviate the pain.
4. Chronic tension headaches may be a symptom of an underlying depression, which may need antidepressant therapy.
5. Stress management courses are currently popular and may help some patients.

Sinus Headache (Nasal Headache)

1. *The most important diagnostic clue* is: a frontal, nonthrobbing headache with tenderness to percussion over the sinus.
2. Sinus headaches are rare without predisposing nasal abnormality (structural defect, allergy, polyps).
3. May be unilateral or bilateral; location depends on sinus involved.
4. Often seasonal, particularly in allergic individuals.
5. Associated with nasal congestion and discharge, fever, malaise, painful teeth.
6. Percussion over sinuses exacerbates pain.
7. Sinus x-ray films show opacification. CT scan or MRI shows the changes much better.

Treatment

1. Systemic decongestant: pseudoephedrine hydrochloride (Sudafed) 60 mg tid or phenylpropanolamine hydrochloride (component of Entex-LA).
2. Topical nasal decongestant: 0.25% phenylephrine hydrochloride (Neo-Synephrine Hydrochloride).
   Caution. Decongestants should be used sparingly as tachyphylaxis and rebound may develop.
3. Antihistamines: The allergic patient usually knows which works best. Terfenadine (Seldane) 60 mg bid is associated with less drowsiness than other agents.

4. Nonnarcotic analgesics such as aspirin, acetaminophen, or ibuprofen.

5. Systemic antibiotics such as ampicillin 250 mg qid or dicloxacillin 250 mg qid, if patient has systemic manifestations such as fever.

6. Intranasal cromolyn sodium (Nasalcrom) bid or qid and/or intranasal beclomethasone dipropionate (Vancenase) bid or qid can be used for long-term prophylaxis.

7. Surgical drainage when chronic and severe.

Posttraumatic Headache

1. Posttraumatic headaches occur after significant head trauma (loss of consciousness) and have both organic and psychological components.

2. May be indistinguishable from chronic, recurring tension headaches.

3. Duration is usually from 6 to 12 months but may persist for years.

4. May be associated with dizzy spells.

5. May be part of postconcussion syndrome, which is characterized by fear, anxiety, fatigue, irritability, and inability to concentrate.

Caution: Symptoms of a subdural hematoma can be insidious and hence a CT scan should be done.

Treatment

1. Nonnarcotic analgesics such as aspirin, acetaminophen, or ibuprofen.

2. Diazepam 5 mg tid may be used to reduce anxiety and restlessness, but dependence may develop and diazepam should never be used for longer than 6 months.

3. Propranolol or amitriptyline (see previous section on migraine) may sometimes be useful for the more severe and prolonged posttraumatic headache.

Caution: The physician should be alerted to emotional factors or to litigation problems in the patient with prolonged or treatment-unresponsive posttraumatic headache.

Post-LP Headache

1. *The most important diagnostic clue* is headache following lumbar puncture that is precipitated by sitting or standing and relieved promptly by lying down.

2. Often frontal or occipital, may be generalized, and may be associated with nuchal pain.

3. Occurs within one to two days of lumbar puncture and is thought to be due to leakage of CSF through the dural hole.

4. Duration varies from one to several days.
5. Predisposing factors may include poor lumbar puncture technique, larger size of needle, and multiple punctures.

Treatment:
1. Strict bed rest with feet elevated; let patient try to sit up every 12 hours to determine if headache reappears.
2. Adequate hydration (about 4 L/day).
3. Analgesics are usually ineffective.
4. With persistent headache, an epidural blood patch (usually done by the anesthesiologist) using the patient's venous blood may be highly effective.

Subarachnoid Hemorrhage Headache

1. *The most important diagnostic clue* is the abrupt onset of a severe occipital or generalized headache in a patient with no previous history of headaches.
2. Usually not localized, but definite localization may suggest the site of an underlying leaking aneurysm.
3. Associated with *stiff neck*, dizziness, nausea and vomiting, irritability, restlessness, convulsions, drowsiness.
4. Altered consciousness is common.
5. Signs of localizing neurologic dysfunction may be *absent*.
6. Papilledema (see Chapter 13) may develop after hemorrhage depending on the location of hemorrhage and degree of impedance to venous return around the optic nerve. *Subhyaloid hemorrhages* are pathognomonic.

Treatment.

CT scan and angiography should be performed as soon as possible, since aneurysms tend to rebleed, leading to fatal outcome. Neurosurgical consultation should be obtained immediately to decide whether the aneurysm can be clipped.

Temporal Arteritis

1. Onset of severe, continuous unilateral head pain in an elderly person is temporal arteritis until proved otherwise.
2. The presence of an elevated erythrocyte sedimentation rate (ESR greater than 40 mm/h).
3. Tender swollen nonpulsatile temporal arteries are often, but not always, present.
4. The typical patient is over age 55 years and female.

5. Polymyalgia rheumatica (generalized muscle aches and pains) is frequently associated with temporal arteritis.

Treatment

1. This is a neurologic emergency because arteritis may involve the ophthalmic or other intracranial arteries, leading to blindness and other focal deficits. Start steroid therapy with prednisone 60 to 80 mg *immediately*. Continue high-dose steroid therapy until the ESR returns to normal. Then gradually reduce the dose to 20 to 30 mg/day and continue for 6 months to 1 year. Monitor the patient for complications of steroid therapy such as gastrointestinal bleeding, intercurrent infection, osteoporosis, or aseptic necrosis of femoral head. Alternate-day therapy may reduce steroid induced complications.

2. Diagnostic temporal artery biopsy should be scheduled within two to three days of presentation. A sufficient length of artery should be taken since the arteritis tends to be focal and may be missed. Therapy should not be delayed since instituting treatment with corticosteroids will not alter the histologic findings for a number of days.

CNS Infection Headache (Abscess, Encephalitis, Meningitis)

1. Any headache associated with fever and altered mentation is CNS infection until proved otherwise.
2. Subacute or acute onset of constant, increasingly severe pain.
3. Usually generalized but may be worse in occipital area.
4. Increases with physical activity.
5. Associated with stiff and painful neck, nausea and vomiting, irritability, restlessness.
6. Altered consciousness may be present.
7. Photophobia, strabismus, ptosis, or pupillary inequality may be present.
8. Lumbar puncture is mandatory for diagnosis and culture of the organism. *Caution*: If an abscess is suspected obtain a CT scan before the LP (see Chapter 14).

Treatment

Treatment depends on culturing the organism and determining antibiotic sensitivity; broad spectrum parenteral antibiotics should be used to treat the patient until the culture result returns. Consider isolation of patient until infectious agent is known (see Chapter 14).

Ocular Headache

Ocular causes of headache include glaucoma, diplopia with accompanying orbicularis contraction, uncorrected refractive errors (such as astigmatism), ocular or retro-ocular inflammations, or orbital tumors.

1. Ocular headache starts as a feeling of heaviness in the eyes, gradually becoming more severe.
2. Absent on awakening, appears in afternoon and gradually worsens.
3. Pain may be dull, bursting, sharp, or throbbing, and is often due to persistent muscle contraction.
4. Bifrontal or periorbital in location.
5. May be associated with prolonged reading or other use of eyes.
6. May be associated with altered visual acuity and/or reduced ocular motility.

Treatment

Measurement of intraocular pressure is necessary. Corrective lenses may be helpful. Obtain CT scans of the orbit if retroocular lesion is suspected.

Trigeminal Neuralgia (Tic Doloureux)

1. Recurrent paroxysmal pain in the distribution of one or more branches of the trigeminal nerve is most probably trigeminal neuralgia.
2. Pain may radiate to jaw or teeth and present as a dental problem.
3. Precipitated by minimal sensory stimuli to the affected side of the face (especially a localized area or trigger point, which may appear as a dirty or unshaven patch).
4. Occurs after age 40 years; suspect multiple sclerosis when onset is earlier.
5. No sensory loss in trigeminal distribution; if there is sensory loss or decreased corneal reflex look for tumors or vascular abnormalities involving the trigeminal nerve.
6. Occasionally associated with multiple sclerosis.

Treatment

1. Carbamazepine (Tegretol) 400 to 1200 mg daily is the drug of choice; the initial dose, 200 mg bid with meals, is increased gradually to the minimal effective dosage.

   Caution: Pretreatment and follow-up blood counts while on carbamazepine are recommended because of rare bone marrow suppression.
2. Phenytoin (Dilantin) 300 to 700 mg/day, adjusted to produce a blood level of 10 to 20 $\mu g/ml$.
3. Lioresal (Baclofen) in doses of 20-80 mg/day may be effective in some patients.
4. Surgical treatment may be considered in resistant cases. Trigeminal gangliolysis by percutaneous radiofrequency technique

(80% chance of pain relief for 1 year), injection of glycerol around the Gasserian ganglion, and suboccipital craniotomy with decompression of trigeminal nerve are some of the techniques used.

Temporomandibular Neuralgia (TMJ Syndrome)

1. Recurrent facial pain associated with tenderness over the temporomandibular joint is most probably temporomandibular neuralgia.
2. Usually unilateral, severe, constant, aching pain around the temporomandibular joint sometimes radiating to the jaws.
3. Pain exacerbated by movement of the lower jaw (chewing, yawning).
4. Patient may report an associated clicking or grating sound.
5. May be associated with bruxism during sleep; depression or insomnia may also be present.
6. Occurs commonly in young women or in elderly patients with severe overbite resulting from the loss of back teeth, or after fracture.
7. Palpation of the temporalis muscle or direct pressure on the temporomandibular joint may result in pain.
8. Special x-ray techniques often reveal asymmetric temporomandibular joints with degenerative changes in the cartilage.

Treatment

Treatment is often unsatisfactory. Correction of dental malocclusion may or may not relieve the pain. Conservative therapy includes heat applied to the affected area, a diet of soft foods, limitation of mouth opening, dental prostheses, mild analgesics, muscle relaxants, or antidepressants.

Toxic Headache

1. Toxic headache has the characteristics of vascular headache.
2. Drugs causing headache include phenacetin, amyl nitrite, reserpine, lithium, dextroamphetamine, ephedrine, disulfiram, digitalis, imipramine.
3. May result following excessive intake of alcohol or coffee.
4. May appear on discontinuation of corticosteroids, barbiturates, ergot, narcotics.
5. Occupational hazards include mechanics and farmers exposed to exhaust fumes (carbon monoxide), refrigerator repairmen exposed to refrigerants, coal miners exposed to mine gases, and individuals exposed to insecticides.

Treatment

1. Headache will subside following removal from toxic exposure.
2. Caffeine withdrawal headaches terminate with administration of caffeine.

BIBLIOGRAPHY

Calahan M, Raskin N: A controlled study of DHE in the treatment of acute migraine headaches. *Headache* 1986; 26:168-171.

Diamond S, Dalessio DJ: *The Practicing Physician's Approach to Headache*. Baltimore, Williams & Wilkins, 1986.

Gascon, G: Chronic and recurrent headaches in childhood and adolescence. *Pediatr Clin North Am* 1984; 31:1027-1051.

Kovanen J, Sulkava R: Duration of postural headache after lumbar puncture. *Headache* 1986; 26:224-226.

Lance JW: Migraine and cluster headache, in Johnson RT (ed): *Current Therapy in Neurologic Diseases*. Philadelphia, BC Decker, 1985, pp 81-85.

MacDonald JT: Childhood migraine. *Postgrad Med* 1986; 80:301-306.

Mathew NT: Indomethacin sensitive headache syndrome. *Headache* 1981; 21:147-150.

Saper JR: *Headache Disorders*. Boston, John Wright-PSG Inc, 1983.

Soloman GD: Comparative efficacy of calcium antagonistic drugs in the prophylaxis of migraine. *Headache* 1985;25:368-372.

Sweet WH: The treatment of trigeminal neuralgia. *N Engl J Med* 1986; 315:174-177.

Vinken PJ, Bruyn JW, Klawans HL, et al: *Headache. Volume 48. Handbook of Clinical Neurology*. Amsterdam, Elsevier, 1985.

IV

DIZZINESS, VERTIGO, AND LIGHTHEADEDNESS: PROBLEMS OF SPATIAL DISORIENTATION

The dictionary definition of *dizziness* is: "a whirling sensation in the head, mental confusion, giddiness." Patients likewise use the word to describe the sensation they feel when they stand upright too quickly, when they look over the edge of a cliff, when they are unsteady on their feet, when they are seasick, or when they generally feel unwell. To some patients dizziness is the sensation one feels after rapidly spinning around or after receiving a severe blow to the head. The differences in these sensations are subtle, and most patients are not eloquent enough to differentiate between them. The term *vertigo* should be limited to a the sensation of movement, either of oneself or of the environment; a clear-cut history of this type of sensation (vertigo), more often than not indicates that the pathologic process is in the peripheral vestibular system.

History and Examination of the Dizzy Patient

A major responsibility of the primary care physician is to identify the commonest causes of dizziness such as postural hypotension, hyperventilation, multiple sensory deficits, and postinfectious vertigo and thus avoid costly and time-consuming evaluations by a specialist. The following historical information should be obtained from the patient:

1. Attempt to define the complaint of "dizziness"; a practical way to do this is to give the patient examples of dizziness mentioned above and let him decide which sensation is closest to his complaint.
2. The duration and description of the *first* attack is usually most helpful. The frequency of subsequent attacks should also be determined.

46

3. Associated symptoms include progressive hearing loss, diplopia, paresthesias of the hands and feet, and tinnitus.

4. Positional factors: dizziness on arising from a sitting to a standing position, dizziness with sudden movement of the head, or dizziness associated with hyperextension or rotation of the neck.

5. Precipitating factors: dizziness associated with stressful situations, excessive or low salt intake, or directly related to meals may be diagnostic.

6. Past medical history: Severe head trauma, antecedent viral infections, diabetes, atherosclerotic phenomena, or psychiatric difficulties are especially helpful diagnostic signs.

7. All present and past medications should be reported; particular attention should be paid to antibiotics (especially streptomycin), anticonvulsants, antihypertensives, and high-dose salicylates.

Examples of Classic Complaints That Are Nearly Diagnostic

Often the etiology of dizziness is strongly suggested by the history, and under these circumstances a physical and neurologic examination should be targeted to a specific hypothesis, some examples:

1. "I'm dizzy when I get up in the morning." (Patients tend to become dehydrated by morning and this is when postural hypotension is most prominent.)

2. "I'm dizzy whenever I'm alone at night." (Hyperventilation is strongly associated with anxiety-producing situations.)

3. "Every time I'm dizzy I see double." (Intermittent diplopia is usually caused by ischemia of the midbrain and this suggests basilar artery insufficiency.)

4. "I can't use the phone in my right ear any more, the right side of my face is numb, and I'm unsteady on my feet." (Unilateral hearing loss without a history of trauma or ear infection is an acoustic neuroma until proved otherwise.)

5. "I suddenly became dizzy, nauseous, and unsteady on my feet, and my left face and right arm felt funny." (Symptoms on one half of the face and one side of the body strongly suggest brainstem disease; in this case infarction in the distribution of the posterior inferior cerebellar artery.)

6. "I've had diabetes many years, I can't read the newspaper because of my cataracts, and my grandchildren tease me about being drunk all the time." (Elderly patients with multiple sensory deficits commonly complain of dizziness.)

7. "I've had fullness in my ear for a week and then suddenly I became so dizzy I had to lie in bed and hold on for fear of falling out." (Ménière's disease presents with a prodrome and dramatic vertigo.)

On examination special attention should be given to the following:

1. A cardiovascular evaluation should be done (blood pressure in both arms, lying and standing, peripheral pulses, carotid bruits, heart murmurs, arrythmias).
2. Examine ears with otoscope looking for impacted cerumen, evidence of infection.
3. Have the patient *hyperventilate* to see if the symptoms are reproduced. The sitting patient should take a deep breath every 2 seconds for three to five minutes. At the end of this time, ask the patient if this is the sensation he is talking about.
4. Cerebellar function can be tested by having the patient tandem walk and perform rapid alternating movements and the finger-to/ nose test.
5. Cranial nerves should be examined carefully. Pay particular attention to nystagmus when testing extraocular movements. Nystagmus is a rhythmic, involuntary eye movement, present at rest or induced by eye movement but persisting after eye movements cease. Usually there is a slow deviation of the eye in one direction with a quick jerk in the opposite direction. Nystagmus is named for the quick component. Table 4.1 may be helpful in differentiating peripheral (labyrinthine) from CNS nystagmus. Specific types of nystagmus include:
    a. *End-point* nystagmus will result if the normal patient gazes too far laterally. Therefore the examiner should have the patient gaze laterally only to the point where in the adducting eye the limbus meets the lacrimal punctum (see Figure 4.1).

Table 4.1.
Differentiating Labyrinthine and CNS Nystagmus

Labyrinthine (Peripheral) Nystagmus	CNS Nystagmus
Horizontal or horizontal-rotary	Often vertical or rotatory
Fatigues	Persistent
Suppressed by visual fixation	May increase with visual fixation
Latency of onset after head motion	Occurs immediately after head motion
Associated with vertigo	Not directly associated with dizziness
Always conjugate	May be dysconjugate

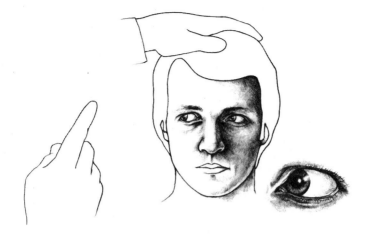

Figure 4.1. When testing for lateral-gaze nystagmus, do not force the limbus of the iris beyond the lacrimal punctum to avoid end-point nystagmus. Nystagmus at this point is usually abnormal.

> b. *Toxic-metabolic nystagmus* is symmetric in both eyes, equal in both directions of gaze, and primarily horizontal.
>
> c. *Asymmetric lateral nystagmus* (absent or reduced in one direction of gaze compared with the opposite direction of gaze) could indicate either CNS or peripheral dysfunction.
>
> d. *Dysconjugate nystagmus*: The abnormal movement is greater in one eye than the other. This always indicates CNS disease.
>
> e. *Upward-gaze, downward-gaze, or rotatory nystagmus* usually indicates CNS disease.
>
> f. *Positional nystagmus* induced by the Nylen-Bárány maneuver often indicates peripheral vestibular disease. The Nylen-Bárány maneuver is performed by seating the patient on the examining table and suddenly lowering him to a supine position with the head held 45 degrees backward over the end of the table and turned 45 degrees to one side (see Figure 4.2).

6. Evaluation of trigeminal nerve (cranial nerve V) function: *Corneal reflex* is a sensitive index of fifth cranial nerve function, and an abnormality may suggest a lesion such as acoustic neuroma.
   Caution: Be sure to touch the cornea and not the sclera and avoid producing a blink by threat reflex (see Figure 4.3).

7. Evaluation of the function of the auditory and vestibular portions of the eighth cranial nerve:

   a. *Auditory acuity* is quickly tested by rubbing the fingers lightly several inches from the patient's ear. If an abnormality is present, perform the Weber's and Rinne's tests.

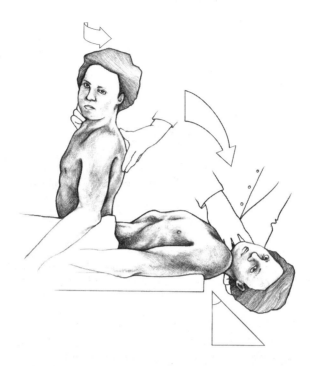

Figure 4.2.Nylen-Bárány maneuver: With the head turned 45° over the end of the table, observe the eyes for nystagmus. The patient is instructed to keep the eyes open. The onset and direction of nystagmus is noted. Note also whether the patient experiences vertigo. This maneuver is repeated with the head turned to the opposite side.

b. *Weber's test*: Place the base of a vibrating tuning fork on the patient's forehead. Ideally, a 512-Hz tuning fork should be used, but often only a 256-Hz tuning fork is readily available. Normally the sound is heard in both ears. With eighth nerve or cochlear destruction (sensorineural deafness), the sound is heard best on the side of normal acuity. With middle ear or outer ear disease (conduction deafness), sound lateralizes to the involved ear (see Figure 4.4).

c. *Rinne's test*: Hold a vibrating tuning fork first in front of the external auditory meatus (air conduction) and then place the base of the vibrating tuning fork firmly against the mastoid process (bone conduction). Ask the patient in which position the sound is loudest (see Figure 4.5). Middle ear disease or plugging of the external canal should be suspected when bone conduction is greater than air conduction. In partial sensorineural loss, air conduction remains louder than bone conduction, but both are diminished. In total unilateral sensorineural loss, air conduction may be absent, while bone conduction is heard by the opposite ear.

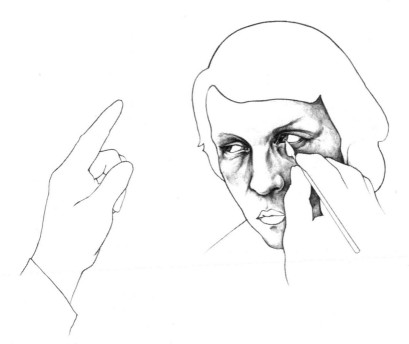

Figure 4.3. Testing the corneal reflex: With the patient looking to one side, bring a wisp of cotton (a few strands pulled out from a cotton-tipped applicator) from the opposite side and touch the *cornea*. The patient should blink.

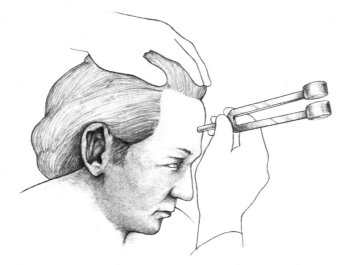

Figure 4.4. Weber's test: Place a tuning fork on the forehead and ask, "Is the sound the same in both ears?"

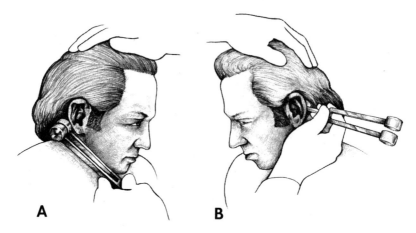

Figure 4.5. Rinne's test: With a lightly vibrating tuning fork, ask the patient if the sound is loudest in position *A* or position *B*.

    d. *Caloric test*: Examine the auditory canal to check that the eardrum is intact and that there is no blood or impacted cerumen. With the patient sitting, tilt the head to one side and inject approximately 2 mL cold water from a syringe equipped with a small-caliber soft polyethylene catheter directed at the posterior wall of the external canal. Start a stopwatch at the beginning of the injection. After 20 seconds, evacuate the water from the ear, tilt the patient's head backward 60 degrees, and have the patient look at the examiner's finger from a distance of approximately 3 feet (see Figure 4.6). Nystagmus may also be observed by visualizing a small-caliber blood vessel with an ophthalmoscope in a darkened room; observed in this way, the nystagmus has a rotary character. In the alert patient the eyes normally drift slowly toward the ear irrigated with cold water with the quick corrective component of the nystagmus back toward the primary position. (Nystagmus, which is named for the quick component, occurs away from the cooled ear). Abnormal responses include the absence of nystagmus or a marked difference in nystagmus between the two ears. (*Note*: Wait 15 minutes after irrigation of one ear before irrigating the other ear.) Instillation of warm water into the ear produces the opposite findings, but is ordinarily not necessary. (For caloric testing in the comatose patient, see Chapter 13).

Laboratory Investigations of the Dizzy Patient

Because the causes of dizziness are so varied, the authors cannot suggest a standard laboratory investigation of all dizzy patients. The choice of laboratory procedures should be tempered by the history and physical examination.

1. A complete blood count, ESR, and analysis of electrolytes and blood components is necessary because dizziness is so often equated with "unwellness."

2. Audiometry should be performed in all patients with significant hearing loss or tinnitus (see Appendix A).

3. Glucose tolerance test: if hypoglycemia is considered in the differential diagnosis.

4. Electrocardiogram: When patient reports palpitations, consider an ECG with carotid sinus massage.

5. Electroencephalography (sleep-deprived, with nasopharyngeal electrodes): when there is a suspicion of complex partial seizures.

6. Brainstem-evoked responses are especially useful in identifying acoustic neuromas and brainstem abnormalities.

7. A CT scan, with and without contrast, with particular attention to the posterior fossa is useful in identifying acoustic neuromas.

8. Magnetic resonance imaging is helpful in the diagnosis of multiple sclerosis and acoustic neuromas.

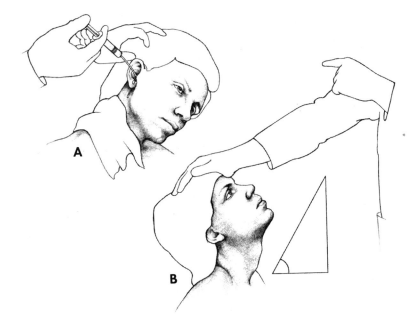

Figure 4.6. Caloric test: A. With the patient sitting in a chair with the head tilted to one side, inject 2 mL of water into the external canal. B. Remove the syringe, tilt head backward 60°, and observe and time the nystagmus. Quick movements will be directed away from the cold ear.

9. Skull x-rays are important with a history of head trauma to identify fractures.
10. Cervical spine x-rays: Hypertrophic osteoarthritis may cause narrowing of vertebral arteries.

DIZZINESS OF PSYCHOLOGICAL ORIGIN

Hyperventilation Syndrome

1. Hyperventilation is a very common cause of dizziness (lightheadedness).
2. It may be associated with circumoral paresthesias, paresthesias of the fingers, and carpopedal spasm (cramps in the hand and foot muscles).
3. Patients with this syndrome frequently are anxious.
4. The diagnosis is usually confirmed when the symptoms are reproduced by having the patient hyperventilate.

Treatment:

1. Explain the cause of the dizziness and reassure the patient. Have the patient breathe into a paper bag (rebreathing) during attacks.
2. Psychologic or psychiatric evaluation is not necessary in most cases.

Psychogenic Dizziness

1. In psychogenic dizziness the patient is inconsistent in regard to history, description of the dizziness, and factors affecting the dizziness; if the dizziness is injury-related or event-related, the circumstances of the injury or events are described in explicit detail.
2. The patient may note dizziness in all body positions.
3. The history may be misleading if the patient has had previous exposure to leading questions by other examiners; sometimes the patient may consciously mislead the examiner.
4. There may be associated symptoms of anxiety or depression; hyperventilation is common.
5. During the examination, there are inconsistencies in many of the tests and often all of the test maneuvers reproduce the symptoms.
6. The sensation of acrophobia or claustrophobia is described by many patients as dizziness.

Treatment:

A psychologic or psychiatric evaluation is indicated.

DIZZINESS AND VERTIGO OF VESTIBULAR ORIGIN

Symptomatic treatment of dizziness of vestibular origin is treated with the following drugs (remember that all of these drugs may cause excessive drowsiness):

1. Transderm Scop Transdermal Therapeutic System (a disc impregnated with scopolamine and placed behind the ear) is the drug of choice for motion sickness and other peripheral labyrinthine disorders. Each disc lasts three days.
2. Promethazine hydrochloride (Phenergan) 50 to 100 mg daily in divided doses for adults and 12.5 to 25 mg bid for children.
3. Meclizine hydrochloride (Antivert) 25 to 100 mg daily in divided doses.
4. Dimenhydrinate (Dramamine) 50 mg q4h may be effective for adults.
5. Trimethobenzamide hydrochloride (Tigan) 100 to 250 mg tid or qid is usually effective for controlling nausea.

Benign Positional Vertigo

1. Recurrent transient vertigo is precipitated by motion. Vertigo occurs with head motion whether the patient is standing or lying.
2. Vertigo is often associated with nausea; auditory symptoms are absent.
3. Examination shows the following:

   a. Nystagmus in the Nylen-Bárány maneuver occurring after a latency period of a few seconds and disappearing after approximately one minute. The phenomenon is less apparent on repetition of the maneuver (fatigable). This finding is virtually diagnostic of benign positional vertigo.

   Caveat: If there is no latency period before onset of nystagmus and if the phenomenon does not become less apparent on repetition, suspect posterior fossa tumor.

   b. Caloric tests are normal in 50% of patients.
4. This is a self-limited benign syndrome, initially severe, but gradually improving over days to weeks.

   Treatment:

   Symptomatic drug treatment.

Post-traumatic Vertigo

1. Skull fractures

   a. A lengthwise fracture through the petrous pyramid often involves structures of the middle ear. The patient often presents with bleeding from the ear.

56

b. Transverse fractures through the petrous pyramid involve the bony and membranous labyrinth; the patient presents with facial paralysis, vertigo, and spontaneous nystagmus.

2. Acceleration-deceleration injuries

a. Severe positional vertigo, especially with the involved ear pointing downward, caused by an inorganic deposit in semicircular canal (cupulolithiasis).

b. Persistent leak of perilymph from oval window to middle ear space.

c. Whiplash injuries may result in dizziness with objective findings referable to the vestibular system.

Treatment

Skull radiographs (tomograms) are necessary to document fractures; brainstem-evoked responses may localize the lesion. A thorough otolaryngologic examination is indicated because of the possibility of surgical correction and because these cases so often end up in litigation.

Ménière's Disease

1. The dramatic, episodic vertigo of Ménière's disease is associated with tinnitus (like a seashell held to the ear) and decreased hearing in the affected ear, lasting from hours to days. Vertigo is severe and explosive in onset.

2. Often preceded by an aura consisting of a fullness or pressure in the affected ear.

3. This is a disease primarily of middle age, affecting one side in only 75% of the cases.

4. Although hearing loss may fluctuate, it is progressive.

5. Some patients note that an attack may be precipitated by heavy salt intake.

6. The disease runs a prolonged course over many years and the vertiginous attacks tend to decrease as the deafness increases. Ultimately the patient will become deaf and the vertiginous attacks will cease.

7. Examination shows the following:

a. Decreased caloric response on affected side.

b. Loss of hearing, especially low tones.

c. Spontaneous nystagmus toward the affected side may be present during the attack.

d. Definitive diagnosis should be made with an audiologic examination requiring specialized equipment.

Treatment:

1. The armamentarium of vasodilators, diuretics, low salt diets,

vitamins, antihistamines, and tranquilizers suggest that no treatment is really effective.

2. When the patient is severely incapacitated, some otolaryngologists suggest a shunt procedure (between the membranous labyrinth and the subarachnoid space).

Note: There is a tendency to overdiagnose Ménière's disease. Other causes of severe acute vertigo include occlusion of the vestibular artery or the posterior inferior cerebellar artery, acute toxic labyrinthitis, and vestibular neuronitis. However, these causes of dramatic vertigo are usually not recurrent.

Acute Toxic Labyrinthitis

1. Acute toxic labyrinthitis is characterized by acute onset of vertigo that peaks in 24 hours and subsides in seven to ten days.
2. It is often associated with a nose or throat infection. Other associations include allergy or ototoxic medication.
3. Vertigo is exacerbated by head motion.
4. Examination shows:
   a. Caloric tests are abnormal in 50% of patients.
   b. Examination of nose or throat may show evidence of infection.
   c. Spontaneous nystagmus may be present.

   Treatment:

   1. Throat culture if clinically indicated
   2. Limitation of movement (bed rest).
   3. Symptomatic drug treatment
   4. Discontinuing drugs that may be vestibulotoxic

Postinfectious Vestibular Neuronitis

1. Postinfectious vestibular neuronitis is symptomatically very similar to acute labyrinthitis. The differentiating feature is that it is associated with the influenza syndrome and may occur epidemically.
2. This disease may have a longer recovery period (2-6 weeks) than acute labyrinthitis.

Motion Sickness

Some normal individuals have an increased sensitivity to the stimulus of motion.

Note: Adults with migraine frequently have a history of motion sickness in childhood.

Treatment:

Symptomatic drug treatment before the patient is in a situation where motion sickness is likely to occur.

DIZZINESS OR VERTIGO OF CENTRAL ORIGIN

Cerebrovascular Disorders (especially those involving the posterior fossa)

Dizziness or vertigo of central origin is a common complaint of patients with many types of cerebrovascular disease. The symptom of vertigo is related specifically to cerebrovascular diseases affecting the blood supply to the brainstem. The diagnosis is rarely easy, unless there are focal neurologic signs during or after the attacks. In many cases of vertebrobasilar TIAs the patient is normal between attacks. A four-vessel cerebral angiogram performed by an experienced neuroradiologist may be necessary for confirmation of the diagnosis.

1. Vertebrobasilar insufficiency: The onset is abrupt and often associated with loss of consciousness. Initial neurologic symptoms may include diplopia, slurred speech, numbness, dysphagia, visual field defects, or motor or sensory losses.

2. The subclavian steal syndrome may include attacks of vertigo, especially upon exercising the arm on the affected side. A clue to the diagnosis is asymmetric blood pressure in the arms. This is a particular type of vertebrobasilar insufficiency in which there is an occlusion proximal to the origin of the vertebral artery.

    Treatment: If an occlusion is demonstrated, surgical correction can be considered, but in many cases the symptoms subside spontaneously.

3. Ischemic damage to vestibular nuclei or their connections often includes damage to other parts of the brainstem. Elderly hypertensive patients with diabetes, heart disease, or hyperlipidemia are likely candidates. Focal neurologic signs are present; caloric response is absent or asymmetric.

4. Lateral medullary syndrome: This is a specific type of ischemic damage to vestibular connections due to infarction in the distribution of the posterior inferior cerebellar artery. The patient presents with vertigo, nausea, hiccups, and dysarthria. Abnormal neurologic signs include ipsilateral loss of pain and temperature sensation in the face, contralateral loss of pain and temperature in the body, ipsilateral cerebellar ataxia, and ipsilateral Horner's syndrome. Note that there is no paralysis of arms or legs. Prognosis for complete recovery is especially good with this type of infarction. These patients usually have a history of hypertension.

Treatment: See Chapter 12.

Acoustic Neuroma (Cerebellopontine Angle Tumor)

1. Suspect acoustic neuroma in any patient who develops insidious unilateral hearing loss unless clearly associated with trauma or infection. This tumor accounts for 10% of all primary intracranial tumors. High-pitched unilateral tinnitus may be an initial symptom.
2. Most common vestibular symptom is unsteadiness; true vertigo is rare. Occasionally symptoms are episodic.
3. As the disease progresses patients develop other neurologic complaints such as facial numbness, facial weakness, clumsiness, and headache.
4. Examination shows one or more of the following on the same side of tumor:
   a. Sensorineural hearing loss (air conduction greater than bone conduction; tuning fork on forehead louder in normal ear).
   b. Decreased caloric response on affected side.
   c. Loss of corneal reflex and sensory disturbance over the face.
   d. Facial weakness involving forehead.
   e. Decreased sensation in external auditory canal.
   f. Ipsilateral cerebellar findings.
   g. Café au lait spots with or without cutaneous neurofibromas suggests neurofibromatosis. This disease has an association with bilateral cerebellopontine angle tumors.
   h. Papilledema may be seen with large tumors.
5. Diagnostic Studies
   a. Brainstem auditory evoked responses and a CT scan with and without contrast (or MRI) should identify virtually all tumors.
   b. Audiometric tests show speech discrimination scores lower than expected for the degree of hearing loss, and asymmetry in pure tone audiograms (Békésy III and IV).

   Treatment:

   When diagnosis is confirmed, surgical exploration is necessary.

Other Posterior Fossa Tumors

Posterior fossa tumors are especially common in children, and although vertigo may be present, cerebellar and brainstem signs, cranial nerve abnormalities, and signs of increased intracranial pressure are usually more prominent. If suspected, referral to a neurologist or neurosurgeon is indicated.

Complex Partial Seizures

Vertigo, dizziness, or a feeling of unsteadiness may be an aura for complex partial seizures. For further diagnostic information and treatment, see Chapter 11.

Note: This type of seizure disorder is not necessarily associated with loss of consciousness or tonic-clonic movements.

Basilar Migraine

Basilar migraine usually occurs in children and young women and lasts minutes. Symptoms may include attacks of vertigo, which can be associated with visual disturbance, ataxia, tinnitus, and sometimes sudden loss of consciousness. For further diagnostic information, see Chapter 3.

Multiple Sclerosis

Patients who later are diagnosed as having multiple sclerosis may present with altered sensation of balance, but this is seldom true vertigo. Dizziness may also be the result of multiple sensory deficits. For further diagnostic information, see Chapter 10.

Multiple Sensory Deficits (Aging Balance System)

1. Elderly patients often have altered sensory input: visual (cataracts) and proprioceptive, touch, pressure (from peripheral neuropathy, often diabetic, or cervical cord involvement in cervical spondylosis). Vestibular abnormalities may occur secondary to basilar artery insufficiency or premature aging of the vestibular nuclei.
2. The diminished sensory input causes dizziness (out of touch with environment) especially when walking or turning.
3. Additional sensory cues, sometimes as simple as carrying a cane, during maneuvers that produce dizziness usually reduces the symptoms.

   Treatment:

   Medications often make this condition worse. If possible, devise ways of increasing sensory input, eg, cataract operation, moving slowly.

DRUGS AS A CAUSE OF DIZZINESS

The vestibular nerve and the vestibular apparatus can be damaged by commonly used drugs. Some drugs produce reversible dysfunction, whereas others produce irreversible destruction. If the patient is taking one of the following drugs, it should be considered as a possible cause of the dizziness:

1. Antibiotics
   a. Aminoglycosides (such as streptomycin)

b. Polypeptides (polymyxin B)

c. Semisynthetic penicillin (ampicillin)

d. Sulfonamides

e. Synthetics (chloramphenicol)

2. Diuretics (furosemide)

3. Salicylates (aspirin)

4. Anti-inflammatory drugs (phenylbutazone)

5. Antimalarials (quinine)

6. Anticonvulsants (phenytoin)

7. Antihistamines

SYSTEMIC DISORDERS CAUSING FAINTNESS, DIZZINESS, AND SYNCOPE

Cardiovascular Disturbances

1. Orthostatic (postural) hypotension: Upon standing, the patient experiences faintness from a fall in blood pressure; the magnitude of the drop in blood pressure is less important than the association of the faintness in moving from a lying to a standing position. The differential diagnosis of possible etiologies is lengthy but includes the following:

a. Hypovolemic states.

b. Peripheral neuropathy (especially if the autonomic nervous system is affected as in diabetes).

c. Lower extremity venous pooling (as in severe varicose veins).

d. Antihypertensive drugs.

2. Cardiac arrhythmias may be recognized by auscultation or routine ECG, but 24 hour Holter monitoring may be required.

3. Carotid sinus hypersensitivity.

a. The patient may relate a history of faintness or syncope with neck motion or pressure on the neck; examples include faintness while backing a car out of a driveway or faintness associated with shaving the neck. This syndrome is most common in children and adolescents and in older patients with atherosclerotic disease involving the carotid bifurcation.

b. The faintness or dizziness disappears rapidly (lasting about 15 seconds).

c. The diagnosis is confirmed by reproducing symptoms by lightly massaging the carotid sinus (do not occlude the carotid artery) and monitoring both the blood pressure and the heart rate (ECG). A pause of more than 3 seconds in the heartbeat or a decrease in systolic blood pressure greater than 50 torr is considered abnormal. Valsalva maneuvers may also precipitate cardiac slowing and a fall in blood pressure (micturition syncope); this can be checked at the same time as the carotid massage.

Caution: Do not massage the carotid artery of patients with known carotid artery or intracranial cerebrovascular disease because of the risk of precipitating stroke. Cardiac arrest may also occur.

4. Hypertension: Patients with severe hypertension in the early phases of hypertensive encephalopathy may experience faintness and dizziness.

Caution: The patient with symptoms of dizziness and rapidly elevating blood pressure may have an expanding mass lesion in the posterior fossa (see Chapter 13).

Vasovagal Phenomena

1. *Common vasovagal syncope*: This is the common fainting that occurs in normal persons and which is often precipitated by emotional stress or warm, crowded conditions. It is preceded by an aura of nausea and sweating. The loss of consciousness may be prevented by assuming a supine position and elevating the legs.
2. *Reflex vasovagal syncope*: This is similar to the common vasovagal syncope, but the fainting spell is precipitated by a stimulus, eg, venipuncture. There may be a family history of similar stimulus-precipitated syncope, breath-holding spells, or migraine. This syndrome must be differentiated from a seizure by lack of postictal sleepiness and tonic-clonic movements.
3. *Breath-holding spells*
   a. A form of vasovagal syncope in children aged 6 months to 6 years.
   b. It may be of two types:
      i. Begins with crying; the child holds his breath and turns blue (cyanotic type).
      ii. After minor startle or sudden painful stimulus, the child turns white and loses consciousness (pallid type).
   c. The period from onset through loss of consciousness usually lasts less than 60 seconds. There may be a few seconds of tonic stiffening at the end of the period of unconsciousness, which may be mistaken for a seizure.
   d. At the termination of the breath-holding spell, the child immediately awakens, usually with no apparent postictal symptoms (no headache, confusion, or lethargy).
   e. If the physician thinks an EEG is necessary, the EEG should be done with monitoring of respiration and ECG to differentiate seizures from

breath-holding spells.

Treatment:

This condition is benign with the child outgrowing the disorder. Breath-holding spells do not lead to epilepsy. Parents should be reassured of the benign prognosis.

OTHER MEDICAL CONDITIONS ASSOCIATED WITH FAINTNESS AND DIZZINESS

Almost any medical condition may be associated with dizziness; this chapter assumes that the general health of the patient is good.

1. Anemia causes dizziness due to hypovolemia or decreased oxygen carrying capacity of the blood.
2. Hypoglycemia, especially common in diabetics.
3. Endocrine disorders, especially thyroid and adrenal insufficiency.
4. Visual disorders, especially after a change in prescription for lenses, during diplopia, or after cataract surgery.
5. Allergies: allergic reactions may cause a sensation of fullness in the head, lightheadedness, or faintness. This diagnosis should be pursued in patients with a strong allergy history. Remember that many of the drugs used to treat allergies also cause dizziness.

BIBLIOGRAPHY

Bucy PG: Vertigo with diseases of the central nervous system. *Arch Otolaryngol* 1967;85:535-536.

Drachman DA, Hart CW: An approach to the dizzy patient. *Neurology* 1972; 22:323-334.

Harner SG, Laws ER: Clinical findings in patients with acoustic neuroma. *Mayo Clin Proc* 1983;58:721-728.

Healy GB: Hearing loss and vertigo secondary to head injury. *N Engl J Med* 1982;306:1029-1031.

Schumacher GA: Demyelinating diseases as a cause for vertigo. *Arch Ontolaryngol* 1967;85:537-538.

Sugrue DD, Wood DL, McGoon MD: Carotid sinus hypersensitivity and syncope. *Mayo Clin Proc* 1984; 59:637-640.

Wolfson RJ, Silverstein H, Marlowe F, et al: Vertigo. *Ciba Found Symp* 1986; 38:2-32

V

SLEEP DISORDERS

It has been estimated that each year, almost 10 million Americans consult their physicians for sleep problems. In order to diagnose and treat sleep disorders successfully, the physician needs to have an understanding of the normal sleep cycle, the pharmacology of hypnotics and related medications, and the various disorders of sleep and arousal.

Normal Sleep Pattern

A. Sleep Stages

    1. On the basis of EEG and other physiologic parameters, two categories of sleep are recognized: non-rapid eye movement (NREM, slow wave, or spindle) and rapid eye movement (REM, active, paradoxical) sleep. NREM sleep is divided into four stages on the basis of the EEG pattern (Table 5.1).

    2. Certain sleep stages may affect underlying medical disorders adversely. Thus during REM sleep angina of coronary heart disease and the pain of duodenal ulcer may be exacerbated. Stage I sleep (the transition between wakefulness and sleep) is most prone to enhance abnormal EEG activity and/or clinical seizures in patients with seizure disorders.

B. Sleep Cycle

    1. In the young adult the normal sleep cycle is made up of 20% to 25% REM, 5% to 10% stage I, 50% stage II, and 20% stages III and IV. Typically, sleep begins with stage I and progresses through Stages II, III, and IV and back through stages II and III. Then, about

TABLE 5.1
SLEEP CYCLE

Category	Stage	Patient Appearance	Physiologic Characteristics	Pathologic Disturbances
REM	REM	Very still, deep sleep; body apparently paralyzed; rapid eye movements	Bursts of REM; irregular respiration; high BMR; inhibited peripheral muscle activity (except diaphragm); dreaming; penile tumescence; bursts of sympathetic nervous system activity	Narcolepsy; nightmares
NREM	I	Drowsiness	Sleep myoclonus	Excessive sleep myoclonus; seizure activity
	II	Light sleep	EEG: sleep spindles	
	III	Deep sleep	EEG: slow waves	
	IV	Deep sleep	EEG: slow waves	Sleepwalking; night terrors; enuresis
			Decreased body temperature, pulse, and respirations; peripheral muscle activity present; increased vagal tone	

REM = rapid eye movement; NREM = nonrapid eye movement; BMR = basal metabolic rate.

70 to 100 minutes after the onset of sleep, the first REM period occurs.

2. This cycle is repeated approximately every 90 minutes with a total of four to six cycles each night. Toward morning the REM periods lengthen and NREM sleep progresses only to stages II and III.

C. Normal Variations

1. There are specific variations in the sleep cycle with age. Thus, a newborn may spend as much as 50% of sleep in REM, with the child reaching adult proportions by the 3rd year. Children have a high percentage of stages III and IV sleep, while the elderly have virtually no stage IV sleep. The elderly also often have frequent and lengthy awakenings.

2. There is also considerable amount of individual variation in the sleep cycle and total duration of sleep. Some individuals can function with very little sleep, while others need much more than the suggested eight hours.

Approach to the Patient with Sleep Disorders

A large number of clinical conditions affect sleep. The major categories include patients with disorders of initiation and maintenance of sleep and those with excessive daytime sleepiness (Table 5.2). Clinical evaluation of the patient with sleep disorders should include the following steps:

1. Interview: The first and most important step in evaluating a patient with a sleep disorder is the interview.

   a. First, it is important to determine whether the sleep-related complaints are real or simply subjective. Patients often tend to overestimate sleep complaints. A bed partner can give valuable information during the interview. A sleep log (written record kept by the patient and the patient's bed partner that charts bedtime, time of onset of sleep, awakenings during sleep, time of awakening, and other sleep habits like snoring, apnea, bruxism, myoclonus, etc) could offer further insight into the sleep pattern of the individual.

   b. Obtain the following information without asking leading questions:

      i. Sleep habits: when, where, how long, naps.

      ii. Sleep problems: difficulty in falling asleep, use of sleep aids; awakening during night, frequency and length; cause of awakenings - dreams, movement, pain, anxiety.

      iii. Daytime somnolence: how often, duration, history suggestive of cataplexy (sudden loss of power in lower limbs while laughing or when emotionally upset).

TABLE 5.2
SLEEP AND AROUSAL DISORDERS

A. Disorders of initiating and maintaining sleep (DIMS, insomnias)
   1. Psychophysiologic: transient, persistent
   2. Psychiatric disorders, eg, affective disorders
   3. Use of drugs and alcohol
   4. Sleep-induced respiratory impairment, eg, sleep apnea
   5. Sleep-related myoclonus and "restless legs"
B. Disorders of excessive somnolence (DOES)*
   1. Psychophysiologic and psychiatric disorders
   2. Use of drugs and alcohol
   3. Narcolepsy
   4. Rare disorders such as idiopathic CNS hypersomnolence, periodic som-
      nolence syndromes (Kleine-Levin syndrome)
C. Disorders of sleep-wake schedule
   1. Transient: ie, rapid time zone change (jet lag), work shift syndrome
   2. Persistent: delayed sleep phase and advanced sleep phase syndrome.
D. Parasomnias
   1. Sleep walking (somnambulism)
   2. Sleep terror
   3. Sleep enuresis
   4. Sleep-related seizures, bruxism, nightmares, etc

*Any condition that causes insomnia can lead to excessive daytime somnolence

---

    iv. Medications and drug history: sedatives, stimulants, street
       drugs, alcohol.
    v. History suggestive of seizure disorders, anxiety neurosis,
      depression, or affective disorders.
    vi. Medical history: any medical condition that may lead to
       disturbances in sleep (eg, cluster headache, asthma, car-
       diac failure, hyperthyroidism, etc).
2. Physical examination: Obesity, hypertension, cardiac abnormalities,
   neurologic deficits, evidence of endocrine dysfunction, such as thyrotoxicosis or hypothyroidism.
3. Investigations
   a. A decision regarding investigations should only be taken after
     detailed consideration of the history and physical findings. Pa-
     tients with transient sleep problems do not need costly inves-
     tigations such as polysomnography.
   b. If an underlying medical disorder such as intracranial disease
     or endocrinopathy is suspected, perform the relevant investi-
     gations (eg, CT scan, EEG, biochemical tests for endocrine dis-
     orders).

c. Patients with persistent sleep disorders often need polysomnography (recording of EEG along with other physiologic parameters such as respiration, EMG, ECG, electro-oculography [EOG], etc). This will require referral to a sleep disorders laboratory (Table 5.3).

Disorders of Initiating and Maintaining Sleep (DIMS, Insomnias)

In evaluating a patient with insomnia, take into account the normal variations as well as the effects of age on the architecture of sleep stages and cycle. Remember that there is significant variation from person to person regarding the optimal duration of sleep; it is important to ascertain whether the patient feels alert and is performing well despite a shorter duration of sleep, which may simply be the normal for that person.

  A. Psychophysiologic Insomnia
     1. Transient and situational insomnia. The characteristic features are:
       a. Insomnia lasting less than 3 weeks.
       b. The presence of a clear, precipitating cause, such as emotional shock (eg, the death of a loved one, divorce); depression or anxiety provoked by circumstances such as change of job, tests, interviews; sleeping in unfamiliar surroundings (eg, the hospital).

TABLE 5.3
LABORATORY INVESTIGATIONS IN SLEEP DISORDERS

TEST	PROCEDURE	INDICATIONS
Multiple sleep latency test (MSLT)	During an 8-9-hour period the patient is allowed to sleep for five 20-min periods; the average sleep latency and any REM-onset sleep are documented	Excessive daytime sleepiness, particularly narcolepsy
Polysomnography	Simultaneous recording of EEG, EOG, EMG, respirations, ECG, and oxygen tension during all-night sleep recordings; may also be combined with video recording of patient activity.	Sleep apnea syndrome, sleep myoclonus, and other sleep related disorders; differentiation of nocturnal seizures from night terrors, nightmares, sleepwalking, and apneic spells

       c. A premorbid personality revealing insecurity and proneness to emotional arousal.

Treatment:

1. Reassurance and, if necessary, crisis intervention by a psychiatrist
2. Temporary use of hypnotics, mainly to ensure rest and to prevent chronic insomnia

2. Persistent or chronic insomnia
   a. When insomnia persists for more than 3 weeks it is considered as chronic insomnia.
   b. May evolve from situational insomnia, or there may be no obvious factors.
   c. Difficulty in falling asleep, frequent awakenings, or early morning awakenings.
   d. Somatization of anxiety and negative conditioning to sleep are considered as underlying factors.

   Treatment:

   1. General measures for sleep hygiene include establishing regular schedules for bedtime and waking, improving sleep environment, late afternoon or early evening exercises, avoidance of alcohol and caffeine-containing drinks in the evening, and stress management.
   2. Hypnotics: Continual use of hypnotics should be avoided because they can be addictive, usually lose their effect within a few days (leading to escalation of dosage), tend to produce rebound insomnia when withdrawn, and may be dangerous if taken in larger than the prescribed amount. Occasional use may be permitted in insomniacs who experience a run of sleepless nights to avoid panic and other psychological problems. Of the hypnotics, benzodiazepine derivatives are considered to be the drugs of choice, with the most safe and effective being flurazepam hydrochloride (Dalmane) 15 to 30 mg, temazepam (Restoril) 15 to 30 mg, and triazolam (Halcion) 0.25 to 0.5 mg at bedtime. Use smaller doses in the elderly.
   3. L-Tryptophan 2 to 4 g at bedtime may be helpful in some patients, particularly when there are frequent awakenings.

B. Insomnia Associated with Psychiatric Disorders

Psychiatric disturbances constitute major causes of insomnia. The underlying condition may be excessive tension with somatization of symptoms, anxiety neurosis, depression, or major psychiatric disorders like schizophrenia.

Treatment:

Treatment should be directed toward the underlying cause (see Chapter 9).

Caution: Do not simply prescribe sedatives or hypnotics without adequate treatment of the underlying psychiatric disorder.

C. Medical Insomnia

Underlying medical problems that disturb sleep may account for insomnia in about 20% of patients. Such conditions include chronic pain from cancer, arthritis, peripheral neuropathy, metabolic disorders like uremia, and endocrine disorders like hyperthyroidism.

Treatment:

The underlying medical problem should be identified and appropriately treated. Sedatives can be used as an adjunctive treatment if necessary.

D. Insomnia Associated with Use of Drugs and/or Alcohol

1. When sedatives or hypnotics such as barbiturates, glutethemide, chloral hydrate, or methaqualone are taken regularly they lose their effectiveness in about 2 weeks, leading to need for increased dosage. Later tolerance develops and sleep becomes disturbed with frequent awakenings. Abrupt withdrawal leads to more marked insomnia.

3. Use of CNS stimulants: Excessive intake of caffeine-containing beverages, excessive use of weight-reducing agents, drug abuse (amphetamines, cocaine), or ingestion of other stimulants (pemoline, ephedrine, etc) can lead to insomnia.

4. Chronic alcohol abuse leads to insomnia, especially during withdrawal.

E. Insomnias associated with nocturnal myoclonus, restless leg syndrome, and sleep apnea syndrome are discussed under disorders of excessive somnolence.

Disorders of Excessive Somnolence (DOES)

These disorders manifest as inappropriate sleepiness while awake, frequent naps, incomplete arousal in the morning and sometimes cognitive dysfunction. Any condition that impairs nocturnal sleep may lead to daytime sleepiness. In addition, there are a number of disorders that lead to periodic or persistent daytime somnolence. The two most important causes of persistent daytime somnolence are sleep apnea syndrome and narcolepsy.

A. Psychophysiologic somnolence
   1. Transient and situational excessive daytime somnolence
      a. Onset related to a specific event such as death of a loved one, divorce, change of job, etc
      b. Lasts from a few days to 2 to 3 weeks
      c. Difficulty in remaining awake, frequent naps, and disturbed nocturnal sleep

      Treatment: Reassure the patient; sedatives or hypnotics may be used at night as a temporary measure.
   2. Persistent excessive daytime somnolence
      a. Excessive sleepiness and tiredness persisting for more than 3 weeks
      b. Tends to occur repeatedly with periods of stress

      Treatment: Psychiatric help for stress management.
B. Persistent excessive daytime somnolence may occur in affective disorders (such as bipolar manic-depressive illness), tolerance to or withdrawal from CNS stimulants, or in alcohol abuse. These conditions are also associated with disturbed nocturnal sleep. Sleepiness resolves with treatment of the underlying disorder.
C. Narcolepsy
   1. The manifestation of an imbalance between wakefulness and sleep in which the REM stage seems to be dominating over wakefulness.
   2. Irresistible "sleep attacks" that occur at any time and usually last less than 15 minutes.
   3. As part of the narcolepsy syndrome, the patient may also experience one or more of the following (11%-14% may show all the features):
      a. Cataplexy: a sudden loss of muscle tone (may fall down without warning) is often precipitated by laughter or any strong emotion. If cataplexy persists for more than 60 seconds the patient may go into actual REM sleep.
      b. Sleep paralysis occurs during the transition between sleep and waking, most frequently at the time of falling asleep, and characterized by an inability to move even though awake.
      c. Hypnagogic hallucinations (vivid visual or auditory perceptions) occur at the time of falling asleep.
   4. Onset is usually in adolescence or young adulthood.
   5. There may be a family history of similar problems.
   6. Diagnosis is confirmed by special studies such as the multiple sleep latency test (MSLT) which shows a reduced sleep latency and REM-onset sleep.

    7. High association with HLA DR$_2$ phenotype.

    Treatment:

      1. Explain the nature of the symptoms to the patient. This is crucial in the long-term management.

      2. Impress upon the patient the need to exercise extreme caution while driving an automobile or operating heavy machinery.

      3. Scheduled naps of 15 minutes in the morning and afternoon may cut down the sleep attacks.

      4. Pemoline (Cylert) 18.75 to 75 mg/day or methylphenidate hydrochloride (Ritalin) 5 to 60 mg/day in divided morning and early afternoon doses may control the irresistible sleepiness. Start with a small dose, eg, methylphenidate 10 mg once or twice a day, and find the smallest effective dose for that particular patient.

      5. Imipramine hydrochloride (Tofranil) 50 to 200 mg/day may benefit cataplexy, sleep paralysis, and hypnagogic hallucinations, but it has minimal effect on irresistible sleep attacks. Protriptyline hydrochloride (Vivactil) 15 to 30 mg/day is an alternative.

      6. Patient information materials may be obtained from the American Narcolepsy Association, P.O. Box 5846, Stanford, CA 94305.

D. Idiopathic CNS Hypersomnolence (NREM narcolepsy, idiopathic DOES)

    1. Idiopathic CNS hypersomnolence resembles narcolepsy in causing recurrent daytime somnolence, but is unassociated with other features of narcolepsy such as cataplexy, sleep paralysis, and hypnogogic hallucinations. The naps are longer, less compelling in onset, and less refreshing than the sleep attacks of narcolepsy.

    2. May account for 12% to 15% of patients with excessive daytime somnolence.

    3. May be familial.

    4. Differentiate from narcolepsy and excessive sleepiness associated with depression. Other conditions to be considered include communicating hydrocephalus and post-head trauma hypersomnolence.

      Treatment: Response to stimulants such as methylphenidate may be poor. Methysergide has been found to be useful in some patients (see Chapter 3 for a discussion of complications of methysergide therapy).

E. Sleep Apnea

    1. Sleep apnea may result from problems with neural control of respiration (central apnea), from obstruction of upper airway (obstructive apnea), or from a combination of the two (mixed apnea). Apneic

episodes are defined as cessation of airflow at the nose and mouth lasting 10 seconds or more. A considerable number of such episodes occur in patients with sleep apnea syndrome.

2. Obstructive apnea is due to sleep-related upper airway obstruction (relaxation of muscles around the upper airway during sleep leads to the obstruction). It occurs predominantly in older males. It is characterized by extreme restlessness during the night with severe snoring, snorting, and frequent respiratory pauses and excessive daytime sleepiness. Once asleep, arousal may be difficult and accompanied by confusion, disorientation, and ataxia. Predisposing factors for sleep-related upper airway obstruction includes enlarged tonsils and adenoids, micrognathia, macroglossia, and endocrinopathies (such as hypothyroidism and acromegaly).

   Note: Sleep apnea syndrome may cause both insomnia and excessive daytime sleepiness.

3. A number of associated symptoms and complications are reported with sleep apnea syndrome: cardiac arrhythmias, right heart failure, hypertension, obesity, night sweats, and morning headache. In children, nocturnal enuresis, learning difficulties, and hyperactivity interrupted by hypersomnolence may be seen.

4. CNS dysfunction which occurs only during sleep leads to lack of respiratory drive in patients with central apnea. Such patients experience frequent nocturnal awakenings. The syndrome may have some overlap with sudden infant death syndrome (SIDS).

5. Consider in the differential diagnosis: intracranial lesions (eg, diencephalic tumor), nocturnal seizures, hypothyroidism, acromegaly, and drug dependence.

6. Confirmation of diagnosis should be done by nightlong polysomnographic recording (Table 5.3).

Treatment:

1. Factors such as the degree of daytime sleepiness, level of oxygen desaturation during the apneic spells, cardiac status, and the type of apnea (central or obstructive) should be taken into consideration in charting out the treatment plan.

2. Weight reduction, alcohol withdrawal, and sleeping in a position other than supine may prove helpful in mild cases.

3. Respiratory stimulants such as theophylline, protriptyline, and progesterone have been tried with varying success.

4. Nasal continuous positive airway pressure (CPAP) is being used more frequently in obstructive and mixed apnea. The positive pressure tends to splint the upper airway, keeping it open during sleep.

5. Some patients with airway obstruction are helped by surgery (ie, tonsillectomy, adenoidectomy, uvulapalatopharyngoplasty, or removal of an intrathoracic goiter).
6. Permanent tracheostomy, which can be kept closed during the day and open at night, gives relief in severe cases with marked upper airway obstruction and cardiac decompensation.
7. No effective treatment has been found for central sleep apnea. In severe cases the feasibility of pacing the diaphragm by electrophrenic stimulation is being evaluated.

   Caution: Do not prescribe hypnotics in sleep apnea, as they will aggravate the apnea and the daytime sleepiness.

F. Sleep-Related Abnormal Movements

1. Sleep-related (nocturnal) myoclonus is characterized by abrupt jerking of feet and legs, which may be frequent enough to cause symptoms.
   a. The myoclonic jerks may be violent enough to awaken the individual fully or partially. Sometimes the patient may not be aware of the movements and the complaint may come from the bed partner.
   b. Both insomnia and excessive daytime sleepiness can result from this disorder.

   Treatment:

   Clonazepam 0.5 to 1.0 mg at bedtime has been found to be helpful, particularly when troublesome insomnia accompanies abnormal movements. Recently temazepam has also been found to be useful.

2. "Restless legs" syndrome is characterized by an indescribable, unpleasant sensation in the legs with an irresistible urge to move the legs.
   a. Movement seems to relieve the discomfort.
   b. Sleep-related myoclonus may also be present; insomnia may be a prominent complaint.
   c. There may be a family history of similar complaints.
   d. Sometimes associated with peripheral neuropathy (eg, uremic neuropathy, diabetes, etc).

   Treatment:

   1. Phenytoin (Dilantin) 300 to 700 mg/day or carbamazepine (Tegretol) 400 to 1200 mg/day may be useful in some patients.

      Caution: Pretreatment and follow-up blood counts while on carbamazepine are recommended because of rare bone marrow suppression.

2. Clonazepam 0.5 to 1.0 mg at bedtime has been tried with varying success.
3. Treatment should be directed at the underlying condition, eg, diabetes, uremia, etc.

G. Periodic Disorders with Daytime Somnolence

Kleine-Levin syndrome

This syndrome of periodic hypersomnia is very rare and is characterized by recurrent episodes of markedly prolonged sleep (several weeks) with intervening periods of normal sleep and wakefulness. It may also be associated with periodic increase in appetite for food and sex. It occurs in adolescence and young adulthood, more commonly in males. Consider lesions (inflammatory and neoplastic) involving the diencephalon or limbic system in the differential diagnosis.

Disorders of Sleep-Wake Schedule

These are disorders of the circadian or 24 hour biological clock.

A. Transient Disorders

1. Rapid time zone change (jet lag) syndrome: The patient's sleep wake schedule does not adjust immediately to the new time zone and hence sleepiness and fatigue occurs during wakefulness and insomnia during the new sleep period. Symptoms last on an average for two days.

   Treatment:

   The morning awakening time is a strong cue to reset the biological clock. Hence, one should adjust the wake-up time to suit the new environment. Use of a hypnotic for the first two nights may also be helpful.

2. "Shift work" change: When the work period is shifted to normal sleeping hours, the person is sleepy, performance suboptimal, and the new sleep period disrupted.

B. Persistent Disorders

1. Delayed sleep-phase syndrome
   a. The person finds it very difficult both to fall asleep and to awaken in the morning, and when allowed to sleep, often sleeps into the early afternoon. Such a patient's biological clock is set differently from the norm, the circadian rhythm being out of phase with socially prescribed bedtime.

b. When on vacation such a person reports sleeping from 4 AM until noon or 2 PM.

Treatment:

Chronotherapy, which involves "resetting the biological clock," consists of going to bed three hours later each day, eg, functioning on a 27-hour "day," until the individual has advanced to the normal 10 or 11 PM bedtime.

2. Advanced sleep-phase syndrome
This is a rare disorder. Sleep onset and awakening times are earlier than desired, without difficulty in maintaining sleep once begun. The main complaint is that the person cannot stay awake in the evening without falling asleep and cannot delay sleep onset by enforcing conventional sleep times.

Parasomnias

The parasomnias include a number of conditions which occur either exclusively during sleep or are exacerbated by sleep.

A. Bed-Wetting (Enuresis)

1. Primary enuresis (child never toilet-trained):
   a. Often due to maturational lag.
   b. Ten to fifteen percent of children 4 to 5 years of age continue to wet the bed; this rarely continues into adulthood.
   c. There is often a family history of this disorder. Enuresis occurs in all sleep stages.

   Treatment:

   1. Advise the parents against overreacting to the situation, and reassure them that children usually outgrow it. Patience and understanding are important.
   2. Rewarding the child for a dry bed is helpful.
   3. Various behavior modification methods can be applied in difficult cases with the aid of experienced child psychologists.
   4. Imipramine (10 to 75 mg at bedtime) is often effective in preventing bed-wetting but is not recommended for prolonged usage.

2. Secondary enuresis (relapse to bed-wetting after a dry period of several months to years):
   a. Often due to psychological factors such as childhood depression.
   b. Organic disease must be ruled out, even if a psychological cause is obvious.

Treatment:

1. Psychological evaluation and family counseling are often necessary.
2. Imipramine hydrochloride (Tofranil), a tricyclic antidepressant, in doses of 0.5 to 2.0 mg/kg/day at bedtime has been shown to be effective in reducing the frequency of bedwetting. It is most effective when childhood depression is associated with the enuresis; with other causes the response is not as good. There is a tendency to relapse when the drug is withdrawn, and it is not recommended for prolonged use.
3. Behavioral techniques, such as bladder control exercises, rewards for dry beds, and wetting alarms frequently improve the enuresis.

Remember: An important organic cause of enuresis is urinary tract infection, and all children with enuresis should have urinalysis and a culture done. Other rare possibilities to consider include seizures in sleep, diabetes, congenital anomalies of the bladder, urethral obstruction, or ectopic ureter.

B. Sleepwalking (Somnambulism)

1. The prevalence of sleepwalking is estimated at 1% to 6%.
2. It occurs mostly in children and usually disappears by 14 to 15 years of age.
3. There is often a family history of sleepwalking.
4. Episodes last several minutes with total amnesia for the incident.
5. Episodes occur during stages III and IV sleep.
6. Sleepwalkers have a high incidence of enuresis.
7. The onset of sleepwalking in older age groups should arouse suspicion of a psychiatric disorder or medication effect. Nocturnal delirium ("sundown syndrome") may manifest as sleepwalking in the demented elderly.

Treatment:

1. Protect the patient from injury by locking doors and windows and avoiding other dangerous situations. Advise parents that children usually outgrow it.
2. Benzodiazepines, such as diazepam (Valium) 2 to 5 mg at bedtime, which suppress sleep stages III and IV, may be helpful for chronic and frequent sleepwalking.
3. In adult sleepwalkers, psychological disturbances are frequent, unless there is a strong family history. Thorough psychological evaluation and treatment are recommended.

C. Night Terrors

1. Night terrors occur early in the night during slow-wave sleep, most frequently at ages 4 to 6 years.
2. Sudden apparent awakening is accompanied by extreme physiologic arousal (increased heart rate, respiratory rate, and sweating), and the child will scream and cry, but cannot be awakened.
3. The incident is usually not remembered, although the child may recall a single frightening image or a sense of doom.

   Treatment:

   1. Advise the parents that children usually outgrow night terrors, and medication is generally not necessary.
   2. Night terrors may be abolished by diazepam 2 to 5 mg for children or 5 to 20 mg for adults. Long-term use is not recommended.
   3. Other medical conditions causing distress and disturbing stage IV sleep may result in night terrors. Correction of this condition may decrease the frequency of night terrors.
   4. Psychiatric referral is indicated for night terrors past age 14 years.

D. Nightmares (Dream Anxiety Attacks)

1. Nightmares are frightening dreams occurring in REM sleep, more frequently toward morning.
2. The degree of physiologic arousal is much lower than in night terrors.
3. Patients often have detailed recall of dream content.

   Treatment:

   1. Usually reassurance is all that is necessary.
   2. In cases where nightmares are frequent and disabling to the patient, psychotherapy and behavioral treatment may be effective.

E. Sleep-Related Epileptic Seizures

1. While seizures may occur predominantly or exclusively during sleep in epileptic patients, conditions like enuresis, night terrors, and sleep-walking may be triggered by seizures originating in the temporal lobe.
2. Nightlong EEG recording along with observation of the clinical phenomena (split-screen video recording) may be necessary to confirm the diagnosis.

   Treatment: Anticonvulsant therapy (see Chapter 11).

Other Medical Conditions Affecting Sleep

A. Patients secrete 3 to 20 times more gastric acid during REM sleep.

   Treatment:
   1. Treatment for sleep problems must not interfere with primary therapy of the underlying medical condition.
   2. Try to minimize sleep disruptions.
   3. Antidepressants, eg, amitriptyline and doxepin, in low dosage may prove helpful for both the sleep disturbance and hyperacidity.

B. Angina is more likely to occur during REM sleep.

C. Bronchial asthma attacks often occur during REM sleep.

   Caution: Do not prescribe hypnotics to patients with bronchial asthma.

D. Hypo- and hyperthyroidism may cause excessive sleepiness or insomnia, which are treated by correcting the thyroid dysfunction.

E. Pregnancy: Sleep time is increased in early pregnancy and decreased in later pregnancy, but normal sleep patterns should be recovered a few weeks after delivery. Drugs should be avoided during pregnancy.

F. Alcohol depresses REM sleep and results in REM rebound during withdrawal. Chronic alcoholics show fragmented shallow sleep. Insomnia is also associated with alcohol withdrawal.

BIBLIOGRAPHY

Association of Sleep Disorders Centers and the Association for the Psychophysiological Study of Sleep: Diagnostic classification of sleep and arousal disorders. *Sleep* 1979;2:5-137.

Cartwright RD, Samelson CF: The effects of a nonsurgical treatment of obstructive sleep apnea. The tongue retaining device. *JAMA* 1982; 248:705-709.

Chaudhary BA, Speir WA Jr: Sleep apnea syndrome. *South Med J* 1982; 75:39-45.

Coleman RM, Roffwary HP, Kennedy SJ: Sleep-wake disorders based on a polysomnographic diagnosis. *JAMA* 1982;247:997-1003.

Drugs and Insomnia: *NIH Consensus Development Conference Summary*. Nov 1983, Vol 4, No. 10.

Guilleminault C, Eldridge FL, Tilkian A: Sleep apnea syndrome due to upper airway obstruction. *Arch Intern Med* 1977;137:296-300.

Hauri P: *The Sleep Disorders. Current Concepts*. Kalamazoo, Mich, Scope Publication, Upjohn, 1982.

Kales A, Kales JD: *Evaluation and Treatment of Insomnia*. New York, Oxford University Press, 1984.

Parkes JD: The sleeping patient. *Lancet* 1977;1:990-993.

Riley TL (ed.): *Clinical Aspects of Sleep and Sleep Disturbance*. Stoneham, Mass, Butterworth, 1985.

Sanders MH: Nasal CPAP effect on patterns of sleep apnea. *Chest* 1985; 86:839-844

VI

DIMINISHED MENTAL CAPACITY AND DEMENTIA

Dementia is a general term for mental deterioration; stupid people are not necessarily demented (they may have been born that way) and people with normal intelligence may become demented (at one time they may have been brilliant). The task of a physician caring for a demented patient is twofold:

1. Identify those dementias that are treatable.
2. Educate and support the family of the patient with incurable dementia.

Diagnosis of Diminished Mental Capacity

Suspect dementia when the patient presents with any of the following:

1. Increasing forgetfulness
2. Confusion as a result of slight provocation such as a change in schedule or surroundings
3. A tendency toward repetition during the process of history-taking
4. Slowness in following commands during physical examination (eg, the examiner may have to demonstrate the tasks of station and gait)
5. Emotional lability, irritability

If dementia is suspected, or if the patient or the family complain of mental deterioration, a mental status evaluation *must* be performed. It should be conducted so that the patient does not become defensive. Usually, it can be worked in during the history and presented in an easy conversational style: "I'm going to ask you some questions that may sound silly, but it's part of my examination." We suggest three options (see Appendix B):

1. The mental status evaluation that has been used by neurologists for many years: The experienced physician gains considerable insight into brain function with this format, but it is not quantified.

2. The Six-Item Orientation Memory Concentration Test: this deceptively simple questionnaire is quantitative and is sensitive to mild dementing processes.

3. Formal neuropsychological evaluation: This must be administered by a trained individual, takes three to four hours to complete, and is relatively expensive.

In addition to the formal mental status examination, specific notation of the following should also be made:

1. Appearance and behavior
   a. Dress and grooming: Clean? Neat? Appropriate?
   b. Attention: Alert? Dull? Apathetic? Distracted?
   c. Movements: Slow? Hyperactive? Restless? Tremor?
   d. Discretion: Inhibited? Discusses intimate topics without restraint?
2. Language abnormalities
   a. Quantity: Talkative? Noncommunicative?
   b. Content: Simple or complex sentence structure? Trouble finding words?
   c. Perseveration: Trouble changing topics? Words from earlier sentence used inappropriately in a new sentence?
   d. Appropriateness: Irrelevant? Illogical?
   e. Comprehension: Follows commands? Answers questions directly?

Caution: Aphasic or schizophrenic patients may appear to be demented. Patients with a motor aphasia have a paucity of speech and difficulty finding words and are aware of their problem. Patients with a sensory aphasia or schizophrenia may produce many words which make no sense (see Chapter 12).

3. Mood
   a. Depression: "I-don't-know" responses. (Degree is important, because many patients with neurologic abnormalities also have depression; see Chapter 9.)
   b. Euphoria: Demented patients seem unconcerned about their problems.

Abnormalities Sometimes Seen in Demented Patients

Caution: These abnormalities do *not* diagnose dementia; but one or more of them are often seen in demented patients. The diagnosis is made on the basis of a *global* decline in intellectual function.

1. Expressionless or masklike facies; facial grimacing.

2. Brun's ataxia: A broad-based gait with short steps and feet placed flat on the ground as if on ice; a tendency to retropulsion increases the risk of falling; occurs in patients with frontal lobe deficits.

3. Athetoid posturing and tremors as seen in chronic or progressive diseases of the basal ganglia (see Chapter 7).

4. Grasp reflex: Lightly stroking the palm of the patient's hand elicits a grasp response and reluctance to let go (see Figure 6.1).

5. Rooting reflex (sometimes incorrectly called suck reflex): patient turns lips toward a stroking stimulus at the corner of the mouth (see Figure 6.2).

6. Snout reflex: patient puckers lips in response to gentle percussion of the lips (see Figure 6.3).

7. Active jaw reflex (see Figure 6.4).

8. Paratonic rigidity (gegenhalten): Advise patient to relax his limbs. Passive manipulation of the patient's arm in unpredictable directions feels as if he is consciously resisting every movement of the examiner (see Figure 6.5).

9. Motor perseveration: When asked to perform a task such as rapid alternating movements, the patient continues for an inappropriate length of time.

10. Motor impersistence (inability to persist in a motor task):
    a. Keeping eyes closed
    b. Keeping tongue out
    c. Fixating gaze
    d. Sustaining "ah" or "ee" sound
    e. Maintaining hand grip

    For example, in position sense testing, demented patients tend to peek (they are unable to sustain eye closure).

Treatable Dementias

Table 6.1 is a list of those disease processes which present as diminished mental capacity and which may either be cured or the progression stopped. This table suggests that the following laboratory studies should be considered in every demented patient:

1. Computed tomographic (CT) scan, with and without contrast: CT scan shows mass lesions, multiple infarcts, normal pressure hydrocephalus, cerebral atrophy.

2. Electroencephalogram (EEG): generalized slowing is seen in toxic metabolic encephalopathies, a periodic complexes pattern in Jakob-Creutzfeldt disease.

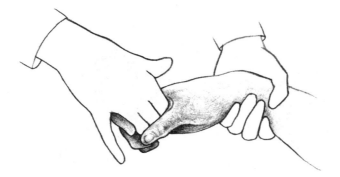

Figure 6.1 A grasp reflex: When the examiner pulls his fingers from the patient's hypothenar eminence to the thumb and forefinger, the patient squeezes the examiner's fingers (a normal response in infants).

3. Endocrine studies: Since hypothyroidism is the most common endocrine cause of dementia, tri-iodothyronine (T_3), thyroxine (T_4) and thyroid stimulating hormone (TSH) levels are recommended. Other studies should be ordered as suggested by the history and physical examination.
4. Lumbar puncture: LP is the only sure way to diagnose indolent infections and tertiary syphilis.
5. Blood chemistries are essential in diagnosing secondary metabolic encephalopathies.

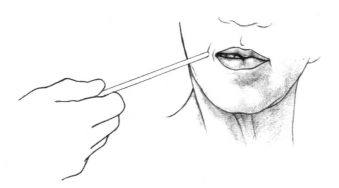

Figure 6.2 Rooting (suck) reflex: Stroking away from the corner of the mouth elicits lip movements and movement of mouth toward stimulus (normal in infants.)

84

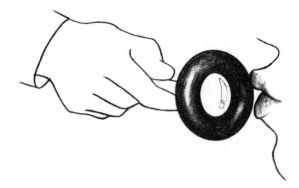

Figure 6.3 Snout: A light tap on closed lips causes lip to pucker.

6. Complete blood count and ESR: Abnormalities may suggest infection, vitamin deficiency, or autoimmune disease.
7. Serum vitamin B_{12} and folate levels are especially important in patients with chronic ulcer disease or postgastrectomy.
8. Urinary toxicology screen (including heavy metals).

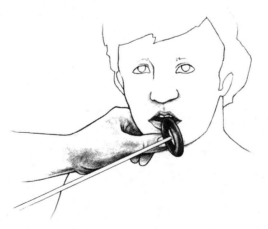

Figure 6.4 Jaw reflex: With the patient's mouth slightly open, examiner places finger on chin and lightly taps the fingers. The jaw closes momentarily.

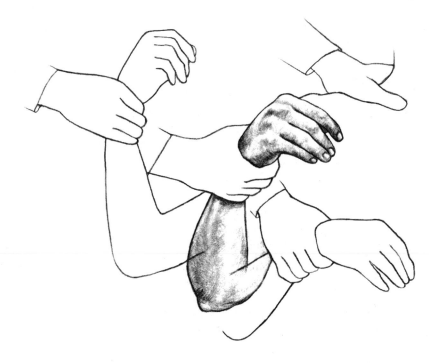

Figure 6.5 Gegenhalten: Ask patient to relax arm "like a rag doll." Examiner moves the arm in unpredictable directions. If the patient has gegenhalten, it feels to the examiner as if the patient is actively resisting movement.

Cerebrovascular Disease

    A. Multi-infarct dementia (Binswanger's disease):
        1. Patients always have a history of chronic hypertension.
        2. History may be one of a "stepwise" progression - periods of stability with sudden decompensation.

TABLE 6.1
Treatable Causes of Dementia

Toxins and Drugs
Nutritional Deficiency States
Metabolic or Endocrine Disorders
Hypoxia
Normal Pressure Hydrocephalus
Intracranial Mass Lesions
Central Nervous System Infections
Atherosclerotic Cerebrovascular Disease

3. CT scan or MRI shows multiple small infarcts just beneath the cortical gray matter.

   Treatment: Progression can be halted by controlling hypertension.

B. Pseudobulbar palsy:
   1. Patients almost always have a history of chronic hypertension.
   2. Patients present with emotional lability; they may burst into tears at a trivial incident, but, when asked, deny they are sad.
   3. Neurologic examination shows generalized hyperreflexia, including a hyperactive jaw reflex.
   4. CT scan shows multiple small infarcts in or near the internal capsule.

      Treatment: Control hypertension; some patients may be helped with tricyclic antidepressants.

C. Multiple cerebral emboli: The most common source of emboli is from the heart: Atrial fibrillation, mural thrombosis, postmyocardial infarct, and mitral valve prolapse are common associated conditions.

D. Occlusive disease of large vessels in the neck: There are scattered reports of improvement in mental status after endarterectomy, presumably because ischemic neurons function improperly. Selection of patients for surgery should be conservative.

Mass Lesions

1. Patients with large brain tumors sometimes may have no symptoms or signs other than dementia, especially if the tumor is slow growing.
2. CT scan and/or MRI easily diagnose these conditions.

Alcoholism

1. The patients usually have a history of drinking more than the equivalent of 150 mL/day of absolute alcohol for many years.
2. Lability of mood is common.
3. Recovery of mental faculties is surprisingly good if alcohol consumption can be stopped.

   Caution: This dementia should be differentiated from Korsakoff's psychosis which is a specific defect in acquiring new information, not a global defect (see Chapter 8).

Drugs

1. Many drugs, even when prescribed in conservative therapeutic doses, may result in diminished mental capacity. Examples include phenobarbital and phenytoin.
2. All demented patients should be given a drug-free period if at all possible.
3. Elderly patients are especially sensitive to medications; tranquilizers and sleep medication should be prescribed with great caution.

Subacute Combined Degeneration (Combined System Disease; Vitamin B_{12} Deficiency)

1. Patients commonly have a history of ulcer disease or gastrectomy; older patients may develop gastric achlorhydria and fail to produce intrinsic factor.
2. Although the patients have four neurologic abnormalities (dementia, corticospinal tract signs, posterior column abnormalities, and peripheral neuropathy), the dementia may be the most prominent finding (see Chapter 15).
3. Other vitamin deficiencies may produce a dementia, but rarely do so in the presence of an adequate diet.

Endocrine Abnormalities

1. Hypothyroidism: Neurologic abnormalities include dementia and slowed relaxation phase of the Achilles reflex.
2. Hypoglycemia: The usual clinical setting is repeated hypoglycemic attacks precipitated by inappropriate doses of insulin. Acute attacks should be treated with IV glucose. The dementia already incurred is permanent, but can be made worse if care is not taken to prevent further hypoglycemic attacks.
3. Both hyperparathyroidism and hypoparathyroidism may present as dementia; three normal fasting calcium levels are necessary to exclude parathyroid disease.
4. Any endocrine abnormality, if severe enough, may cause mental slowness; this includes Cushing's syndrome and panhypopituitarism.

Secondary Metabolic Encephalopathy

The abnormality is usually obvious on general physical examination, multichannel chemistries, and blood gas determinations. Common causes include chronic obstructive pulmonary disease, and hepatic and renal failure. The EEG often shows generalized slowing.

Chronic Infection

1. Tuberculous and fungal meningitis may produce dementia both by destroying the brain parenchyma and by thickening the posterior fossa meninges and causing an obstructive hydrocephalus. The patient may have no other signs of infection, such as fever, and diagnosis can be excluded only by examining the CSF (see Chapter 14).
2. Tertiary CNS syphilis: The presence of typical pupillary abnormalities (Argyll Robertson pupil) may suggest the diagnosis. The blood VDRL test may be non-reactive; the diagnosis is made with certainty only with a CSF VDRL test.

Normal Pressure Hydrocephalus

1. The diagnosis of normal pressure hydrocephalus should be entertained with a subacute (months) onset of dementia associated with ataxia and urinary incontinence.
2. Many patients have a history of a previous subarachnoid hemorrhage or meningitis.
3. The neurologic examination shows very hyperactive reflexes in the lower extremities (sometimes with a Babinski reflex) and normal reflexes in the upper extremities.
4. The CT scan shows large ventricles with little or no space between the skull and the surface of the brain. The gyri are not prominent.

   Treatment: A few patients show dramatic improvement after a shunt procedure. Considering the seriousness of the disease, a shunt is recommended for all patients with the "classic" CT scan changes.

Pseudodementia

1. The term *pseudodementia* refers to a major depressive disorder (see Chapter 9) in the elderly.
2. Often mistaken for Alzheimer's disease (Table 9.2 may help in distinguishing the two).
3. Vegetative signs such as sleep disturbance (early morning awakening), motor slowness, and lack of energy are often present.

   Treatment: Antidepressant and/or electroshock therapy often results in dramatic improvement.

Progressive Dementias

Alzheimer's Disease (Presenile and Senile Dementia)

1. Alzheimer's disease accounts for over 50% of all dementias over the age of 40 years.
2. The *probable* diagnosis is made on gradual, progressive global cognitive changes (language use, perception, acquisition of skills, judgment, problem solving, abstract thinking) with no disturbance of consciousness and the absence of systemic disorders or other brain diseases that cause dementia.

   Caution: Diagnosis of Alzheimer's disease can be made only by brain autopsy or biopsy. A wrong diagnosis of Alzheimer's disease may deprive the patient of treatment for a curable dementia.
3. Associated symptoms sometimes include depression, sleep disturbances, paranoia, agitation, and aggression.

4. Hereditary tendency, especially if mother or father had relatively early onset of the disease (before age 65 years).

   Note: All patients with Down's syndrome past the age of 40 years develop Alzheimer's disease.

5. Except for the dementia, the routine neurologic examination is normal: cranial nerves, reflexes, sensation, and station and gait.

6. Most patients show "intrusion" -- incorporation of a previous response in a later, irrelevant context. For example, after correctly naming the month of "January", the patient asked to name his children, might say "Bill, January, Erik."

7. CT scan shows progressive atrophy, but this is *nonspecific* and the atrophy does *not* correlate well with the degree of dementia.

Management:

   1. After diagnosis, sympathy, support, listening, education, and referral to appropriate support agencies are very important to both the family and the patient. The book *The 36-Hour Day* (see Bibliography) may be very helpful. More information may be obtained from: Alzheimer's Disease and Related Disorders Association, 70 East Lake St, Chicago, IL 60601 (telephone: 312-853-3060 or 800-621-0379).

   2. Protect the patient from unproven and often expensive therapies (lecithin, megavitamins, etc).

   3. If depression is present, low-dose antidepressant medication, such as imipramine (25 mg qhs), may be useful.

   4. Use psychotropic medications in very low doses, if at all; Alzheimer's disease patients seem to be more sensitive than the average patient to side effects.

   5. Ergoloid mesylates (Hydergine), 1 mg PO tid, does not help memory difficulties but, if initiated early, may enable the patient to accomplish the activities of daily living with greater ease.

Jakob's Disease (Jakob-Creutzfeldt Disease)

1. Any patient with dementia and generalized myoclonus has a high probability of Jakob's disease.

2. The course is generally more rapid than Alzheimer's disease, and death usually occurs in 1 to 2 years.

3. The infectious agent is related to the agent of sheep scrapie and transmissible mink encephalopathy and has been called a prion; the only proven mode of transmission is direct contact between the nervous tissue of an infected patient and an open wound of a recipient.

Note: Transmission has occurred through use of incompletely decontaminated neurosurgical equipment, corneal transplants, human pituitary-derived growth hormone injections, and patch grafts prepared from human dura.

4. The EEG often shows characteristic periodic complexes.
5. Brain biopsy is rarely necessary, but will show typical spongiform alterations.

   Caution: Formaldehyde does not inactivate the responsible infectious agent. Pathologists and neurosurgeons are at particularly high risk for infection. A correct diagnosis is important for protection of these physicians, as well as for epidemiologic studies. Organ donations should not be permitted from affected individuals.

Huntington's Disease

Dementia may precede the choreoathetosis and psychosis by many years. The correct diagnosis is most strongly suggested by a family history of dominantly inherited psychosis or dementia (see Chapter 8).

Pick's Disease

1. Pick's disease may be difficult to distinguish from Alzheimer's disease.
2. Initial symptoms are prominent alterations in emotion, affect, and behavior.
3. Pick's disease progresses to death within several years, whereas Alzheimer's disease generally progresses at a slower rate.
4. CT scan may show frontal and temporal lobe atrophy which is out of proportion to the atrophy in the rest of the brain.
5. Twenty percent of cases have a pattern of autosomal dominant inheritance.

   Management: Same as for Alzheimer's disease

BIBLIOGRAPHY

Benson DF, Blumer D: *Psychiatric Aspects of Neurologic Disease*. New York, Grune & Stratton, 1975, pp 123-147.

Gajdusek DC, Gibbs CJ Jr, Asher DM, et al: Precautions in medical care and in handling materials from patients with transmissible virus dementia (Creutzfeldt-Jakob disease). *N Engl J Med* 1977; 297:1253-1258.

Heston LL, White JA: *Dementia: A Practical Guide to Alzheimer's Disease and Related Illnesses*. New York, W.H. Freeman & Co., 1983. Jenike MA: Alzheimer's disease: clinical care and management. *Psychosomatics* 1985; 27:407-416.

Katzman R: Alzheimer's disease. *N Engl J Med* 1986; 314:964-973.

Katzman R: Validation of a short orientation-memory concentration test of cognitive impairment. *Am J Psychiatry* 1983; 140:734-739.

Khachaturian ZS: Diagnosis of Alzheimer's disease. *Arch Neurol* 1985; 42:1097-1105.

More NL, Robins PO: *The 36-Hour Day: A Family Guide to Caring for Persons with Alzheimer's Disease*. Baltimore, Johns Hopkins Press, 1982.

Rappaport EB: Iatrogenic Creutzfeldt-Jakob disease. *Neurology* 1987; 37:1520-1522.

VII

MOVEMENT DISORDERS

Accurate observation and description are essential for classifying movement disorders. The patient's abnormal movements and postures can often be observed during the interview -- one look is worth a thousand words.

Types of Abnormal Movements

Tremor: Involuntary, rhythmic movement across a joint. The movement may be present at rest (static tremor) or only apparent with motion or a specific posture (intention or postural tremor).

Chorea and *athetosis:* Chorea is sudden, nonrepetitive movement which usually involves the extremities and the face; athetosis is a slow, sinuous movement. In some cases the distinction between these two types of movement is unclear and the term choreoathetosis is used.

Myoclonus: Spontaneous, shocklike contractions of one or more muscles, usually causing movement across a joint (think of the jerk-like movements often seen in dogs and cats as they go to sleep).

Tics: Irregular, stereotyped movements, usually complex and very often involving the face.

Focal motor seizures: Relatively rhythmic movements, usually involving multiple joints and often persisting in sleep (tremors, choreoathetosis, and tics disappear during sleep).

Clonus: Rhythmic tremor precipitated by sudden stretching of a muscle. This is most commonly seen at the ankle, and is associated with upper motor neuron lesions.

Fasciculations: Very brief twitches of a group of muscle fibers, all innervated by the same anterior horn cell. Best seen where subcutaneous fat is thinnest, eg, the back. Generally, fasciculations do *not* cause movement across a joint, but they may occasionally cause tremor of the fingers.

Dystonia: A sustained abnormal or inappropriate posture.

HISTORY AND EXAMINATION OF THE PATIENT WITH A MOVEMENT DISORDER

History

1. Many movement disorders are *familial*.
2. Drug and alcohol history: Alcoholism may cause cerebellar degeneration and alleviate familial tremor; phenothiazines may cause Parkinson's syndrome or tardive dyskinesia; excess thyroid hormone (endogenous or exogenously administered) may result in a metabolic tremor.
3. Medical history: Liver disease may cause asterixis; Sydenham's chorea is associated with streptococcal infections.
4. A description of the movement disorder should include age of onset, rate of progression, symmetry, and exacerbating or alleviating factors (stress, drugs, sleep).

Neurologic Examination

1. Have the patient draw a spiral or connect dots as a permanent record of the motor dysfunction; later this can be used to monitor the efficacy of treatment.
2. Muscle tone: *Hypotonia* may be seen as floppiness of joints or an excessive number of swings after the patellar reflex is elicited when the patient is sitting on the examining table (see Figure 7.1). *Hypertonia* may be appreciated by passive movement of the arm, especially when the patient is distracted as when the contralateral arm is engaged in some activity such as drawing an imaginary figure eight in the air.
3. Instruct the patient to point index fingers (see Figure 7.2) to differentiate proximal and distal tremors.
4. Abnormal postures are most often appreciated during station and gait testing.

   Caution: Never make the diagnosis of a movement disorder on the basis of a single finding. Table 7.1 illustrates this point by showing the overlapping features of Parkinson's syndrome, cerebellar tremor, and essential tremor. Also note that on the finger-to-nose test, both cerebellar tremor and essential tremor have an intentional component (see Figure 7.3).

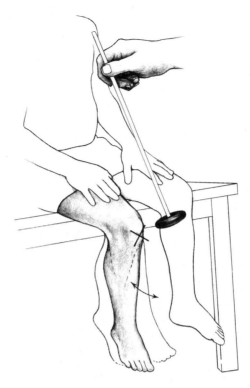

Figure 7.1 The patient with cerebellar disease may have an abnormal number of swings of the leg when the patellar reflex is tested.

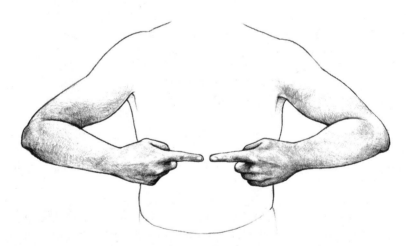

Figure 7.2 Having the patient point (but not touch) his index fingers as illustrated may differentiate between a proximal and distal tremor. With a proximal tremor there is flapping of the arms; with a distal tremor the fingers are constantly in misalignment.

Table 7.1
Overlapping Features of Various Types of Tremor

Feature	Parkinson's Syndrome	Cerebellar Tremor	Essential Tremor
Present at rest	Yes	No	Yes
Increased tone	Yes	No	No
Decreased tone	No	Yes	No
Postural abnormality	Yes	Yes	No
Head involvement	Yes	Yes	Yes
Intentional component	No	Yes	Yes
Incoordination	No	Yes	No

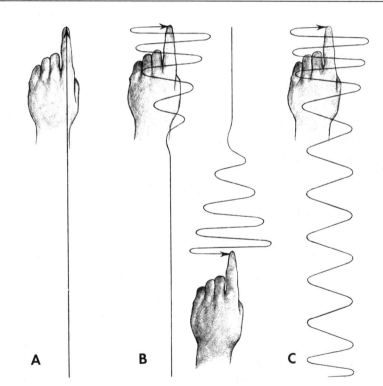

Figure 7.3 Finger-to-nose test. A. The normal person is able to point to a target accurately and smoothly. B. The patient with cerebellar hemisphere disease shows a tremor that increases in amplitude as the target is approached. C. The patient with essential tremor shows a tremor throughout the range of motion. Note the increase in amplitude as the target is approached. B and C are easily confused.

Parkinsonism

Parkinson's *disease* is an idiopathic disorder resulting from a progressive loss of neurons in the midbrain substantia nigra; Parkinson's *syndrome* involves entirely different pathophysiologic processes and is associated with dozens of other neurologic diseases (eg, repeated head trauma, Alzheimer's disease, and acute effect of neuroleptics). In a relatively mild case of parkinsonism, suspect Parkinson's *syndrome* (and refer to a neurologist) if:

1. Reflexes are abnormal (hyperactive, in ALS-dementia-parkinsonism complex or olivopontocerebellar degeneration).
2. Significant dementia is present (Alzheimer's disease).
3. Downward gaze is impaired (progressive supranuclear palsy).
4. Postural hypotension is present (Shy-Drager syndrome).
5. The patient does not respond to combination carbidopa-levodopa (repeated head trauma).

Early Symptoms

1. Voice changes (decrease in volume and loss of melody): These are often not apparent to the examiner but are quite obvious to the family and close friends of the patient.
2. Sleep disturbances: frequent nocturnal awakenings, possibly secondary to loss of automatic motor movements during sleep; considerable relief may be obtained from sleeping on satin sheets.
3. Wet pillows: Saliva often is not swallowed during sleep even if there is no such problem during waking.

Late Signs and Symptoms (see Figure 7.4)

1. *Tremor*
   a. Present at rest, worse with emotional stress or when the examiner calls attention to it.
   b. A "pill rolling" motion with the index finger flexing and extending in contact with the thumb, at approximately 4 to 10 Hz. May involve the arm with rhythmic flexion-extension, abduction-adduction, pronation-supination, or a combination thereof.
   c. Present most commonly in the hands and fingers; often begins unilaterally and distally and spreads proximally and to the other side over a period of months or years.
2. *Rigidity*: Passively move the extremities; instruct the patient to relax the arm ("like a rag doll") and then passively move the arm. Increased tone (rigidity) is appreciated as increased resistance throughout the range of movement (the so-called lead pipe rigidity); tremor may also be felt during this movement (the so-called cogwheel phenomenon).
3. *Postural changes* are observed during testing of station and gait. These include stooping of shoulders and slight flexion of back. In starting to

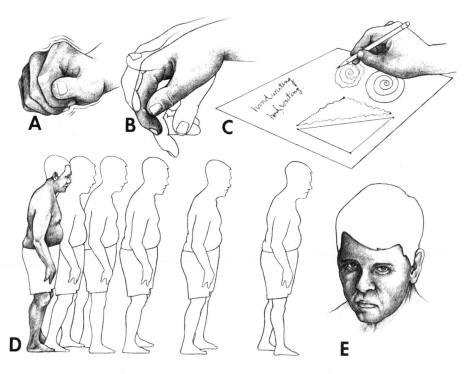

Figure 7.4 The parkinsonian syndrome. A. The "pill-rolling" tremor. B. Tremor that may become worse with emotional stress. C. Handwriting abnormalities, which include micrographia. D. Typical posture and gait, which becomes faster (festination). E. Lack of facial expression as well as "stare" from decreased blinking.

walk, steps at first are slow and small (the so-called *marche á petit pas*) and then rapidly increase. In turning, the motion is not fluid but is done in a rigid whole-body fashion *(en bloc)*.

4. *Bradykinesia* is a major problem manifested as difficulty in initiating movements (including bowel), and as slowed movements and slowed thought processes (sometimes referred to as a "constipated mind"). Typically the family will notice the patient's lack of interest or involvement in many usual activities (this may be confused with depression or dementia).

5. Handwriting is slow and small with letters tightly bunched together (micrographia).

6. The basal ganglia are a center for automatic motor functions such as walking, maintenance of posture, maintenance of facial expression, clearing of saliva from the mouth, swallowing, arising from a chair, regaining balance; most of the symptoms of Parkinson's syndrome can be explained in this context (ie, a dysfunction of automatic motor behavior).

Treatment:

1. Treatment is directed toward relieving the symptoms of tremor and rigidity; none of the drugs is a "cure." Initial doses should always be small and built up slowly. Do not treat unless the patient is symptomatic and is significantly inconvenienced by the disease.

2. Patient education materials may be obtained from the United Parkinson Foundation, 360 West Superior St, Chicago, IL 60610 (telephone: 312-664-2344) or the National Parkinson Foundation, 1501 NW 9th Ave, Miami FL 33136 (telephone 305-547-6666 or 800-327-4545).

3. Drugs of choice for initial treatment:

   a. Benztropine mesylate (Cogentin): Start at a dose of 0.5 mg/day and increase until the tremor is subdued or dosage of 6 mg/day is reached.

      Caution: Anticholinergic drugs may exacerbate constipation and result in urinary retention (especially in males with prostatic enlargement).

   b. Amantidine hydrochloride (Symmetrel): Start with 50 mg qd and gradually increase to 100 mg bid. Mental changes are common at higher dosages (capsules are available only in 100 mg sizes; a syrup is available which contains 10 mg/mL).

4. When amantidine and/or benztropine provides insufficient relief, the physician should begin carbidopa-levodopa (Sinemet) and bromocriptine mesylate (Parlodel) *simultaneously*. Drugs should be started at the lowest possible dose and gradually be increased over a period of *months*. Levodopa is converted to dopamine in the substantia nigra, while bromocriptine acts directly on brain dopamine receptors.

   a. Sinemet: A combination of levodopa (L-dopa) and carbidopa (to inhibit peripheral dopa decarboxylase and allow smaller effective doses of L-dopa with fewer side effects). The average patient needs approximately 100 mg/day of carbidopa to inhibit peripheral dopa decarboxylase; smaller amounts limit dose effectiveness, while larger amounts are not necessary and may cause undesirable side effects. The average initial dose is one 25/100 tablet tid; dosage of L-dopa greater than 500 mg/day is usually not recommended. The patient should also be instructed to receive the majority of his dietary protein in the evening since many dietary amino acids will compete with the L-dopa for transport across the blood-brain barrier.

   b. Bromocriptine: Start at 2.5 mg bid and gradually increase as necessary to a maximum of 30 mg/day.

Caution:

1. Patients with advanced Parkinson's disease respond poorly to L-dopa because there are no longer sufficient cells in the substantia nigra to convert it to dopamine. Patients with Parkinson's syndrome respond poorly or not at all because the defect is at the postsynaptic receptor.
2. Toxic amounts of dopamine cause abnormal movements most frequently involving the tongue (buccal-lingual dyskinesia). In this circumstance the L-dopa dose should be reduced.
3. The "on-off" phenomenon: Some patients, especially those receiving L-dopa for a long period of time, may have symptoms which change dramatically from hour to hour. One moment they may be virtually immobile and unable to walk, while the next they may be mobile but suffer from abnormal movements. The measures to combat this disabling condition include giving the same total daily dose of L-dopa but in smaller and more frequent doses and adding more bromocriptine.

Essential Tremor (Benign, Familial, Hereditary, or Senile Tremor)

1. Tremor
   a. Coarse, rhythmic, usually symmetric, present at rest, most noticeable in the fingers, but also involving the hands and head, seldom affecting the legs.
   b. Persists throughout the range of voluntary activity and increases in amplitude as the limb approaches an object (finger-to-nose test) (see Figure 7.1) (like a cerebellar tremor).
   c. Characteristically increases with attempts to write or to bring liquids to mouth to drink.
   d. Increases markedly under stress (like a parkinsonian tremor).
   e. Often attenuates or disappears with a small amount of alcohol. (This feature, if present, is almost diagnostic.)
2. Onset may be in adolescence or early adult years; often called senile tremor if it develops late in life.
3. Autosomal dominant inheritance can be identified in most families.
4. Tremor increases in amplitude with age and may eventually interfere with fine movements.
5. Neurologic examination is normal except for tremor. Distinguish from parkinsonism by lack of rigidity and bradykinesia; distinguish from cerebellar lesion by lack of hypotonia and ataxia.

6. Cerebellar and parkinsonian tremors rarely involve the head. Tremor similar to essential tremor may be seen in individuals with thyrotoxicosis and patients receiving lithium, epinephrine, or terbutaline sulfate. Fatigue and anxiety may cause a similar fine rapid tremor.

Treatment:

1. Reassurance is often all that is necessary. If the tremor interferes with social adjustment or activities of daily living, drug treatment may be necessary.
2. Propranolol hydrochloride (Inderal) is often effective. The long-acting form at an initial dose of 80 mg is convenient.
3. Some patients respond to primidone (Mysoline). The initial dose should be 125 mg qhs and increased by 125 mg weekly until the tremor is controlled.
4. Alcohol is often the most effective agent, but is not recommended for chronic use. In fact, chronic alcoholism may occur in patients with essential tremor who attempt this form of treatment. Wine with dinner occasionally may be used for elderly patients with symptomatic senile tremor.

Cerebellar Tremor

1. Cerebellar tremor is noted only during movement. It may be unilateral or bilateral and indicates disease of the cerebellar hemisphere.
2. In the finger-to-nose test tremor increases as the finger nears the target and is less between targets (see Figure 7.3).
3. Other signs of cerebellar hemispheric disease include the following:
   a. Ipsilateral (same side) difficulty with rapid alternating movements (have patient rapidly alternate pronation and supination of hand against thigh).
   b. Hypotonia manifested as a limp "rag doll" arm with passive motion and as a pendular patellar reflex (see Figure 7.1). Hypotonia may also be manifested by hyperextension of the fingers (see Figure 7.5).
   c. Rebound is commonly elicited by having the patient flex his arm against resistance from the examiner, and then having the examiner suddenly let go of the arm; normally the arm remains relatively stationary, but with cerebellar disease, the arm will rebound and tend to strike patient's face.

      Caution: The examiner must place his arm or hand so as to guard patient's face (see Figure 7.6).

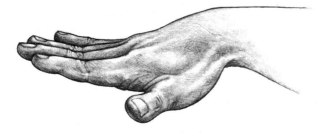

Figure 7.5 "Spooning" of hands as illustrated is occasionally seen in cerebellar disease. Hyperextension of fingers in this manner may also exacerbate an essential tremor.

    d. Occasionally speech abnormalities occur, which consist of loss of normal speech melody. Speech tends to have an explosive quality (ataxic dysarthria or scanning speech).

Note: Disease of midline cerebellar structures may cause only difficulty in tandem walking (gait ataxia) with no abnormalities of finger-to-nose testing and no tremor or other signs of cerebellar hemisphere disease. Commonly this is seen in chronic alcoholism, as a remote effect of carcinoma, or with phenytoin intoxication. In children, medulloblastoma or a midline cerebellar tumor cause similar abnormalities.

Treatment:

Therapy must be directed at the underlying cerebellar disorder. Lesions of the cerebellum including cerebellar atrophy may be demon-

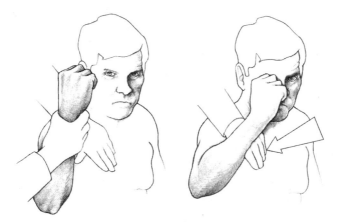

Figure 7.6 Testing for rebound. Request the patient to pull against resistance, then suddenly release the arm without warning. *Caution*: If not protected by the examiner's arm, the patient with cerebellar disease will strike himself.

strated with CT or MRI scans. Cerebellar tremor is commonly seen in patients with multiple sclerosis or brainstem strokes.

Asterixis

1. Asterixis denotes a movement disorder brought out primarily when the patient extends the arm in front with the wrist also extended. Irregular sudden flexion at the wrist (from gravitational pull) is followed by extension of the wrist back to the original position (see Figure 7.7).
2. Although originally described in hepatic disease ("liver flap"), it occurs in patients with a wide variety of metabolic disorders (such as renal failure, pulmonary insufficiency, malabsorption syndromes).

Treatment:

Treatment of the underlying metabolic disorder is indicated.

Huntington's Disease (Huntington's Chorea)

1. Huntington's disease is a dominantly inherited disorder with progressive dementia, usually occurring after age 30 years.
2. Initial symptoms may include clumsiness of movement, slowness of finger movements, or a tendency to drop objects. Abnormal movements at first may be converted to seemingly purposeful movements in order to conceal the abnormality.
3. The abnormal movements are irregular rapid jerky movements of the

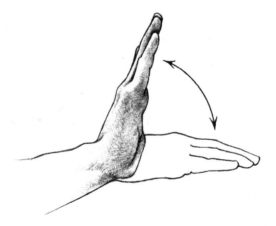

Figure 7-7 Asterixis. The patient is unable to maintain wrist extension; intermittently there is a sudden loss of tone, causing the hand to flap in a bye-bye gesture.

fingers and wrists associated with slower dystonic movements of the upper limbs.

4. The gait is unsteady with a tendency to bob and weave.

5. Facial grimacing with involuntary movements of the tongue are common; this produces a dysarthria.

6. Sustained activity such as clenching a fist or protruding the tongue may result in an exaggeration of the abnormal movements in other body parts.

7. Patients commonly present with subtle signs of intellectual deterioration, personality change, or frank psychosis. Depression and suicide attempts are frequent. The movement disorder may not be evident until many years later.

8. Family history is a very important diagnostic clue but may be exceptionally difficult to elicit; the family history may include mental deficiency, alcoholism, suicide, psychosis, and behavior disorders.

Treatment:

1. There is no cure for Huntington's disease; genetic counseling is necessary. Provocative tests for young, asymptomatic patients are available, but their role in the diagnosis is controversial. The genetic locus of this disease has been identified on the short arm of chromosome 4, and in utero diagnosis may soon be available.

2. For improvement of the abnormal movements:
   a. Haloperidol 3 to 6 mg/day may initially be effective for the movement disorder and for behavior control.
   b. Phenothiazines such as chlorpromazine (up to 150 mg/day), perphenazine (10-16 mg tid), or trifluoperazine hydrochloride (2 mg tid) are alternative treatments.

3. If serious depression is present, suicide precautions may need to be taken.

4. Educational materials for patients and information about local support groups may be obtained from Huntington's Disease Society of America, 140 West 22nd St, New York, NY 10011 (telephone: 212-242-1968 or 800-345-HDSA).

Spasmus Nutans

1. Spasmus nutans is a rhythmic nodding or rotatory tremor of head associated with pendular nystagmus.

2. It occurs in infants between 4 and 18 months of age.

3. It must be differentiated from the head tremor associated with congenital nystagmus (due to reduced visual acuity).

4. The tremor disappears when infant is lying down.

Treatment:

This disorder is rare, but it is important to recognize because it is self-limited and disappears by the age of 2 years. Further workup is not necessary. The parents need reassurance.

Sydenham's Chorea (Infectious or Rheumatic Chorea)

1. Sydenham's chorea occurs in children and adolescents aged 5 to 15 years. It is more common in females. It is often associated with rheumatic fever and a β-hemolytic streptococcal infection, which may precede the onset of chorea by days to months, but is important to recognize because Sydenham's chorea has the same cardiac implications as rheumatic fever.

2. May begin as an apparent restlessness, clumsiness, and behavior disorder characterized by involuntary movements, incoordination, and weakness.

3. Choreic movements are nonrepetitive, abrupt, jerky, and purposeless; present at rest and accentuated by posturing; are usually seen in the face and hands; and may involve only one side of the body (hemichorea).

4. Facial grimacing, dysarthria, and explosive speech are common.

5. When asked to sustain a grip on the examiner's fingers, the patient will exhibit a "milking grip"; the patient cannot maintain a protruded tongue ("darting tongue sign").

6. There may be decreased resistance to passive movements; reflexes may be hypoactive, delayed, or pendular.

7. Duration is usually 4 to 6 weeks; complete recovery is frequent, but residua may be evident.

8. The patient may have an elevated ESR. Serum calcium and phosphorus levels should be obtained to rule out hypocalcemia. ECG changes or other features consistent with the Jones criteria for rheumatic fever should be sought. Throat culture for β-hemolytic streptococcal infection and serum ASO titers should be performed.

Treatment:

1. Bed rest with a tranquil environment.

2. Haloperidol at an initial dose of 0.5 mg, gradually increased until movements are controlled.

3. Streptococcal infections should be treated with penicillin.

4. Prevent rheumatic complications by prophylactic *lifelong* antibiotics (additional antibiotics may be necessary in situations where there may be bacteremia, eg, dental work). Pencillin G benzathine is the recommended drug at the following dosages:

AGE (YEARS)	DOSAGE (UNITS/MONTH)
< 6	600,000
6 - 12	900,000
> 12	1,200,000

5. Frequent examinations are necessary to detect early signs of cardiac involvement.

Chorea Gravidarum

1. Chorea gravidarum occurs in approximately one in every 2000 to 3000 pregnancies. It occurs more commonly in first pregnancies and may recur in subsequent pregnancies. The etiology is unknown.
2. Its average duration is 1 to 2 months; chorea usually subsides spontaneously during pregnancy or shortly after delivery.

Treatment:

Termination of pregnancy is rarely required. If the chorea is incapacitating, sedatives or phenothiazines may be used to control the movements, but use of such medications may pose a risk to the fetus.

Kernicterus

1. Kernicterus is related to the combination of hyperbilirubinemia and cerebral ischemia/hypoxia in the newborn with resultant deposition of unconjugated bilirubin in the brain (primarily the basal ganglia). This form of "cerebral palsy" is now rare because most infants are effectively treated early for hyperbilirubinemia.
2. A jaundiced newborn at two or three days of age may show symptoms such as listlessness, poor sucking, fever, hypotonia, weak cry, and Moro reflexes and deep tendon reflexes that are difficult to elicit.
3. Permanent symptoms appear after 18 months of age and may include choreoathetosis, dystonia, rigidity, tremor, upward gaze paralysis, mental retardation, spasticity, and hearing impairment.

Treatment:

An attempt should be made to prevent kernicterus by treating newborn hyperbilirubinemia using techniques such as phototherapy and exchange transfusion.

Gilles de la Tourette Syndrome

1. A syndrome of axial (neck and face) tics with onset usually between 7

and 15 years of age; more common in males. Childhood hyperactivity may precede the onset of tics.

2. Initial symptoms include facial tics and facial grimaces followed (in months and years) by sudden involuntary movements of the head, neck, shoulders, trunk, or legs. These movements may be repeated several times a minute and become worse with stress.

3. Frequently movements are accompanied by respiratory tics which initially are grunts, snorts, or yells, but eventually may develop into repeated obscenities yelled in a loud voice with no provocation (coprolalia). Vocal tics are a hallmark of the disease.

4. The character of the abnormal movements may change over the years.

Treatment:

1. Patients may gain some voluntary control of the tics, but must, from time to time, "let it out." It should be emphasized that this is purely a social disability, and has not prevented many patients with this disease from leading productive lives.

2. Haloperidol, at a recommended dose of 2.5 to 10 mg daily, may result in improvement. Careful dose adjustment is important for long-term therapy.

   Caution: Long-term use of a neuroleptic such as haloperidol may result in tardive dyskinesia.

3. Clonidine, 0.05 mg/kg/day, increased by 0.05 mg/kg every 2 weeks to a therapeutic dose ranging from 0.1 to 0.9 mg/kg, is often effective in controlling the behavioral disorder sometimes associated with the syndrome.

4. Educational material for patients and information about local support groups may be obtained from the Tourette Syndrome Association, Inc, 4240 Bell Blvd, Bayside, NY 11361 (telephone: 718-224-2999 or 800-237-0717).

Hemiballismus

1. Hemiballismus is a rare disorder caused by a lesion of the subthalamic nucleus, usually as a result of hemorrhage or infarction. The patient frequently suffers from chronic hypertension.

2. It is characterized by violent involuntary movement (unilaterally and contralateral to the lesion), mainly of the arm; the appearance is similar to a baseball pitcher's windup.

3. Onset is sudden; movement is worsened by stress.

Treatment:

1. There is usually spontaneous recovery.

2. For long-term control of movement, oral diazepam alone or diazepam supplemented with reserpine or haloperidol has been used with variable success.

Caution: This disorder should not be confused with focal motor seizures (see Chapter 11).

Myoclonus

Myoclonus resembles the muscular twitching seen in dogs and cats as they drop off to sleep. Causes of myoclonus include CNS degenerative disorders, benign hereditary myoclonus, cerebral anoxia, and metabolic disorders. The movement is indicative of a CNS disorder, but from a neurologic point of view, has poor localizing value. For severe persistent myoclonus, pharmacotherapy (such as with clonazepam) is available.

Caution: A demented patient with myoclonus very likely has Jakob's disease (see Chapter 6). The brains of such patients harbor an infectious agent.

Dystonia

Dystonia is a sustained abnormal posture. The most common form is spasmotic torticollis with persistent contraction of the sternocleidomastoid. Patients may also have sustained closure of the eyes (blepharospasm). Medical treatment for dystonia is often ineffective and patients may require such drastic measures as cervical rhizotomy. Causes of dystonia include cerebral anoxia, birth injury, head trauma, or the rare syndromes of dystonia musculorum deformans and hepatolenticular degeneration (Wilson's disease).

Movement Disorders Associated with Neuroleptics

A. *Acute Parkinsonism*: The symptoms of acute parkinsonism often are dramatically relieved with diphenhydramine hydrochloride (Benadryl) 50mg IV.
B. *Tardive dyskinesia*
   1. Tardive dyskinesia is a very common syndrome that develops in a significant number of patients receiving long-term treatment with neuroleptic drugs (especially the more potent phenothiazines and haloperidol).
   2. Symptoms include an oral-buccal-lingual dyskinesia involving tongue protrusion, lip smacking, and facial grimacing. Abnormal movements of limbs and trunk may be seen.
   Treatment:
   1. In many patients, tardive dyskinesia remains refractory to all forms of treatment. Symptoms may be relieved by reinstating

the offending drugs, but this practice is generally considered self-defeating.

2. A therapeutic trial of reserpine at an initial dose of 0.25 mg bid increased to 2 to 8 mg/day may relieve symptoms in some patients.

3. The best treatment is preventive, ie, prescribing neuroleptics only for serious psychiatric disorders and monitoring patients carefully for the side effects.

C. *Akathisia.* Akathisia is a *reversible* motor restlessness which is often confused with psychotic agitation. It is seen acutely with treatment with neuroleptics and with some antihistamines or as part of the tardive dyskinesia syndrome.

Other Medications Associated with Movement Disorders

1. CNS stimulants (amphetamine or methylphenidate) may produce tics.

2. Antihistamines, oral contraceptives (similar to chorea gravidarum of natural pregnancy), anticonvulsants, and chloroquine occasionally produce involuntary choreoathetosis.

3. The meperidine analog MPTP (1-methyl-4-phenyl-1,2,3,6-tetrahydropyridine), an illicit "designer" drug, damages the substantia nigra and produces parkinsonism.

BIBLIOGRAPHY

Calne DB: Progress in Parkinson's disease. *N Engl J Med* 1984; 310:523-524.

Calne DB, Burton K: Pharmacology of Parkinson's disease. *Neurol Clin* 1984; 2:461-472.

Carter CO, Evans KA, Baraitser M: Effect of genetic counseling on the prevalence of Huntington's chorea. *Br Med J* 1983; 286:281-283.

Fahn S, Jankovic J: Practical management of dystonia. *Neurol Clin* 1984; 2:555-569.

Gusella JF, Wexler NS, Conneally PM, et al.: A polymorphic DNA marker genetically linked to Huntington's disease. *Nature* 1983; 306:234-238.

Jankovic J, Fahn S: Physiologic and pathologic tremors. *Ann Intern Med* 1980; 93:460-465.

Klawans HL, Goetz CG, Perlik S: Presymptomatic and early detection in Huntington's disease. *Ann Neurol* 1980; 8:343-347.

Koller WC, Biary N: Metaprolol compared to propranalol in the treatment of essential tremor. *Arch Neurol* 1984; 41:171-172.

Kotter WE, Royse VL: Primidone for essential tremor. *Neurology* 1986; 36:121.

Marsden CD, Schachter M: Assessment of extrapyramidal disorders. *Br J Clin Pharmacol* 1981; 11:129-151.

Muenter MD: Should levodopa therapy be started early or late? *Can J Neurol Sci* 1984; 11:195-199.

Nutt J: Effect of cholinergic agents in Huntington's disease: A reappraisal. *Neurology* 1983; 33:932-935.

Shoulson I: Care of patients and families with Huntington's disease, in Marsden CD, Fahn S (eds): *Movement Disorders*. London, Butterworth, 1982.

Shapiro A, Shapiro E, Eisenkraft GJ: Treatment of Gilles de la Tourette Syndrome with pimozide. *Amer J Psychiatry* 1983; 140:1183-1186.

Swaiman KF: Myoclonus. *Neurol Clin* 1985; 3:197-208.

Vonsattel JP, Myers RH, Stevens TJ, et al: Neuropathological classification of Huntington's disease. *J Neuropathol Exp Neurol* 1985; 44:559-577

VIII

NEUROLOGIC COMPLICATIONS OF ALCOHOLISM

In the United States, alcohol abuse accounts for a substantial percentage of hospital admissions, highway deaths, and psychiatric disturbances, yet alcoholic beverages are readily available and accepted by many Americans as a routine adjunct to social interaction. Identifying all pathologic users is one of the most common and difficult challenges facing the physician.

Establishing the Diagnosis of Alcohol Abuse

1. Table 8.1 may be used as a basis for the patient interview. Positive responses in several categories make it likely that the patient is alcohol-dependent.
2. The CAGE questionnaire consists of only four questions, and has been proved to be a specific and sensitive tool in the diagnosis of alcoholism. The acronym comes from cutting down, annoyance by criticism, guilty feelings, and eye openers. Put in conversational terms:
   a. Ever felt the need to cut down drinking?
   b. Ever felt annoyed by criticism of drinking?
   c. Ever had guilty feelings about drinking?
   d. Ever take morning eye openers?

   Positive answers to two or more of these four questions correlates highly with alcoholism.
3. The diagnosis of alcoholism is associated with social stigmata: patients from lower socioeconomic classes more often have the diagnosis on their

110

TABLE 8.1
Suggested Questions for Use in Establishing the Diagnosis
of Alcohol Dependence

PREOCCUPATION

What are the occasions on which you have had a drink this past week (month)?
When do you think about drinking?
When during the day do you sometimes feel you need a drink?
How often during the past week (month) did you crave a drink in the morning?

INCREASED TOLERANCE

How often during the past week (month) have you been able to drink more
than others and not show it?
Has anyone ever commented on your ability to "hold your liquor?"
Why do you think you are able to do this?
How does this make you feel?

GULPING DRINKS

What strength drinks do you prefer?
How long does it take you to finish your first drink?
How many drinks do you usually have before going out to dinner or a party?

DRINKING ALONE

When in the past week (month) did you have a drink alone?
Where were you when you had a drink alone? (At home? In a bar?)

USE AS A MEDICINE

What are some of the reasons you drink? (Calm nerves? Reduce tension? As
a night cap to get to sleep? Relieve physical discomfort? Relieve feelings of
inadequacy or depression?)
Do you enjoy parties or dances if there is nothing to drink?

BLACKOUT

When during the past week (month) have you been unable to remember what
happened the night before?
When during the past week (month) have you been unable to remember how
you got home after a night's drinking?

PHYSICAL

What reasons have doctors given for you to cut down or stop drinking?
Where have you been hospitalized for drinking or a complication from drinking?

SOCIAL

How many of your friends drink?
How has your group of friends changed since you began drinking?
How have your hobbies and interests changed since you began drinking?
How often in the past week (month) have you been ashamed of what you did while you were drinking?
What kinds of things have you done that you were ashamed of while you were drinking?
How do you act while you are drinking?

FAMILY

Is there anyone in the family who is or was an alcoholic?

---

medical chart than do more affluent patients from higher socioeconomic classes (unfairly). A clear medical diagnosis of alcoholism may be a powerful incentive to reform.

4. Many alcoholics are extremely skillful (consciously or subconsciously) in camouflaging their addiction.

5. Any patient with a physical disability secondary to alcohol *is* an alcoholic (peripheral neuropathy, cirrhosis, dementia, cerebellar degeneration).

6. Any patient with withdrawal symptoms from alcohol abstinence *is* an alcoholic.

7. The quantity of alcohol consumed does not necessarily define an alcoholic; body weight, nutrition, ethnic background, medical condition, and medical therapy all influence a patient's sensitivity to the acute and chronic effects of alcohol.

8. In making a diagnosis of alcoholism, the physician must make every effort to be *objective*; the alcoholic physician makes the diagnosis too seldom, and the teetotaler makes it too often.

Clinical Clues to Alcohol Abuse

1. *Physical Examination:* On the general physical examination the following signs may indicate a diagnosis of alcoholism:

   a. Excessive sweating, tachycardia, flushed face (withdrawal syndrome)

   b. Bruises, cigarette burns, or other trauma often incurred with severe drunkenness

   c. Signs of liver disease: palmar erythema, vascular spiders, jaundice

   d. Neurologic abnormalities: coarse hand tremor, peripheral neuropathy, forgetfulness, emotional lability

   e. Poor hygiene, dehydration, poor nutrition

   f. Persistent or recurrent infections

    g. Odor of alcohol on breath at the time of examination

2. *Laboratory Findings:* On the laboratory profile the following abnormalities may indicate a diagnosis of alcoholism:

    a. A blood alcohol level of 150 mg/dL in a rational patient strongly suggests tolerance to alcohol, implying heavy and persistent alcohol ingestion.

    b. Blood count showing a mean corpuscular volume (MCV) greater than 97 with round macrocytosis.

    c. Elevated serum uric acid levels without history of gout.

    d. Elevation of serum glutamic pyruvic transaminase (SGPT), serum glutamic oxaloacetic transaminase (SGOT), and gamma-glutamyl transpeptidase (GGT).

Stupor and Coma in Alcoholic Intoxication

This diagnosis should *only* be made with a blood alcohol level greater than 300 mg/dL and *without* other cause for coma. *Most* comatose patients with an "odor of alcohol" on their breath will have some other cause for coma, such as diabetic ketoacidosis or another drug. Subdural hematoma, particularly bilateral subdural hematomas without localizing signs, must be suspected or ruled out in all cases of stupor or coma in an alcoholic.

    Treatment:

1. The physician must look for some other cause of coma and treat that cause appropriately.

2. Immediate measures as in treatment of any coma: Ensure clear airway, treat shock, check blood glucose levels, administer glucose and thiamine (see Chapter 13).

3. Gastric lavage is unnecessary; the bladder should be emptied and drainage instituted.

4. Check vital signs frequently; mechanical ventilation may be necessary.

5. In addition to blood levels for blood alcohol, obtain blood levels for other sedative drugs.

Alcoholic Blackouts

Alcoholic patients with blackouts may be suffering from seizures or may be having *simple alcoholic blackouts.*

1. Alcohol blackouts are periods of amnesia during which the patient apparently functions normally but later has no recall for that period; they are related to the acute effect of alcohol.

2. Blackouts are not necessarily correlated with blood alcohol level.

3. They are usually of short duration.

4. Blackouts often are an early neurologic symptom of potential alcoholism.
5. They may rarely occur paradoxically in the nonalcoholic individual who consumes a large quantity of alcohol.
6. A related phenomenon is pathologic intoxication in which relatively small amounts of alcohol produce irrational and combative behavior for which the patient may later be amnesic.

Alcohol Withdrawal Syndrome

Chronic consumption of alcohol results in physical dependence. There are at least four withdrawal syndromes:

A. Tremulousness
B. Alcoholic hallucinosis
C. Withdrawal seizures
D. Delirium tremens

Withdrawal symptomatology (listed separately here but often occurring in various combinations) usually begins at any time during which there is a falling blood alcohol level and may occur as late as seven days after cessation of alcohol intake. Prolonged or late withdrawal syndromes may occur in patients who abuse other drugs along with alcohol, or in patients who are receiving tranquilizers or sedatives in a treatment program. The severity of the syndrome is affected by a variety of factors including associated illness, other drug use or abuse, and environmental factors as well as the amount of alcohol consumed and the duration of alcohol abuse.

In all of the withdrawal syndromes, treatment with atenolol is recommended in addition to the other therapy. The maximum dose is atenolol 100 mg/day, with no drug given if the heart rate is less than 50/min and 50 mg given when the heart rate is 50 to 70/min. This regimen significantly reduces the duration of the withdrawal syndrome.

A. *Tremulousness:*
   1. The ''shakes'' or ''jitters'' often occur the morning following a few days of excessive alcohol consumption and are frequently responsible for early morning alcohol consumption to relieve symptoms.
   2. Tremulousness is associated with general irritability and gastrointestinal (GI) problems (especially nausea and vomiting). There may also be overalertness, flushed facies, tachycardia, anorexia, or insomnia.
   3. A tendency to startle, uneasiness, jerkiness of movement, and insomnia may persist for as long as 2 weeks.

   Treatment:
   In severe reactions benzodiazepines (such as diazepam 5 to 10 mg

PO q2h prn) may be instituted and can be withdrawn over several days.

B. *Alcoholic hallucinosis*

1. The patient complains of terrifying hallucinations with no disorientation. Generally these are auditory hallucinations, lasting a brief period of time. Visual hallucinations are less common.

2. May be related to REM rebound, since alcohol is known to suppress REM sleep.

Treatment:

1. Hospitalization is usually necessary; if the patient is not hospitalized, close supervision is necessary.

2. Diazepam 5 to 10 mg PO q2h prn may be used for sedation.

3. Institute a high-protein diet, supplemented with multiple vitamin therapy including thiamine 50 mg bid PO.

4. Make every attempt to keep the patient oriented to reality by having a sympathetic individual present who can reassure the patient that the hallucinations are not real.

5. Occasionally, patients with alcoholic hallucinosis may enter a chronic stage of hallucinosis following the clearing of the alcohol withdrawal process. Such a condition may require neuroleptic treatment.

6. During the phase of acute and remitting alcoholic hallucinosis, the patient may need treatment with a neuroleptic, which can be discontinued following remission of symptoms and a successful withdrawal regimen.

C. *Withdrawal Seizures ("Rum Fits")*

1. Withdrawal seizures are characteristically brief generalized convulsions with loss of consciousness.

2. They may be preceded by an aura of "fear" (anticipation of doom).

3. About one-third of patients with alcohol withdrawal seizures develop delirium tremens.

4. In patients with preexisting epilepsy, alcohol withdrawal may increase the frequency and intensity of seizures.

5. Alcoholics frequently have cortical scars from repeated head trauma, and these scars may trigger seizures during alcohol withdrawal.

Treatment:

1. Usually anticonvulsant medication is *not* necessary since seizures cease before medication becomes effective; diazepam 5 to 10 mg PO q2h prn for treatment of other associated withdrawal symptoms may be preventive.

2. Rarely, a "rum fit" may result in status epilepticus, which should be handled as described in Chapter 11.

3. An alcoholic with epilepsy who continues to consume alcoholic beverages should probably not be given anticonvulsants, since compliance is usually poor. If compelled to use long-term anticonvulsants due to frequent seizures, phenytoin is the drug of choice. Phenobarbital should not be used since abrupt withdrawal may cause seizures even in patients who are not epileptic.

D. *Delirium Tremens*

1. Delirium tremens is characterized by profound confusion, delusions, extremely vivid visual hallucinations, tremor, agitation, and insomnia, as well as signs of increased autonomic nervous system activation (ie, fever, tachycardia, profuse sweating).

2. The patient is suspicious, restless, very disoriented, and difficult to distract; he carries on imaginary conversations or activities and may shout for hours or mutter inaudibly.

3. The peak incidence is between 72 and 96 hours following cessation of alcohol consumption.

Treatment:

1. *This is a medical emergency, since mortality may reach 15% in the untreated state.*

2. Maintenance of fluid and electrolyte balance is the most important consideration.

3. Treat with diazepam 5 to 20 mg PO q2h prn or diazepam 10 mg IV immediately, then 5 mg IV q15 minutes until the patient is quiet, but not asleep.

4. Carefully record all intake and output.

5. Administration of large quantities of IV fluids are necessary. Usually 6 L of IV fluids are required per day:
   a. Glucose (at least 5%) must be included in each IV solution.
   b. Thiamine 50 mg must be included in each liter of IV solution.
   c. A therapeutic multivitamin preparation must be included in the first IV solution.
   d. Potassium, sodium, calcium, and magnesium must be added to the IV solutions based on the patient's laboratory determinations.

6. Restraints are almost always necessary, but a patient adequately sedated with diazepam may need less restraint.

7. Search for associated injury or infection (especially cerebral laceration, subdural hematoma, pneumonia, and meningitis).

8. Seizures require treatment *if* they are repeated, continuous, or life-threatening. Anticonvulsants need not be continued past the withdrawal period, unless there was a preexisting seizure disorder.

9. Pancreatitis, cirrhosis, and renal disease frequently complicate the course of delirium tremens.

Caution: The symptoms of delirium tremens resemble those of carbon dioxide narcosis. Carbon dioxide narcosis may occur in patients with delirium tremens who also have chronic obstructive pulmonary disease and have been given sedatives that may depress respirations.

Nutritional Diseases Secondary to Alcoholism

Wernicke-Korsakoff Syndrome

This is an acute, subacute, or chronic disease of CNS injury related to thiamine deficiency.

A. *Wernicke's syndrome* is the *acute* disorder, and is characterized by:

1. Nystagmus associated with ataxia and a confusional state
2. Followed by paralysis of extraocular muscles in any combination

Treatment:

This is a neurologic emergency and should be treated *immediately* with thiamine 100 mg IV. Prompt treatment will reverse the neurologic deficit.

B. *Korsakoff's psychosis* results if Wernicke's syndrome is not treated.

1. The outstanding feature of the mental disturbance is the inability to form new memories despite relatively intact immediate recall and relatively preserved remote memory. In effect, it is as though the patient's intellectual life was arrested at the moment of the onset of the pathology.

2. In conversation, the patient may discuss situations or give answers which sound very plausible but have little basis in reality (part of the mental aberration known as confabulation). For example, when asked what was served for breakfast, the patient will describe a sumptuous feast when in reality there was no meal that day.

Treatment:

Thiamine 50 mg bid should be administered to patients with Korsakoff's psychosis even though the disease is generally considered irreversible.

Peripheral Neuropathy Associated with Alcohol

1. Peripheral neuropathy is usually the earliest neurologic symptom of chronic alcoholism.

2. The disorder is primarily a sensory neuropathy with the patient complaining of burning or painful feet (see Chapter 15).

3. Very hypoactive or absent ankle reflexes are usually evident on examination before the patient notes any symptoms, and should alert the physician to the diagnosis of alcoholism. Evidence of summation on sensory examination (see Chapter 1) as well as subjective symptoms of sensory loss are apparent later.

4. The patient's feet may have thin, atrophic skin devoid of hair.

5. Peripheral neuropathy is often seen in association with the Wernicke-Korsakoff syndrome.

Treatment:

May respond to thiamine 50 mg bid, as well as abstinence from alcohol.

Alcoholic Dementia

1. Cerebral atrophy by CT scan and deterioration of intellectual function is well documented in chronic alcoholics.

2. Alcohol abuse is one of the common causes of dementia. Fortunately *substantial recovery* of function may occur if the patient ceases alcohol consumption.

Alcoholic Cerebellar Degeneration

1. Alcoholic cerebellar degeneration is characterized primarily by truncal ataxia and difficulty in tandem walking with lesser degrees of abnormality seen on finger-to-nose testing (see Chapter 7).

2. Subacute onset is over several weeks or months

3. Pathology is degeneration of midline cerebellar structures.

4. Not clearly related to thiamine deficiency.

Treatment:

Abstinence from alcohol and oral thiamine 50 mg bid supplementation is recommended but is of no clear benefit.

Alcoholic Myopathy

1. The chronic form of alcoholic myopathy presents with proximal muscle wasting and weakness; creatine phosphokinase (CPK) is mildly elevated; muscle biopsy shows type II muscle fiber atrophy, necrosis, and other anatomical abnormalities.

2. The acute form presents with severe weakness, myoglobinuria, and rhabdomyolysis. This constitutes a medical emergency and should be treated with vigorous diuresis to prevent renal failure from the myoglobinuria; additionally, serum potassium levels must be closely monitored to prevent hyperkalemia.

Treatment

Alcoholic myopathy is potentially reversible if the patient abstains from alcohol.

Neurologic Disorders Due to Liver Dysfunction

There are two syndromes of hepatic encephalopathy:

1. *Acute hepatic encephalopathy* is a progressive state of altered consciousness, ataxia, dysarthria, asterixis, lethargy, and finally coma. During this progression, characteristic EEG abnormalities can be detected. This syndrome is reversible with appropriate treatment of the liver disease. The degree of coma does not necessarily correlate with the degree of hyperammonemia.

2. *Chronic hepatic encephalopathy*: After repeated episodes of hepatic coma with recovery, a chronic progressive dementia develops.

   Treatment

   Treatment should be directed at the underlying liver disease.

Chronic Alcoholism

The treatment of alcohol abuse (chronic alcoholism) has the goals of sobriety and amelioration of the psychological problems underlying the alcohol abuse. The "cure" rate is low, but no worse than that of bronchogenic carcinoma. Sadly, many physicians treat only the complications of alcoholism, not the disease itself.

1. Alcoholics Anonymous (AA), a worldwide informal fellowship of recovering alcoholics, has been shown to be the most effective therapy for alcoholics. The philosophy is embodied in a series of steps to guide the alcoholic to recovery. There are also associated groups for the spouses (Al-Anon) and for teenage children (Al-Ateen). It is generally agreed that alcoholics should be encouraged to attend AA meetings on a regular basis. Each physician should identify a local resource person in AA to contact should the need arise. Alcoholics Anonymous information may also be obtained from the General Service Office of AA, Box 459, Grand Central Station, New York, NY 10017 (telephone: 212-686-1100).

2. Some alcoholics may need supportive individual therapy. For others, group therapy and/or family therapy may be most effective. It is very important to encourage family support and employment when appropriate and realistic. When a mental disorder is associated with alcoholism, the most likely condition is an affective disorder, either bipolar or unipolar depression, and referral to a psychiatrist is necessary. If there is lack of social support, or if deemed necessary by a psychiatrist, live-in programs, such as in halfway houses, may be appropriate. The physician must be aware of the current facilities available in the commu-

nity, such as programs administered by local mental health centers and other local agencies.

3. A source of information on alcohol for both physicians and patients is the National Clearinghouse for Alcohol, P.O. Box 2345, Rockville, MD 20852 (telephone: 301-468-2600)

BIBLIOGRAPHY

Ewing JA: Detecting alcoholism. The CAGE questionnaire. *JAMA* 1984;252:1905-1907.

Kraus ML, Gottlieb LD, Horwitz RI, et al: Randomized clinical trial of atenolol in patients with alcohol withdrawal. *N Engl J Med* 1985; 313:905-909.

Martin F, Ward K, Slavin J, et al: Alcoholic skeletal myopathy, a clinical and pathological study. *Q J Med* 1985; 55:233-251.

Noori SS, Adelstein J: Evaluating and treating chronic alcoholism. *Penn Med* 1978; 81:33-36.

Reuler JB, Girard DE, Cooney TG: Wernicke's encephalopathy. *N Engl J Med* 1985; 312:1035-1039.

Victor M: Alcoholism, in Baker AB, Joynt RJ (eds): *Clinical Neurology*. Hagerstown, MD, Harper and Row, 1986.

Victor M, Adams RD, Collins GH: *The Wernicke-Korsakoff Syndrome*. Philadelphia, FA Davis Co, 1971

IX

PSYCHIATRIC DISORDERS IN NEUROLOGIC DISEASE

Psychiatric and neurologic abnormalities often occur concomitantly in the same patient. Diseases once thought to be "emotional" now unquestionably have an organic basis: these include schizophrenia and manic-depressive psychosis. The boundary between psychiatry and neurology is becoming less and less distinct. If a physician is able to recognize the common psychiatric disturbances, diagnosis of many "neurologic" problems is facilitated and unnecessary diagnostic tests and referrals will be avoided. Psychiatric conditions should never be diagnosed by exclusion. Positive evidence must be gathered from the history and physical examination, and inconsistencies with known patterns of anatomy and physiology are major diagnostic clues. Unfortunately for the diagnostician, the presence of mental, emotional, or behavioral disturbances does not preclude the existence of an underlying organic abnormality. In order to convince a physician of the seriousness of the presenting complaint, patients sometimes considerably embellish symptoms. Psychiatric diagnosis should not be made lightly, because such labels may preclude investigation of organic symptoms at a later date. The intent of this chapter is to illuminate the interrelationship between common neurologic and psychiatric disorders, not to be a definitive psychiatric text.

DEPRESSION

Depression is so pervasive in the population of ill adults that physicians may unwittingly accept it as the norm. The depression may be the basic underlying illness, the result of a chronic disease process or disability, or drug-induced.

    1. Grief Reaction (Bereavement, Reactive Depression)

        This is the sadness which is a natural human emotion following personal loss. It is especially common in patients who have chronic diseases which in some way result in the loss of normal functional abilities and activities. It may also result from the death of or separation from a loved one. This type of depression does not usually respond to drug therapy.

Treatment:

1. Grief reaction is potentially a life-threatening situation, eg, the man who has just lost his wife and children in an automobile accident may commit suicide.

2. The patient needs the opportunity to discuss feelings and requires sympathetic support; this may be accomplished through a pastor, close friend, or professional counselor. If the family physician assumes this counseling responsibility, the physician must be available to the patient if things are not going well.

3. Drugs are not indicated; the disorder is self-limited and will gradually fade with time.

2. Major Depression (Endogenous Depression).

 a. The depressed patient has an ''emptiness'' that is out of proportion to any life crises experienced. If questioned carefully, these patients will reveal that their mood alteration is different in quality from the sadness experienced after personal misfortunes, bereavements, and tragedies.

 b. Major depressions may seem to be precipitated by some life event, but this is coincidence and not causation. In addition, positive changes in life circumstance do not improve the depression.

 c. Although patients with either major depression or grief reaction may have a variety of psychological symptoms, it is the physiologic symptoms characteristic of major depression (see Table 9.1) that often cause a patient to seek the physician's help. Common presentations include headaches, chronic pain, sleep disturbances, eating disturbances, confusion, and memory disturbances.

 d. Major depression is the result of an alteration of CNS biochemistry and thus responds to drug therapy. Usually the condition is idiopathic, but occasionally the major depression may have a demonstrable cause.

Treatment:

The patient with major depression often may be successfully treated by the primary care physician, if the depression is not severe and if the following guidelines are followed:

1. Take time to form a supportive relationship with the patient. Explain the nature of the illness, the fact that the medication may take 2 to 3 weeks to become effective, and even then the

Table 9.1.
Symptomatology of Depressive Illness

Physiologic (Biologic, Vegetative)	Psychological (Behavioral)

Sleep disturbance
  Delayed insomnia
 	
  Frequent awakening
	Dysphoric mood, unhappiness, sadness, crying spells

Somatic complaints
  Headaches
  Abdominal pain
  Dizziness
  Vague aches and pains
  Blurred vision
	Cognitive negatives
	  Negative feelings about self (low self-esteem, self-deprecation)
	  Negative feelings about relationships or friendships (or paranoia)
	  Negative feelings about the future (pessimism, hopelessness)

Alimentary tract disturbance
  Eating disorder (increase in or loss of appetite)
  Constipation
	Irritability, anger, poor frustration tolerance, temper outbursts

Weight change (loss or gain)	
Fatigue	
	Social withdrawal
Diminished sexual function (loss of libido)	

Psychomotor disturbance
  Increased body activity (agitation or hyperactivity) or decreased body activity (retardation)
  Increased or decreased mental activity (including impaired concentration and confusion)
	Guilt

Non-reactivity to surrounding events (including inconsolability or nonreactivity to cheering efforts)	Loss of interest or pleasure in usual activities (including loss of interest in school)
Diurnal variation in mood and symptoms (usually worse in the morning)	Preoccupation with death and/or suicidal thoughts, threats, or attempts

effect may not be magical. Schedule frequent return visits to discuss any problems, including troublesome side effects of the drugs and possible suicidal ideation.

2. Take suicidal thoughts and gestures seriously. Patients who talk about suicide will often attempt suicide. Clear suicidal ideation or attempts are stark testimony to the existence of a suicidal state. Such patients should be hospitalized with appropriate psychiatric evaluation and treatment.

3. Involve family members in the treatment; insist that they accompany the patient on office visits. The family may be very helpful in assessing the efficacy of the drug and may notice improvement in the patient's condition before the patient does. Families are an excellent source of information with regard to compliance, side effects, and suicidal thoughts.

4. Be familiar with drug side effects. Patients will have a dry mouth, some grogginess, especially in the mornings, and some constipation. Orthostatic hypotension, blurring of vision, tachycardia, and minor memory difficulties may also be troublesome. The patient should be told that the side effects often subside with time.

5. Initiate therapy gradually with amitriptyline hydrochloride or imipramine hydrochloride at a single dose of 25 to 50 mg at bedtime. Gradually increase the dose to a therapeutically effective level (150-200 mg/day) during the next week or so. Occasionally a patient who is unusually sensitive to side effects may require a smaller starting dose (10 or 20 mg/day). Serum drug levels may be obtained to monitor the dosage. Once remission is attained, the dosage may be gradually lowered to a maintenance level, which is usually about 10% to 20% lower than the maximum dose reached. Remember that these drugs are potentially lethal when taken as an overdose and not more than 500 mg should be dispensed at any time to a patient when there is any possibility of suicidal risk.

6. Encourage the patient to continue with usual activities, but to make as few important decisions as possible while in the depressed state. Irretrievable steps such as resigning from a job, divorcing a spouse, or selling property should be expressly discouraged while the patient is depressed.

7. Discontinue the drug gradually over a period of several weeks after the patient has been asymptomatic for at least 6 months.

8. Recognize anticholinergic psychosis characterized by restless agitation, confusion, disorientation, and perhaps seizures. The patient may have dry and sometimes flushed skin, tachycardia, dilated pupils, constipation, and urinary retention. This occurs especially in elderly patients who are taking other drugs such

as benzodiazepines, antihistamines, and phenothiazines in addition to the tricyclic antidepressants.

3. Drug-Induced Depression

In otherwise normal individuals (as well as in individuals susceptible to depression), the following drugs may induce depression: alcohol, reserpine, propranolol, ∝-methyldopa, benzodiazepines (such as diazepam), barbiturates, clonidine, corticosteroids, and oral contraceptives.

Treatment:

Withdrawal of the above drugs will often, but not always, result in remission of the depression. Concomitant pharmacotherapy for major depression is sometimes necessary.

4. Depression with Neurologic Disorders

Neurologic diseases commonly accompanied by depression are:

a. Huntington's disease
b. Parkinson's disease
c. Multiple sclerosis
d. Stroke syndrome (especially the right hemisphere)
e. Myotonic dystrophy

Treatment:

Physicians often identify with the depressed patient with neurologic disease ("I'd be depressed too, if I were that crippled"). However, if such patients have symptoms of major depression, a therapeutic drug trial is indicated and will often be successful. Antidepressant pharmacotherapy usually makes the neurologic disease more amenable to treatment.

5. Organic Disease Disguised as Depression

a. *Dementia* (see Chapter 6): Especially in elderly patients, depression (depressive pseudodementia) may be virtually indistinguishable from dementia. Clinical clues for distinguishing these two entities are shown in Table 9.2.

b. *"Silent" brain tumor*: With severe frontal and/or right parietal lobe damage, the patient may present with only an alteration in mood. Paresis and alteration in reflexes may be subtle or absent. Such patients usually do not have a history of mood fluctuation; differentiation from dementia and depression may be made by:

i. An elevated CSF protein,
ii. Focal neurologic findings
iii. Abnormal neuropsychological test results
iv. CT scan abnormality

Table 9.2.
Features Distinguishing Depression and Dementia

Feature	Dementia	Depression
Onset	Gradual	History of mood fluctuation
Appetite	Normal	Decreased
Constipation	Rare	Frequent
Motor activity	Relatively normal	Often decreased (may be agitated)
Mental status	Errors frequent	Tasks performed slowly but accurately

    c. *Pseudobulbar palsy:* Such patients will easily cry with minimal provocation, but will deny a feeling of sadness or emptiness. They have bilaterally increased deep tendon reflexes and an active jaw reflex. This is most frequently seen in elderly patients with a long history of hypertension (see Chapter 6).

ANXIETY

Anxiety is a common accompaniment of many illnesses, but sometimes may be the underlying illness itself. When the anxious patient walks into the office, the following features may be observed:

1. A hesitant or inappropriately hurried gait
2. Rigid posture, often with excessive fidgeting.
3. Poor eye contact
4. Excessive decoy activity (eg, lighting a cigarette)

The history will often include the following:

1. Gastrointestinal disturbances (anorexia, nausea, vomiting, diarrhea, constipation)
2. Genitourinary dysfunction (urgency, frequency, dysmenorrhea, impotence)

On examination, the following may be noted:

1. Dilated pupils, tremulousness
2. Excessive sweating
3. Elevated blood pressure, rapid pulse

Recognition of anxiety is important in the following conditions:

1. Headache (see Chapter 3): Especially important with tension headache.

2. Low back pain (see Chapter 17).
3. Alcohol and drug abuse: Anxiety may be an early symptom of alcohol withdrawal (see Chapter 8), or amphetamine or cocaine abuse.
4. Excessive use of coffee, caffeine-containing soft drinks, and tobacco.
5. Vertigo: Especially the hyperventilation syndrome (see Chapter 4).
6. May be one of the presenting symptoms of a serious depression.

   Note: Prescription of benzodiazepines may aggravate the underlying depression.
7. Patients on neuroleptics may develop an inward restlessness and fidgety legs and hands (akathisia). This is not a symptom of anxiety but a manifestation of neuroleptic toxicity and an increase in the neuroleptic will only increase this toxicity.
8. Symptoms ɪesembling anxiety may be seen in the following medical conditions: hypoglycemia, thyroid disorders, pheochromocytoma.

Treatment:

1. Identify the cause of anxiety, eg, stressful occupation or home situation, phobias. A supportive physician patient relationship is often a sufficient treatment; occasionally psychological or psychiatric counseling is indicated.
2. Withdraw all drugs or toxic substances that may be related to anxiety.
3. Pharmacologic treatment of anxiety.
   a. Pharmacologic treatment should be avoided if possible. Drugs should never be used as a substitute for a supportive physician-patient relationship. All antianxiety drugs become ineffective after a few months.
   b. Never prescribe barbiturates in anxiety states. The risk of dependency is too great, and overdosing is more lethal than with other drugs.
   c. Benzodiazepines are sometimes recommended in the treatment of anxiety, but a paradoxical reaction may worsen the anxiety in some patients and may cause drowsiness or ataxia. If benzodiazepines are used, the patient should be monitored closely and the length of treatment should be limited.
   d. Never combine antianxiety drugs, and be sure to obtain a drug history before prescribing any medication. Patients with a history of heavy use of alcohol, tobacco, and nicotine should be given antianxiety agents with caution. The risk of dependency in such patients is high.
   e. The largest dose of an antianxiety drug may be given at bedtime to exploit its sedative properties. Diazepam (Valium) is

the most frequently prescribed antianxiety drug; the dose is 5 to 10 mg tid.

   f. Propranolol (Inderal), 10 mg PO qid, will alleviate many symptoms but should be prescribed with caution because occasionally it will induce a depression.

HYSTERICAL DISORDERS

There are two major categories of hysterical disorders:

1. Patients with factitious illness as in malingering or Munchausen's syndrome.

2. Patients with signs and symptoms that have no organic basis, but the patient is not deliberately attempting to mislead the physician.

   Caution: The diagnosis of hysteria should be established on the basis of positive evidence, not the fact that all tests are negative. Also, even if the patient has an obvious hysterical disorder, a serious organic illness may still be present. Sooner or later all hysterics die. However, many medical diagnostic tests carry serious risks, and hysterical patients should not be subjected to tests unnecessarily.

A. Factitious Disorders (Malingering; Conscious, Nonphysiologic Disorder)

   1. The patient consciously feigns an illness in order to obtain something perceived as valuable.

   2. Often the examination is inconsistent with the complaint; for example, weakness of an extremity or side of the body will not be associated with any change (increased, decreased, or pathologic) in tone or reflexes. When testing muscle strength, the patient may give way with a ratchetlike quality.

   3. Some patients make malingering a lifelong occupation. These individuals feign illness with remarkably clever and complex histories, inflicting self-injury or administering drugs to produce abnormal signs consistent with the reported disease process. For example, such a patient will instill atropine into one eye to produce a fixed, dilated pupil, and then present with neurologic symptoms suggesting intracranial disease.

   Treatment:

   1. Confrontation is usually of no benefit. A cure most frequently occurs when legal matters are settled or when the patient realizes that a secondary gain is not obtainable.

   2. The physician should attempt to determine the underlying gratification the patient obtains from the illness. Occasionally the patient will have had an organic disability that has resolved; however, because of the adverse social and/or legal repercus-

sions of improvement, the patient must maintain the appearance of illness.

B. Conversion Disorder (Unconscious, Nonphysiologic Disorder with Apparent Neurologic Dysfunction)

1. Conversion symptoms have no physiologic or pathologic substrate. *Remember:* These patients are asking for help, but in an inappropriate way.
2. Conversion symptoms often occur in mentally defective individuals or in adolescents as a way of coping with the environment (albeit inadequately).
3. Common presentations include blindness, deafness, paresis, sensory disturbances, ataxia, seizures, and unconsciousness.
4. The following is a list of some conversion reactions with suggestions on how they may be recognized during the neurologic examination.

    a. *Bilateral blindness:* The patient will commonly avoid injury when walking and will blink to u..expected threat. Pupillary reactions are normal and opticokinetic nystagmus (nystagmus induced by rotating a striped drum in front of the patient's eyes) is normal. In organic blindness, pupillary reflexes and opticokinetic nystagmus are frequently abnormal. A hysterical field defect, when plotted out on a tangent screen, will not change with varying distance between the patient and the screen.

    b. *Unilateral blindness:* If there is an organic basis, the lesion must be anterior to the optic chiasm, and the pupillary reaction is usually abnormal. The Marcus Gunn phenomenon is especially useful in evaluating unilateral blindness (see Chapter 10).

    c. *Paralysis of the legs:* Reflexes are normal, and there is no atrophy. A useful test is as follows:

       i. With the patient supine, the examiner places both palms beneath the heels of the patient.
      ii. The patient is then asked to lift the nonparalyzed leg. The patient will unconsciously increase the pressure on the palm of the hand in the paralyzed leg.
      iii. The patient is then asked to press down with both heels. If pressure is not applied as it was when the patient lifted the nonparalyzed leg, a conversion reaction can be suspected (see Figure 9.1).

    d. *Hemiparesis:* A patient with a paralyzed leg and arm may incorrectly assume that there will also be difficulty in turning the head toward the paralyzed side (see Figure 9.2). Pronation drift and hemiplegic posturing are also absent on station and gait.

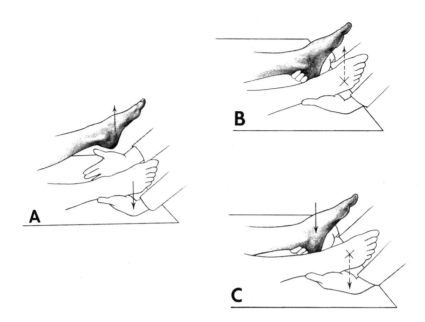

Figure 9.1 Distinguishing true paralysis from hysterical paralysis of the leg. Place both hands under the heels and ask the patient to raise the *good* leg: A. The examiner will feel increased downward pressure by the ''paralyzed'' leg. B. Ask the patient to lift the paralyzed leg; there is little or no response. C. Then ask the patient to bear down with both heels; if the same pressure noted in maneuver A cannot be exerted, ''something is rotten in the state of Denmark.''

e. *Reduced level of consciousness*: In a conversion reaction the pupillary and corneal reflexes and plantar responses will be normal. Often, when the patient's hand is held and dropped over the face, it will swerve to avoid striking the face. A patient with an organically caused reduced level of consciousness will usually have pupillary abnormalities and other positive neurologic signs (see Figure 9.3).

f. *Deafness*: The patient with a conversion reaction may startle to loud noise and can be awakened from a sound sleep by a loud noise.

g. *Sensory disturbance*: Conversion reactions that involve only the sensory systems are difficult to prove. Organic sensory losses make anatomical sense, while conversion reaction sensory disturbances will follow the patient's perception of body anatomy:

i. Patients with organic sensory disturbances are able to appreciate a vibrating tuning fork placed on either side of the

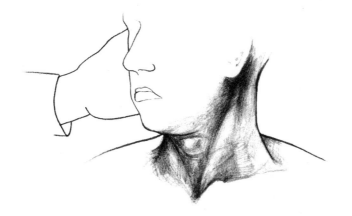

Figure 9.2 The *left* sternocleidomastoid muscle turns the head to the *right*, as illustrated. Patients with a psychogenic *left*-sided weakness will often show weakness when turning toward the left (or vice versa).

head and on either side of the sternum due to the conduction of the vibration through the bone. In a conversion reaction, the sternum or head is split, ie, vibration is perceived on one side of the midline of the forehead or sternum but not on the other (see Figure 9.4).

ii. If anesthesia is present, instruct the patient to close his eyes,

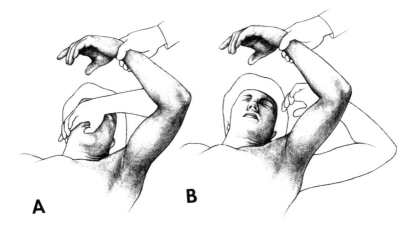

Figure 9.3 A. A hand dropped over the face of a comatose patient will strike the face. B. In psychogenic coma, a hand held over the face and then dropped often swerves to the side.

and then instruct the patient to answer "yes" if he feels the pinprick or "no" if he does not. (Obviously the only appropriate answer is silence when the supposedly anesthetic area is touched.) *Remember*: Many of these patients have limited intelligence.

iii. If a sensory disturbance involves the hands, have the patient make a fist as illustrated in the diagram (Figure 9.5), and then quickly touch the fingers for differences in sensation. In this position, most patients cannot tell the difference between their right and left hands.

h. *Pain syndrome.* The conversion reaction patient has a very vivid description of the pain, but the pain usually does not interfere with the "pleasures of life." Analgesics, even narcotics, have little effect on the pain. Often the patient is addicted to narcotics. The patient with pain from an organic disorder will usually receive some relief from narcotics, and the pain will interfere with such pleasures of life as sleeping.

Treatment:

1. Confrontation of the patient is usually not helpful since the patient often develops other symptoms and will "doctor-shop." Such patients usually find psychiatrists very threatening, and often will refuse a psychiatric interview.

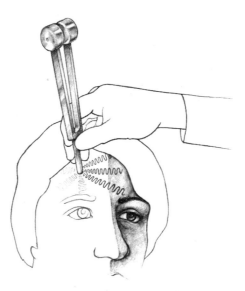

Figure 9.4 Even with an anesthetic face, the vibrations from a tuning fork will be transmitted via bone to the opposite side.

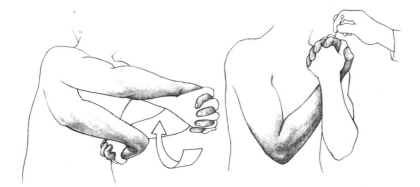

Figure 9.5 After having first demonstrated a sensory deficit in one hand, have the patient perform this maneuver and then quickly test sensation in the fingers again. This maneuver seriously distorts a person's sense of which hand is which, and accurate responses are extremely difficult unless sensation is truly disturbed.

2. Rather than confront the conversion reaction patient, the physician may emphasize that the symptoms are not medically serious (eg, "I'm so happy to be able to tell you that you do not have cancer or a brain tumor"). From that point on, try to substitute a discussion of life problems and interpersonal relations. It is important that the physician not reject or become angry with the hysteric patient. Limited, precisely scheduled visits and telephone calls on a regular basis are often helpful. With time, the physician may learn what goal or conflict is producing the conversion reaction. Administration of the Minnesota Multiphasic Personality Inventory (MMPI) and hypnosis in the hands of a skilled specialist may be helpful in establishing the diagnosis.
3. Once the diagnosis is made, the major goal is to avoid unnecessary hospitalization and surgery.
4. Drugs of any kind should be avoided in conversion states.

SCHIZOPHRENIA

Schizophrenia and the following neurologic problems occasionally cause diagnostic confusion:

1. *Basal ganglia disease.* As a side effect of neuroleptic therapy, the patient may develop a restlessness, especially in the legs (akathisia). These patients are usually more "inwardly" restless than is immediately apparent. Neuroleptics may also produce a parkinsonian syndrome (see Chapter 7).

2. *Dementia* (see Chapter 6). Catatonic patients may appear to be demented. Schizophrenia causes a disorder of thought, but memory is spared.

3. *Aphasia* (see Chapter 12): The patient with parietal or temporal lobe damage may have a speech disturbance in which speech melody is normal, but the words make little sense. This damage may be caused by tumor, infarct, or hemorrhage. Specific testing for aphasia will distinguish aphasia from schizophrenia.

4. *Complex partial seizures* (see Chapter 11): The onset of symptoms may begin and end abruptly. An EEG with nasopharyngeal leads may reveal a spike focus in the temporal lobe. Patients with complex partial seizures have a distinctive personality profile, perhaps because of a disturbed limbic system, and this profile may be confused with schizophrenic personality profiles.

5. *Illicit drugs*, such as lysergic acid diethylamide (LSD), amphetamines, and phencyclidine (PCP) may produce states closely resembling schizophrenia. A history of drug abuse and a subacute onset will usually be distinguishing features. Prescribed medications such as thiazides, steroids, and disulfiram may also cause a disturbance of thinking resembling schizophrenia.

6. *Delirium tremens* may produce hallucinations and an agitated state (see Chapter 8). The hallucinations with delirium tremens are usually visual, while those of schizophrenia are generally auditory.

7. *Wernicke-Korsakoff syndrome* (see Chapter 8). This is an acute or subacute onset of extraocular muscle paralysis and mental changes that may resemble schizophrenia. When this syndrome is suspected immediately give thiamine 100 mg IM or IV. Schizophrenics do not have abnormal eye movements.

8. *Diffuse CNS vascular disease,* such as that seen in hypertensive encephalopathy, tertiary syphilis, or collagen vascular disease, may produce acute or chronic disturbances in thought processes that resemble schizophrenia.

9. *Endocrine dysfunctions*, especially those associated with thyroid and adrenal disorders, on occasion produce striking changes in mentation.

10. *Hereditary neurologic disease*, especially Huntington's disease, may produce schizophrenic symptoms years before the movement disorder becomes obvious.

To differentiate true schizophrenia from the preceding schizophrenic-like states, it is essential to take a careful history with a special regard to:

1. Mode of onset (acute, subacute, or chronic)

2. Past history of similar disturbances

3. Drugs, licit and illicit

4. Alcoholic intake

5. Head trauma, seizures, or headache

6. Temperature intolerance, weight change

7. Family history

8. History of viral encephalitis, especially *Herpes simplex* encephalitis

On a screening neurologic examination, pay particular attention to focal neurologic signs, abnormal movements, and posture.

Minimal laboratory tests that should be performed include the following:

1. CBC with ESR

2. Serum Na, K, BUN

3. Serum test for syphilis

4. Thyroid function tests

Consider also the following tests:

1. Lumbar puncture

2. CT scan

The following points may help the primary care physician to recognize a schizophrenic patient. Florid schizophrenia is seldom seen, but borderline or subclinical schizophrenia, schizophrenia in remission, and schizophrenics on treatment with phenothiazines are relatively common.

1. Schizophrenic patients may be described as having "sunburned minds." That is to say, they are extremely sensitive to criticism, stress, emotional closeness, and rejection.

2. Onset of symptoms is usually before the age of 40 years.

3. The patient has a disorder of thought processes with an inappropriate rate, flow, or content of thinking, but the sensorium is clear. When a patient has delusions or hallucinations, there is no disorientation or memory disturbance.

    Caution: The presence of delusions, hallucinations, paranoid ideation, or catatonic symptoms should not automatically lead to the diagnosis of schizophrenia. These symptoms are almost as common among manic-depressive patients.

4. Often there is a blunted, shallow, inappropriate affect and/or bizarre motor behavior. Unfortunately, physicians often have little sympathy for emotional reactions in schizophrenic patients.

5. Patients are often single and have poor premorbid social adjustments or work history.

6. Frequently there is a family history of schizophrenia.

Treatment:

1. Acutely disturbed schizophrenics are usually best treated at inpatient mental health facilities with antipsychotic medications.

2. When the primary care physician is following a schizophrenic in remission on a phenothiazine or other major tranquilizer, it is important to recognize that akathisia may be a symptom of phenothiazine or other major tranquilizer toxicity; the symptoms of akathisia are often mistakenly interpreted as being due to anxiety and the dose of the phenothiazine or other major tranquilizer may be increased, when actually the proper treatment is to decrease the dose or discontinue the drug.

RECOGNIZING PERSONALITY TYPES AS AN AID TO PATIENT MANAGEMENT

The primary care physician should be able to recognize the common personality types and disorders in order to avoid letting the physician's own emotional reactions interfere with the doctor-patient relationship.

Remember: Every patient has a personality! Different personality types often need different approaches in management. For example, if the therapeutic goal is to have a patient remain at bed rest, the independent, machismo young male should be told, "Staying in bed like this is a tough job, and a lot of my patients can't do it, but I know a person with your determination and will power certainly won't disappoint me." On the other hand, if the patient is a passive dependent male, one would say, "Just lie there in bed, and don't worry about a thing because we will care for you completely." Some of the more common personality types are listed in Table 9.3.

BIBLIOGRAPHY

American Psychiatric Association: *Diagnostic and Statistical Manual of Mental Disorders,* (ed 3.) Washington, American Psychiatric Association, 1980.

Benson DF, Blumer D: *Psychiatric Aspects of Neurologic Disease.* New York, Grune & Stratton, 1975.

Black JL, Richelson E, Richardson JW: Antipsychotic agents: a clinical update. *Mayo Clin Proc* 1985;60:777–789.

Table 9.3.
Characteristics of Common Personality Types

Personality Type	Description	Practical Suggestions
Passive-dependent	Chronic inability to adjust to life demands; completely dependent upon others; longterm hospitalization or institutionalization common	"I'll take care of you"
Passive-aggressive	Stubborn obstructionist who makes intentional errors; follows directions poorly; intolerant of authority; blames others for any bad outcomes	"I know you are tough enough to do it"
Antisocial	Selfish, callous, with no loyalty or trustworthiness; no sense of guilt; low frustration tolerance with frequent interpersonal difficulties; antisocial behavior	These are extremely difficult patients to treat (see Cleckley's *The Mask of Sanity*)
Obsessive-compulsive	Excessive concern about standards, morals, image; excessive inhibitions; frequently isolated and usually chronically unhappy	Give patient orders, lists, and schedules
Paranoid	Suspicious, blames others for all problems; frequently involved in lawsuits; feels self-important and entitled to better	Explain all procedures in a simple, straight forward manner
Hysteric	Immature behavior; sexually seductive in most interactions; dependent, but avoids meaningful interpersonal relationships	Avoid seduction; recognize dependency needs; do not become angry and punitive towards these patients
Schizoid	Isolated, secretive, eccentric; avoids interpersonal relationships of all kinds	These patients are threatened by the natural warmth and closeness of many physicians; on the other hand, the door to communication must be left open because these patients are also very sensitive to rejection

138

Cleckley H: *The Mask of Sanity.* St Louis, CV Mosby Co, 1976.

Goodwin DW, Guze SB: *Psychiatric Diagnosis,* ed 3. New York, Oxford University Press, 1984.

Herskowitz J, Rosman NP: *Pediatrics, Neurology, and Psychiatry — Common Ground.* New York, Macmillan, 1982.

Jacobs JW, Bernhard MR, Delgado A, et al: Screening for organic mental syndromes in the medically ill. *Ann Intern Med* 1977;86:40-46.

Richardson JW, Richelson E: Antidepressants: a clinical update for medical practitioners. *Mayo Clin Proc* 1984;59:330-337.

Winokur G, Clayton P (eds): *The Medical Basis of Psychiatry.* Philadelphia, WB Saunders, 1986.

X

MULTIPLE SCLEROSIS

Multiple sclerosis (MS) is commonly diagnosed by physicians, in part because it is common, and in part because the disease is often emphasized in medical school neuroscience curricula. Curiously, in some surveys, primary care physicians list multiple sclerosis as a "symptom" along with headache and dizziness. In the authors' experience, multiple sclerosis is *over*diagnosed; as many as half of the patients referred to a multiple sclerosis clinic either do not have the disease or have very doubtful evidence to support the diagnosis. Once the patient has been incorrectly labeled with the diagnosis of multiple sclerosis, such a label is often difficult to remove. In addition, all subsequent neurologic deterioration is attributed to multiple sclerosis and evaluation for treatable diseases is neglected.

History

1. Transient blurring of vision in one eye (retrobulbar neuritis) is very common. Vision is often normal by the time the patient is examined by a physician.
2. Double vision.
3. Transient clumsiness of one arm (cerebellar involvement).
4. Urinary urgency and/or frequency and male impotence (spinal cord involvement).
5. Excessive fatigue unrelated to focal symptoms.
6. Paralysis of a leg or arm.
7. Symptoms usually begin in the third decade of life (but cases have been reported in children and in the sixth decade).

8. Patients often note that symptoms recur when they are overheated, eg, hot shower, fever.

Caution: Most patients have repeated exacerbations and remissions of symptoms, but 10% of patients with MS may have a gradually progressive course without readily apparent exacerbations or remissions.

Examination

Because any part of the CNS white matter may become demyelinated, *any* neurologic abnormality is possible. The following are common findings in MS patients:

1. The optic nerve often shows temporal pallor as a residuum of retrobulbar neuritis. A Marcus-Gunn pupil is frequently seen; this indicates damage to the optic nerve anterior to the chiasm from any cause (see Figure 10.1).
2. Internuclear ophthalmoplegia -- especially if bilateral -- is highly suggestive of MS (see Figure 10.2). Incomplete forms exist such as pronounced nystagmus in the abducting eye and mild nystagmus in the adducting eye. Rare causes include brainstem infarcts, tumors, or myasthenia.
3. Intention tremor and incoordinated rapid alternating movements are common because of cerebellar peduncle involvement.
4. Tingling or electric shocklike paresthesias on neck flexion (Lhermitte's sign).
5. Impaired recognition of objects by touch alone (astereognosis).
6. Motor involvement: increased or asymmetrical reflexes, Babinski reflex.

Caution: Multiple sclerosis affects *only* the CNS; absent reflexes, muscle atrophy, and sensory loss in the distribution of a peripheral nerve make the diagnosis unlikely. The presence of significant dementia, papilledema, or symmetric proximal muscle weakness also make the diagnosis unlikely.

Laboratory Studies

In the modern era, the diagnosis of MS should be confirmed by laboratory studies:

1. *Magnetic resonance imaging*: The presence of multiple, predominantly periventricular plaques in a young patient with exacerbations and remissions of neurologic symptoms strongly supports the diagnosis of MS and further tests probably need not be done.

Caution: Many patients with few symptoms have extensive demyelination, and a normal MRI is occasionally seen in patients with severe disability.

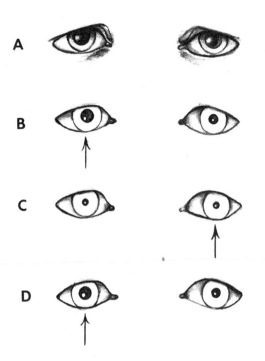

Figure 10.1. Marcus-Gunn pupil: The pupil that paradoxically dilates with direct light. A. Both pupils initially are equal. B. Direct light into the affected eye (*arrow*) causes minimal constriction; the opposite pupil constricts equally because of consensual reflex. C. Direct light into the normal eye causes significant constriction of both pupils, direct and consensual. D. Swinging the flashlight back to the affected eye causes it "paradoxically" to dilate due to removal of strong consensual reflex.

2. *Evoked responses*: Visual, somatosensory, and brainstem auditory evoked responses are abnormal in a majority of patients.

3. *Lumbar puncture* (see Chapter 2): Routine studies show a normal or slightly increased cell count, normal or slightly increased protein, and an increased gamma-globulin level. Tests more specific for MS include:

   a. IgG synthesis calculated by the formula:

$$\frac{CSF\ IgG/serum\ IgG}{CSF\ albumin/serum\ albumin} \quad \text{(normal } < 0.7)$$

   b. Oligoclonal bands

   c. Myelin basic protein (normal < 1.0 ng/mL)

Computed tomography, EEG, EMG, myelography, and isotope scans are of little or no use in establishing a firm diagnosis of MS.

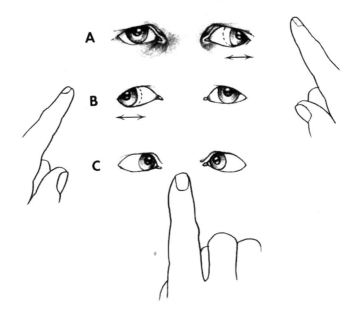

Figure 10.2. Bilateral internuclear ophthalmoplegia: When looking to either side, the adducting eye does not go beyond the midline, the abducting eye shows nystagmus (A and B). This looks somewhat like a bilateral medial rectus palsy; however, the patient is able to converge and focus on a near object (C).

Specific Treatment

Experts agree that MS is associated with an altered immune response, possibly triggered by an unspecified viral agent. In very severe cases, progression may sometimes be halted by high-dose IV cyclophosphamide and ACTH, but this treatment should be reserved for severely ill patients in tertiary care centers. Many centers currently are conducting clinical trials with a variety of agents that affect the immune system, and it can be reasonably expected that in the near future a safe medication that will prevent the development of new plaques will be available.

Physician Advice

1. Because of the exacerbations and remissions and chronicity of the disease, MS patients are particularly prone to quack treatments. Advise patients to use only Food and Drug Administration-approved medications or to participate only in drug trials sponsored by respectable scientific agencies.

2. Most patients are initially upset with their diagnosis. The positive features of the disease should be emphasized: one third of patients have a relatively benign course and the recovery rate from individual attacks is 80% or more.

3. Stress is generally recognized as a precipitating factor for attacks. This includes infections.

4. Avoid situations where the body temperature is raised (hot baths, saunas, prolonged exposure to hot sun) as this may cause a temporary recurrence of old symptoms.

5. Bladder hygiene should be emphasized, and self-catheterization should be taught if residual urine is present.

Symptomatic Drug Therapy

1. Antispasticity agents

   Caution: In some patients, spasticity is beneficial for weight supporting, and these patients will be made worse by such drugs.

   a. Baclofen (Lioresal) at an initial dose of 5 mg bid up to 20 mg tid. Dose should be slowly titrated for maximal benefit.

   b. Dantrolene (Dantrium): Begin with 25 mg daily; every three or four days increase the dose by 25 mg until the therapeutic goal is obtained. Doses as high as 100 mg tid occasionally are necessary. If this drug is used, liver function tests should be performed at regular intervals since hepatitis and liver failure have been reported.

2. Amantadine hydrochloride (Symmetrel): Fatigue is a most bothersome symptom to MS patients; some patients improve dramatically with 100 mg once or twice a day.

3. Steroids (prednisone and ACTH): These drugs should never be used on a chronic basis. Occasionally, short-term therapy (1 week) may be used to shorten the duration of the attack. These drugs have *no* effect on the eventual outcome of the disease.

4. Amitriptyline hydrochloride: In MS patients with major depression or with emotional lability, the tricyclic antidepressants, specifically amitriptyline 50 to 150 mg/day, may ameliorate the symptoms.

Rehabilitation

1. Physical therapy is indicated for patients in remission with residual motor disability. Ideally, this is best carried out in a rehabilitation center.

2. Occupational therapy assists patients with a fixed disability in adjusting to the activities of daily living.

Patient Education

The National Multiple Sclerosis Society is a good source of information: National Multiple Sclerosis Society, 205 East 42nd St, New York, NY 10017 (telephone: 212-986-3240 or 800-637-6303). In addition, most cities have a local MS society and support groups which are invaluable sources of education and emotional support

BIBLIOGRAPHY

Hauser SL, Dawson DM, Lehrich JR, et al: Intensive immunosuppression in progressive multiple sclerosis. *N Engl J Med* 1983; 308:173-180.

International Federation of Multiple Sclerosis Societies: *Minimal Record of Disability for Multiple Sclerosis*. New York, National Multiple Sclerosis Society, 1985.

Johnson KP, Belediuk G: Use of cyclosporine in neurological autoimmune disease? *Arch Neurol* 1985; 42:1043-1044.

Markowitz H, Kokmen E: Neurologic diseases and the cerebrospinal fluid immunoglobulin profile. *Mayo Clin Proc* 1983; 58:273-274.

McFarlin DE, McFarland HF: Multiple sclerosis. *N Engl J Med* 1982; 307:1183-1188,1246-1251.

Poser CM: *Diagnosis of Multiple Sclerosis* New York, Thieme, Inc, 1984.

Scheinberg LC (ed): *Multiple Sclerosis. A Guide for Patients and Their Families*. New York, Raven Press, 1983.

Stewart JM, Howser OW, Baker HL, et al: Magnetic resonance imaging and clinical relationships in multiple sclerosis. *Mayo Clin Proc* 1987; 62:174-184.

Wilson H, Olson WH, Gascon GG, et al: Personality characteristics and multiple sclerosis. *Psychol Rep* 1982; 51:791-806

XI

SEIZURES AND EPILEPSY

A seizure is a sudden change in body functioning due to abnormal, excessive electrical discharges of neurons in the brain. Epilepsy is a symptom complex in which there is a tendency to have repeated seizures. It follows that not everyone who has seizures has epilepsy, but everyone who has epilepsy has seizures. Neither seizures nor epilepsy are a final diagnosis but are symptom complexes requiring a search for underlying etiologic factors.

Frequently, only generalized tonic-clonic movements are recognized as seizures, but consideration of seizures should arise whenever a patient presents with loss of consciousness or any sudden brief change in functioning with or without loss of consciousness. Paroxysmal changes in consciousness, sensation, emotion, or thought processes all may be manifestations of a seizure disorder. A diagnosis of a seizure disorder is especially likely if such changes are repetitive, stereotyped, and preceded by a premonition or warning (aura) or followed by (postictal) confusion, exhaustion, or headache.

The physician's initial task when a patient presents with what might be a seizure is to determine whether indeed the episode was a seizure, or some other episodic, periodic, or recurrent paroxysmal event that is nonepileptic, such as syncope, migraine, pseudoseizures, transient ischemic attacks (TIAs), or narcolepsy. When the diagnosis of a seizure is made, the patient should be evaluated for common toxic-metabolic or structural abnormalities. These commonly include hypoglycemia, infection, alcohol or drug withdrawal, stroke, or tumor.

Patients with recurrent seizures over a long period of time (epilepsy syndrome) most likely have either no structural abnormality or a static abnormality such as a glial scar. Recurrent seizures with neurologic deterioration require evaluation for inborn errors of metabolism, chronic infection, or tumor. Patients with recurrent seizures and an anatomically normal brain or a non-progressive lesion require only symptomatic treatment with anticonvulsants. If the seizures are secondary to a generalized systemic medical condition or a progressive brain lesion, then the patient requires specific treatment in addition to symptomatic treatment with anticonvulsants.

Summary:

1. Seizure or nonseizure?
2. If seizure, classification of seizure type (see Appendix C).
3. Acute medical or neurologic condition or epilepsy?
4. Symptomatic or specific treatment? or both?

In the primary epilepsies no focal brain lesions are found, there is often a family history of epilepsy, and the neurologic examination is normal. They often begin in childhood, and the response to anticonvulsants is usually very good. In the secondary epilepsies neurologic abnormalities may be present, a family history of epilepsy is usually lacking, and the response to anticonvulsants is variable to poor.

History

The history is the single most important part of the diagnostic evaluation and management of seizures. It should include:

1. An accurate description of the onset of the seizures. (If the patient cannot give a history, attempt to interview an eyewitness.)
   a. Bilaterally symmetrical onset without warning (primary generalized seizure) versus focal, partial, or unilateral. For example, arm jerking on one side suggests a lesion in the frontal lobe of the opposite hemisphere.
   b. Dynamic character of seizures (march of movement, focal movement becoming generalized, etc).
2. A review of symptoms suggesting seizures, eg, loss of memory; strange, unexplained smells or other sensations; visual hallucinations; distortions in visual, auditory, or time sensation; feeling of having experienced events before; previous staring episodes (absences); previous undiagnosed nocturnal seizures with bed-wetting; rolling out of bed; awakening exhausted with muscle aches and pain.
3. A family history of seizures. (In primary generalized seizure disorders the familial incidence is as high as 25%.)
4. Previous head trauma or other CNS damage.

Specific seizure syndromes tend to occur with highest frequency at certain ages (see Table 11.1).

Minimum Laboratory Studies

The laboratory examination will be directly based on the clinical history and type of seizure and will be different for each type of seizure and each age group.

Electroencephalogram (EEG). The EEG measures the electrical activity of cortical surface neurons. The EEG is a finite sample of activity in time. Remember that the recording is often done between seizures (interictal) and may or may not reveal epileptiform abnormalities. The reliability of the EEG also depends on the competence of the EEG technologist doing the recording and the expertise of the electroencephalographer. Routine activation techniques such as hyperventilation, photic stimulation, and sleep deprivation, and use of nasopharyngeal leads may add more information. In specialized referral centers continuous monitoring by video-EEG techniques and ambulatory cassette recording are now available for refractory epilepsies or when diagnostic difficulties arise.

Caution: A normal EEG does not rule out the diagnosis of a seizure, and rarely patients may have abnormal EEGs with no clinical symptoms.

Table 11.1.
Age Correlation with Seizure Syndromes

Age	Seizures	Etiology
Newborn (0-3 wk)	Poorly defined seizures; generalized tonic, focal and multifocal clonus, myoclonus	Hypoxia, hemorrhage, congenital malformations, hypoglycemia, hypocalcemia
Infants and toddlers (3 wk - 3 yr)	Simple febrile seizures, infantile spasms, Lennox-Gastaut syndrome	Inborn errors of metabolism, no specific cause (as in febrile seizures), hypoxic brain damage
Children (3-12 yr)	Petit mal, benign centrotemporal epilepsy	Familial
Adolescents (13-24 yr)	Generalized tonic-clonic	Familial
Adults (21-60 yr)	Complex (and simple) partial or secondarily generalized	Head trauma, tumor
Elderly (>60 yr)	Partial or secondarily generalized	Postinfarction (vascular)

Neonatal Seizures

Newborns, unlike older infants, do not have well-organized, symmetric tonic-clonic seizures. Seizures in premature infants are even less organized. Suspect seizures when there are unexplained autonomic, respiratory, or motor changes.

1. Subtle seizures: eye blinking, tonic eye deviation, sucking, lip-smacking, drooling, swimming movements, pedaling movements, apnea.
2. Tonic seizures: usually extension of all limbs.
3. Multifocal clonus: usually associated with perinatal asphyxia.
4. Focal clonus: hypocalcemia, focal brain contusion.
5. Myoclonus: multiple or single flexion jerks of upper or lower extremities.
6. Generally there is an underlying cause, such as neonatal hypoxia-ischemia, trauma, intracranial hemorrhage, meningitis, hypocalcemia, or rarely, inborn errors of metabolism (pyridoxine dependency, phenylketonuria, maple syrup urine disease, galactosemia). Ultrasound imaging or CT scan of the head may demonstrate anatomical abnormalities (hemorrhage, developmental brain anomalies). Blood and urine chemical analysis may detect metabolic disturbances.
7. Generally, the best prognosis is seen with focal clonic jerking and the worst prognosis with fragmentary multifocal clonic seizures. Prognosis for normal neurologic development and recurrent seizures relates ultimately to etiology and response to treatment of underlying cause. Reversible metabolic disorders (hypocalcemia) have the best prognosis.

Treatment:

1. Prevention and/or early detection with adequate treatment of the underlying disorder(s) is the best approach to neonatal seizures.
2. If seizures occur frequently, then do the following:
   a. Draw blood for glucose, calcium, magnesium, and electrolytes, and leave the needle in place for IV line.
   b. Inject the following solutions (if there is an immediate response, the cause of the seizures will have been determined):
      i. 50% glucose 1 to 2 mL/kg
      ii. Calcium gluconate 200 mg/kg
      iii. Pyridoxine 50 mg
3. If the seizures still do not stop, then phenobarbital 15 to 20 mg/kg should be infused IV slowly over an hour. Subsequent IV phenobarbital dosages can then be ordered according to serial serum phenobarbital levels, attempting to keep the blood level between 20 and 30 μg/mL. If seizures continue, phenytoin 15 to 20 mg/kg IV (never IM) can also be used. Phenobarbital can be continued orally for

long-term maintenance, but oral phenytoin is poorly absorbed in infants and is not recommended for long-term maintenance.

4. If seizures stop in the neonatal period, it is accepted practice to continue anticonvulsants for 3 months and then discontinue them gradually.

Simple Febrile Seizures

1. Simple febrile seizures are the most common cause of seizures in infants and toddlers; the greatest incidence is between ages 18 and 36 months.
2. Onset with fever (often during rapidly rising or falling stage of temperature); fever is often not detected until after seizure occurs.
3. Brief (less than ten minutes) generalized seizure; seizure has almost always stopped by the time patient arrives at physician's office.
4. EEG is normal by 2 weeks after the seizure.
5. Family history of simple febrile seizures in early childhood supports the diagnosis of simple febrile seizure.

Caution: If the seizure is focal or prolonged or if the neurologic examination shows focal abnormalities, it is *not* a simple febrile seizure and a search must be made for underlying pathology, especially infection. It is also unusual for the *first* simple febrile seizure to occur before 6 months or after 3 years of age.

Treatment:

1. If CNS infection is suspected, patients should have a lumbar puncture and CSF examination.
2. Parents should be reassured that the condition is benign (not associated with brain damage and highly unlikely to develop into epilepsy).
3. If the aim is to prevent future febrile convulsions, anticonvulsants are *not* beneficial if given intermittently, ie, with fevers. *Phenobarbital* is effective (phenytoin is not) prophylactically, but enough must be given to produce therapeutic blood levels (15-30 g/mL). The usual dosage of 3 to 5 mg/kg/day can be given as a single evening dose.
4. Valproic acid is the only other effective prophylactic anticonvulsant for simple febrile seizures, but is probably contraindicated because of potential hepatotoxicity.
5. Since simple febrile seizures are so benign and since anticonvulsants may have significant side effects, many physicians do not treat them; however, the physician may find it difficult to resist pressure from parents to treat the child.

Complicated Febrile Seizures

1. Fever lowers the seizure threshold, ie, fever of any cause may trigger seizures in individuals with underlying epilepsy, or fever and seizures may be associated with CNS infection such as meningitis or encephalitis.
2. These seizures occur in all age groups, but are a diagnostic problem especially in children under the age of 5 years.
3. Thorough neurologic evaluation is necessary if it is the patient's first seizure. The risk of febrile seizures developing into an epileptic disorder is increased by: neurologic abnormalities by history or examination, developmental delay, focality or long duration of the seizure, multiple seizures with each febrile episode, prolonged seizures (greater than 15 minutes), family history of epilepsy, and epileptiform abnormalities in the EEG.

Treatment:

1. Diagnostic lumbar puncture and appropriate antibiotic treatment are necessary for meningitis or encephalitis (see also Chapter 14).
2. Reducing or preventing the fever with antipyretics (aspirin or acetaminophen) will reduce the likelihood of seizures.

   Caution: Although its role is still undetermined, aspirin has been associated with Reye's syndrome, particularly when the underlying cause of fever has been influenza or chickenpox.

3. For maintenance give anticonvulsants to prevent further febrile and/or afebrile seizures: phenobarbital 3 to 5 mg/kg/day is the drug of choice; if seizures recur after adequate blood levels, phenytoin 5 to 7 mg/kg/day may be added. Once the phenytoin level is therapeutic, phenobarbital is gradually withdrawn. Blood levels of the anticonvulsants must be obtained to determine the adequacy of the dosage.

Infantile Spasms

This epileptic syndrome, consisting of massive myoclonic seizures in the first year of life, developmental arrest, and a hypsarrhythmic EEG, is the most devastating seizure syndrome and should be treated with great concern.

1. Massive myoclonic seizures last a second or so and consist of sudden bending forward at the waist with the arms and legs extended in the posture of prayer (hence "salaam seizures"). Less common are extensor spasms, with arching of the back and extension of the neck. Rarely there are hemispasms, involving only one half of the body.
2. The spasms occur in flurries, usually upon awakening, many times daily.
3. Often misdiagnosed as "colic," particularly if noticed during feeding times.

4. Usual onset is between age 3 and 12 months.

5. Associated with developmental arrest and subsequent moderate to severe mental retardation in greater than 90% of these children.

6. The EEG shows hypsarrhythmic pattern consisting of disorganized background activity, multiconfigurational and multifocal discharges during the waking state. Sleep tracings may mimic "burst-suppression" patterns.

7. Etiologies are:

    a. Symptomatic: previous static encephalopathies or (rarely) progressive CNS disease, or neurocutaneous syndromes, particularly tuberous sclerosis.

    b. Cryptogenic: normally developing babies suddenly have the syndrome, and no CNS disease is found.

8. Seizures may be difficult to control, and may evolve into other seizure syndromes (see Lennox-Gastaut syndrome below).

Treatment:

1. Early treatment of the seizures alone is not sufficient. Search for an underlying etiology with neurometabolic urine screen and CT scan (for developmental brain malformations, such as agenesis of the corpus callosum).

2. After obtaining baseline EEGs, treat with ACTH 100 units/m^2/day (usually 80 units) for 3 to 4 weeks. Clinical improvement usually does not occur before ten to 14 days, and may be preceded by EEG improvement.

3. After this initial course, follow with ACTH gel IM every other day until the patient is spasm-free for 1 month. Monitor for steroid toxic side effects, the most important of which is hypertension.

4. If spasms persist or evolve into other seizure types, clonazepam at 0.5 mg bid can be started and then increased. Valproic acid can be substituted if clonazepam is only partially effective or ineffective.

5. Genetic counseling is necessary if a genetic syndrome can be identified.

6. Families should be offered assistance in managing the young retarded child (see Chapter 16).

Lennox-Gastaut Syndrome

1. The Lennox-Gastaut syndrome is similar to infantile spasms but presents in a later age group, usually age 2 to 5 years; akinetic and myoclonic seizures (drop spells), absences, and generalized convulsions occur, often many times daily.

2. Associated with mild to moderate mental retardation, hyperactivity, and behavior disturbances.

3. Characteristic EEG changes consist of poorly developed background activity, and multifocal slow (less than 3 Hz) spike-wave complexes.
4. Since both the infantile spasms and Lennox-Gastaut syndrome are clinically devastating, initial management is probably best handled by someone experienced with these disorders, such as a pediatric neurologist, epileptologist, or a pediatrician with specialized training and experience with epilepsies.

Treatment:

1. Total control of seizures is difficult to achieve. Management usually includes use of the major anticonvulsants such as barbiturates (be careful not to make a hyperactive child worse), clonazepam, valproic acid (see Table 11.2) but might include ACTH and ketogenic diet. Protective helmets (football or hockey type) help prevent head injury from drop spells.
2. If the subsequent course shows persistent myoclonic seizures, and persistent developmental arrest, or developmental regression, suspect a progressive CNS disease (such as the ganglioside storage diseases) and refer the patient to a pediatric neurologist.

Benign Centrotemporal Epilepsy

Benign centrotemporal epilepsy (rolandic epilepsy, sylvian seizure syndrome,

Table 11.2
Drugs Used in Treatment of Seizures

Drug	Dosage		Therapeutic Blood Level (μg/mL)	Plasma Half-Life (hours)
	Adults (mg)	Children (mg/kg)		
Phenobarbital	100-180	3-5	15-30	72-96
Phenytoin	300-400	4-7	10-20	12-24
Primidone (partially metabolized to phenobarbital)	750-1500	10-25	6-12	3-12
Carbamazepine	800-1600	10-30	6-12	7-18
Ethosuximide	750-2000	20-30	40-100	24-48
Clonazepam	1.5-20	0.01-0.2	0.02-0.07	18-50
Valproic acid	1000-3000	15-50	50-100	7-15

lingual seizures) is a relatively common, but often unrecognized and misdiagnosed epileptic disorder. Making the correct diagnosis is important because of the benign prognosis, excellent response to anticonvulsants, and "outgrowing" the disorder by mid- or late adolescence.

1. This is a focal or partial seizure syndrome not associated with focal structural CNS lesion.
2. Often presents as nocturnal generalized convulsions in school-aged children. These are actually secondarily generalized convulsions.
3. The partial onset, seen easily after institution of anticonvulsants and incomplete control of the seizures, consists of localized tongue or oral paresthesias, dysarthria, drooling, and facial twitching, with preservation of consciousness. A careful history for this initial onset of the seizures will give the diagnosis.
4. The EEG shows characteristic central and midtemporal spikes or sharp waves. These are best seen in a sleep EEG.

Treatment:
1. The treatment of choice is phenytoin (keep blood level between 15 and 20 μg/mL) until adolescence.
2. Phenobarbital is also effective (keep blood levels at 25 $\pm$ 5 μg/mL).

Primary Generalized Epilepsies

The most common clinical types of primary generalized epilepsies are *grand mal* and *petit mal*. The following features apply to all generalized seizures:

1. Onset is almost always in childhood or adolescence.
2. From the onset the seizures are generalized, with immediate alteration of consciousness. Motor manifestations are symmetric and bilateral.
3. EEG discharges are generalized and bilaterally synchronous from the start of a recorded seizure.
4. Neurologic examination and CT scan of brain are normal interictally.
5. The EEG background activity is normal, interrupted by generalized, bilaterally synchronous, symmetric spike-wave or poly-spike-wave complexes. These occur spontaneously, or are activated by hyperventilation, intermittent photic stimulation, or sleep.
6. No previous history of brain injury.
7. Family history of seizures is often positive.
8. Good response to appropriate antiepileptic drugs.
9. Relatively good prognosis. Next to benign centrotemporal epilepsy, the primary generalized epilepsies have the best long-term prognosis for seizure control, as well as for intellectual, cognitive, and emotional functioning.

10. Previous terms commonly used that are synonymous with primary generalized epilepsy are "idiopathic" or "centrencephalic" epilepsy.

A. *Petit Mal Epilepsy*

The term *petit mal* is probably the most misused term applied to seizures by the general physician. It does *not* denote any minor seizure that falls short of being a generalized convulsion. *Petit mal* epilepsy (italics for emphasis) is a *specific* clinical and EEG syndrome and has a *specific* therapy.

1. The usual onset is between age 3 and 10 years.
2. Petit mal is characterized by *absences* lasting 2 to 30 seconds associated with a characteristic EEG abnormality (3 Hz spike-wave discharges activated by hyperventilation).
3. Absences clinically appear as staring spells during which the patient is momentarily unresponsive; they may be associated with eyelid fluttering. Often the eyes will roll upward; less commonly there may be automatisms of lip-smacking, chewing, or other purposeless repetitive mouth or hand movements.
4. Absences occur frequently in flurries during the day; the child may be called a "day dreamer", "absent-minded" or "inattentive"; absences may be recognized as transient pauses during eating, speaking, or any other activity.
5. Petit mal is distinguished from complex partial seizures (psychomotor, temporal lobe) by lack of aura, brief duration, and lack of postictal confusion, drowsiness, or headache.
6. Absences can be brought out by hyperventilation, which can be done as an *office test*: Have the patient hyperventilate for three minutes under observation. During an absence, the hyperventilation will stop while the typical features of absence are observed, and then hyperventilation will resume immediately.
7. Petit mal may be complicated by other seizure phenomena: myoclonic jerks (sudden increase in muscle tone *throwing* patient forward or backward), and atonic-akinetic seizures (drop or *slumping* of head or body due to sudden decrease of muscle tone).
8. Petit mal responds readily to treatment unless complicated by other seizure phenomena, in which case there is a risk for later generalized convulsions.
9. Petit mal status consists of continuous absence seizures, and may appear as a confusional state. The EEG shows continuous 3-Hz spike-and-wave activity. It usually occurs:
   a. As a withdrawal syndrome (suddenly from anticonvulsant drugs)

    b. As previously undiagnosed and untreated petit mal epilepsy occurring in adolescence or early adulthood

    c. Incorrectly treated petit mal (eg, using phenobarbital or phenytoin, rather than valproate or ethosuximide).

    Treatment:

      1. The drug of choice is ethosuximide 20 to 30 mg/kg/day in two to three divided doses to maintain a blood level of 40 to 100 μg/mL.

      2. Valproic acid in doses of 10 to 30 mg/kg/day to maintain a therapeutic blood level of 50 to 100 μg/mL is also effective. Valproate is probably preferable as a single drug if generalized convulsions occur concomitantly with absences.

      3. Barbiturates and/or phenytoin may be necessary to control other associated seizure phenomena or generalized convulsions, but should not be used alone.

B. *Grand Mal Epilepsy*

    1. Onset is most frequent during childhood and adolescence.

    2. Seizures, usually tonic-clonic seizures, are bilaterally symmetric from the onset. Typically the patient loses consciousness and the body becomes rigid (tonic phase) followed by jerky movements (clonic phase) and postictal confusion or prolonged sleep.

    3. Interictal EEG may be normal in as many as one-third of patients.

    4. Mental retardation and psychiatric disturbances are *not* usually associated with this disorder.

    5. A family history of seizures is often elicited.

    6. Neurologic examination and CT scan of brain normal.

    Treatment:

    See comments concerning anticonvulsants later in this chapter.

Seizures of Focal Origin (Partial Epilepsy)

    1. Onset at any age.

    2. The features of these partial seizures depend on the site of the lesion, and site of the epileptogenic foci that result from the lesion, and the pattern of spread of the ictal discharge.

    3. Seizures of focal origin may produce simple symptomatology (eg, focal motor) or may lead to a complex picture (eg, complex partial) or result in a convulsion due to secondary generalization (here the aura is the clue to focal onset).

4. A localized ictal EEG discharge is present at seizure onset.

5. An abnormal interictal CT scan and neurologic examination is obtained in many cases.

6. Interictal EEG with localized spikes or spike-and-wave activity with possible abnormalities of background activity focally or regionally.

7. Variable response to antiepileptic drugs.

A. *Focal Motor Seizures*
Focal motor seizures manifest as clonic movements usually involving the arms or the legs. Sometimes the seizure may start in the thumb or the big toe and or spread to involve the more proximal parts (Jacksonian seizure). A new-onset focal seizure suggests a structural lesion.

B. *Complex Partial Seizures (Psychomotor or Temporal Lobe Seizures)*

1. Complex partial seizures consist of various automatisms -- complex, coordinated but purposeless motor movements (eg, lip smacking or walking in a circle) with a blank stare or stereotyped verbal responses; any repeated stereotyped behavior may be a complex partial seizure.

2. Preceded by auras (these may be only some type of difficult-to-describe feeling of strangeness); typical auras include the following:
   a. Déjà vu -- the feeling of having experienced an event previously.
   b. Abdominal or epigastric sensations (often a rising sensation).
   c. Unexplained sudden fear with an urge to run.
   d. Visual, auditory, or olfactory hallucinations, which are usually complex, vivid and unpleasant.

   Note: Unpleasant olfactory hallucinations (called uncinate auras) are commonly associated with brain tumor.

3. Seizures last about one minute with a postictal state of confusion, headache, and exhaustion. Combativeness and violent behavior may occur during this postictal confusional period (especially if well-meaning observers attempt to help or restrain the individual).

4. Seizures may generalize secondarily with loss of consciousness and tonic-clonic convulsive activity.

5. Most common form of seizures in adults.

6. Routine awake EEG shows abnormality in less than 50% of patients; optimal records (about 65% showing temporal lobe spike discharge) are obtained with nasopharyngeal leads (during natural sleep) performed after 24 hours of sleep deprivation. EEG-activating procedures and long-term monitoring further increase the yield of positive tracings.

7. Personality, behavior, and cognitive disorders frequently complicate the picture and may produce severe psychosocial disability.

8. Complex partial status epilepticus may present as a state of confusion or stupor. The EEG shows continuous 5 to 6 Hz high-voltage, rhythmic theta waves or temporal spikes.

Treatment:

See comments regarding anticonvulsants later in this chapter.

Late-Onset Epilepsy

Up to the age of 30 years or so, primary generalized epilepsies (previous section) may still present de novo. After that, however, seizures presenting for the *first time* are overwhelmingly due to either acute progressive or acquired static lesions of the brain. Acute lesions include meningitis, encephalitis, cortical contusions from head injury, arterial or venous infarction, or tumors. The acute disturbance may also be a functional, potentially reversible encephalopathy. These include hypoglycemia, hepatic or uremic encephalopathy, hypertensive encephalopathy, or withdrawal syndromes from drugs or alcohol.

Old static lesions are most commonly a result of head injury (posttraumatic epilepsy) or stroke (postinfarction epilepsy), rarely congenital hamartomas or mesial temporal sclerosis. Slowly progressive tumors may mimic old static lesions.

The most common seizure types are partial or focal seizures, which often generalize secondarily, and which usually result from lesions of the temporal lobe (complex partial seizures). Generalized convulsions begin focally and then spread to involve both sides of the body, rather than involving the body bilaterally and symmetrically from the onset.

Minimal studies in adults presenting with a first seizure should include EEG (preferably sleep-deprived) and CT scan of brain (with and without contrast enhancement). Cerebral angiography and CSF studies may be needed when vascular malformations or an infective etiology is suspected.

Therapy should be directed toward management of the underlying cause as well as symptomatic treatment of seizures.

General Comments on Anticonvulsants

1. The vast majority of patients should be treated with only *one* drug; once a particular drug *at therapeutic levels* clearly does not completely control the seizures, another drug should be added; as soon as this drug reaches therapeutic levels, the first drug should be gradually discontinued.

2. For grand mal epilepsy, partial epilepsy, and complex partial epilepsy, the drugs of choice are carbamazepine, phenytoin, primidone,

valproic acid, and phenobarbital (Table 11.3). Carbamazepine is effective when other drugs are not, but it must be taken in at least three daily divided doses, is expensive, has some initial side effects (such as ataxia and confusion), and (rarely) has been associated with aplastic anemia. Phenytoin is less expensive, can be taken once daily, has fewer initial side effects, but long-term use may result in cerebellar atrophy and decreased mental capacity. Phenobarbital also causes chronic psychomotor retardation.

3. Phenobarbital is contraindicated in hyperactive children (administration of this drug may make an uncomfortable situation unbearable).

4. Phenytoin produces hirsutism, gum hypertrophy, and coarse facies, and thus should be avoided in young girls.

5. Therapeutic drug levels must be obtained and the dose adjusted based on blood level determinations (see Table 11.2). Trough serum levels should be obtained when there is poor response to dosage regimen, intermittent illness, and when noncompliance is suspected.

6. Knowledge of the elementary clinical pharmacokinetics of the anticonvulsant drugs will make the physician a more skilled therapist. After beginning a maintenance dosage regimen, it takes about five half-lives

Table 11.3.
Drugs of Choice in Treatment of Epilepsy

Seizure Type	Drugs of Choice*
Grand mal, focal motor, complex partial	Carbamazepine Phenytoin, valproic acid Primidone Phenobarbital
Petit mal	Ethosuximide Valproic acid
Benign centrotemporal epilepsy	Phenytoin Carbamazepine Phenobarbital
Neonatal seizures	Phenobarbital
Febrile seizures	Phenobarbital Valproic acid
Infantile spasms, Lennox-Gastaut syndrome	ACTH Clonazepam

*Drugs are listed in order of preference

of the drug before steady state is reached. Therefore the first blood levels for monitoring purposes should not be taken before that time (see Table 11.2 for half-lives). Trough levels (blood drawn just before a scheduled dose, preferably the first morning dose) should be assessed if seizure control or compliance is in question. If toxicity is the concern, a peak level (blood drawn shortly after a scheduled dose) should be assessed. Drugs with long half-lives (phenobarbital and phenytoin) can be given once a day, making compliance easier. Drugs with short half-lives (carbamazepine, valproic acid) need to be given in divided doses daily.

7. Generic carbamazepines and phenytoins, made by different pharmaceutical companies, have different pharmacologic properties. Therefore switching from one brand of generic drug to another may radically alter anticonvulsant blood levels and precipitate seizures.

Phenytoin

1. The usual dosage is 5 to 7 mg/kg/day (up to about 400 mg/day).
2. Phenytoin should be administered in one to two divided doses daily, since the average serum half-life is 24 hours.
3. The usual therapeutic blood level 10 to 20 μg/mL, but it is preferable to keep the levels between 15 and 20 μg/mL.
4. Dose-related side effects are:

Blood Level(μg/mL)	Side Effect
1-10	Undertreatment
10-20	Therapeutic dose range (nystagmus in some patients)
20-30	Nystagmus
30-40	Diplopia, dysarthria, ataxia

5. Side effects that are *not* dose-related include gum hypertrophy, coarsening of features, and hirsutism in approximately 40% of patients, and exacerbation of acne. These side effects are especially noticeable in adolescents and may lead to noncompliance in females.
6. Phenytoin rarely may cause a delayed hypersensitivity reaction consisting of fever and pruritic mucocutaneous maculopapular rash with subsequent desquamation, which can be serious or fatal (Stevens-Johnson syndrome).
7. Long-term use may cause organic brain syndrome.
8. Oral dosage forms are 30 mg and 100 mg capsules and 50 mg chewable scored tablets.

   Note: Oral suspensions with concentrations of either 25 mg/mL or 6 mg/mL are available, but use of the oral suspension should be avoided since it provides uneven doses due to the difficulty in achieving uniform mixing of the suspension.

9. Phenytoin is not well absorbed in the neonatal and toddler age group and therefore should be avoided in such patients.

10. The parenteral dosage form is a solution of 50 mg/mL. The solution is highly alkaline and will precipitate if mixed with most other parenteral solutions. The solution should be injected, as much as possible, directly into the vein; saline may be used to flush the IV tubing. Intravenous injection of phenytoin must be at a slow rate (no more than 50 mg/min in adults; no more than 1 mg/kg/min in infants) to prevent cardiac arrhythmias.

> *Caution*: Intramuscular injection should *never* be used since the phenytoin precipitates in muscle, producing necrosis and sterile abscesses, along with unpredictable serum levels of the drug.

Carbamazepine

1. Effective in partial seizures, particularly complex partial seizures, and generalized seizures.

2. Related structurally to the tricyclic antidepressants, and often effective in ameliorating the behavioral and emotional disturbances that accompany some complex partial seizure disorders.

3. Has been known to produce bone marrow depression; all patients have a transient fall in white blood cell count on initiation to the drug. Since aplastic anemia is rare, some experts obtain blood studies only if the patient experiences excessive bleeding or infection.

4. Common initial side effects include ataxia, and clouding of consciousness.

5. The usual starting dose in adults is 200 mg tid (20-30 mg/kg/day in children).

6. Keep therapeutic level at 6 to 10 μg/mL.

7. Dosage forms available are 200 mg scored tablets, 100 mg scored chewable tablets, and a 20 mg/mL suspension.

Valproic Acid

1. Valproic acid is highly effective in absence seizures, both the typical and atypical varieties, and the various forms of myoclonic epilepsies. It is also useful in grand mal and in focal seizures when there is secondary generalization. It is the drug of choice when there is a combination or primary generalized convulsions and absences, myoclonus, of akinetic seizures.

2. Valproic acid is the only drug, besides phenobarbital, proved to be effective in prophylaxis of simple febrile seizures.

3. Relatively few side effects, though gastrointestinal upset is frequent in infants and toddlers.

4. Requires periodic monitoring with CBC and liver function tests for the rare occurrence of bone marrow or hepatic toxicity.

   Caution: Fatal hepatotoxicity has been reported in infants receiving multiple anticonvulsants including valproic acid.

5. Usual dose is 250 mg tid in school children (up to 30 mg/kg/day in younger children).

6. Blood levels should ordinarily be between 75 and 100 μg/mL although in some difficult cases, such as Lennox-Gastaut syndrome, blood levels may need to be kept between 100 and 150 μg/mL (as long as there is no toxicity).

7. Available as 250 mg capsules, as a syrup containing a concentration of 50 mg/mL, and in enteric-coated tablets containing 125 mg, 250 mg, or 500 mg.

Primidone

1. Primidone is effective for both generalized and complex partial seizures.

2. Since it is partially metabolized to phenobarbital, serum determinations for monitoring drug levels should specify both primidone and phenobarbital levels.

3. Since it is relatively short-acting, should be given in divided doses daily.

4. Children taking this drug may develop irritability and personality changes; therefore it is desirable to avoid its use in children if possible.

5. The usual starting dose in older adolescents or adults is 250 mg tid, but start lower if drowsiness ensues, titrating to toxicity if necessary.

6. Usual therapeutic blood level of primidone is 6 to 12 μg/mL.

7. Dosage forms available include 250 mg scored tablets, 50 mg scored tablets, and suspension containing 50 mg/mL.

Phenobarbital

1. The usual dosage 3 to 5 mg/kg/day (up to about 100-180 mg/day for adult males).

2. May be administered as a single daily dose, since the average serum half-life is about 100 hours.

3. Usual therapeutic blood level is said to be 15 to 30 μg/mL, but the levels aimed for should be 25 $\pm$ 5 μg/mL. Most patients will be drowsy when levels are over 40 μg/mL.

4. Will produce hyperactivity in many children, particularly if the child has a previous tendency to be hyperactive or is mentally retarded.

5. Can exacerbate depression (affective disorder) in susceptible individuals and may be used in overdosage in suicide attempts.

6. Of increasing concern is the issue of whether phenobarbital decreases school performance in children, even at therapeutic dosages.

7. Long-term use may cause mental slowing.

8. Rarely may cause a delayed hypersensitivity reaction consisting of fever and pruritic mucocutaneous maculopapular rash with subsequent desquamation, which can be serious or fatal (Stevens-Johnson syndrome).

9. Oral dosage form is tablets of 15 mg, 30 mg, 60 mg, or 100 mg and syrup of 4 mg/mL; in general, crushed tablets are preferred over the syrup in children, since accurate measurement of dose is difficult with the syrup, and its taste is not pleasing to most children.

Ethosuximide

1. Used when absences of the primary generalized type (petit mal epilepsy) are the sole kind of seizure.

2. Less effective when absences are accompanied by other kinds of phenomena (such as myoclonic seizures or primary generalized seizures). Usually not effective in complex partial absences.

3. Gastrointestinal upset is the most frequent initial side effect.

4. Needs periodic monitoring with CBC and liver function tests for possible bone marrow and hepatic toxicity.

5. Starting dose is usually 250 mg tid.

6. Keep therapeutic level between 50 and 100 μg/mL.

7. Dosage forms available are 250 mg capsules and a syrup containing 50 mg/mL.

Clonazepam

1. A diazepam derivative indicated primarily for myoclonic seizures.

2. Can be used as an adjunct in other primary generalized seizures, such as akinetic seizures.

3. Drowsiness is a frequent initial side effect, so begin with a low dose and build up slowly, using 0.5 mg tablets.

4. Be careful when using in combination with valproic acid: may result in absence status ("electrical status" or "spike-wave stupor").

5. Because of its antispasticity action, may make patient hypotonic.

6. Therapeutic blood levels are usually 0.02 to 0.05 μg/mL, but sedation may be the limiting factor in dosage.

7. Available as scored tablets of 0.5 mg, 1.0 mg, and 2.0 mg.

Initiating Anticonvulsants

When the diagnosis of epilepsy is established, anticonvulsant treatment should be instituted promptly. The appropriate anticonvulsant should be chosen based on the type of seizure (see Table 11.3).

1. Only *one* drug should be started at a time and given to its maximum therapeutic effect.

2. The medication should be initiated at about one half the suggested therapeutic dosage for 1 week. If no adverse side effects have appeared by that time and the patient has tolerated it well, the full therapeutic dosage should be given. Patients who experience adverse side effects from an excessive initial dose are likely to be poorly compliant in the future. Since it takes four or five half-lives to obtain a steady state, after approximately that elapsed time (see Table 11.2 for half-lives), obtain a serum anticonvulsant level.

3. The process of instituting anticonvulsant therapy is essentially a clinical titration. Serum levels are titrated against desired therapeutic effects (lessening or abolition of seizure), keeping in mind that undesirable side effects may limit attainment of the end point. The physician therefore needs accurate observations on the kinds, frequency, and duration of seizures from the patient. The physician can help the patient make these observations by requiring the patient to mail monthly progress reports, in which seizures are charted. The patient should be encouraged to write down a description of the seizure as soon as possible after its occurrence.

4. Monotherapy: Patients should be treated as far as possible with a single anticonvulsant drug to avoid drug interactions which may affect efficacy and toxicity. If a single drug is ineffective or only partially effective, a second drug should be added. Then five half-lives later, if the blood level is within the therapeutic range and the seizures are controlled, the first drug should be withdrawn by one dose every five half-lives.

Weaning from Anticonvulsants

When a patient should be weaned from anticonvulsants depends on the duration of the seizure-free period, seizure type, age of onset, and the presence or absence of EEG abnormalities.

Neonates

The best data regarding neonatal seizures indicate that if seizures have stopped with anticonvulsants, the drugs can be withdrawn at age 3 months. Whether seizures will recur later depends on the degree of cortical damage and underlying etiology for neonatal seizures. Severe CNS damage suggests high risk for developing the infantile spasms syndrome later in the first year of life.

Childhood and Adolescence

1. Recent data indicate that in childhood epilepsy (exclusive of neonatal seizures, infantile spasms, or the Lennox-Gastaut syndrome), if a 2 year seizure-free period is obtained, approximately 75% of children will remain seizure-free for at least a 2 to 3-year follow-up period.

2. The EEG is a good predictor; those with no slowing and no spikes are most likely to remain seizure-free. Those with both slowing and spikes are most likely to recur, while those with either slowing or spikes are intermediate in likelihood of recurrence.

3. The clinical variety of the seizure is also a factor for prognosis regarding recurrence of seizures following drug withdrawal. The primary generalized epilepsies and benign centrotemporal epilepsy probably have the best prognosis and are likely to be "outgrown" (successful weaning of anticonvulsants with no recurrence) in adolescence. This outcome occurs in approximately half of children with petit mal epilepsy by early adolescence, and most of the other half by the end of adolescence.

Late-Onset (Adult Onset) Epilepsy

If epilepsy is defined as at least two or more seizures recurring, it is unclear whether the 2-year seizure-free criterion, or any other criterion, is applicable in adult-onset epilepsies. It is likely that in the majority of these patients, lifelong prophylactic anticonvulsant therapy is a necessity. Even though the medical indications for continuing drugs after "good control" are hazy, many social factors conspire to adhere to anticonvulsants, such as the necessity not to have seizures in order to continue having an automobile driver's license, and the fear of losing jobs if the individual has seizure recurrences. Finally, many patients prefer to feel "safe" rather than "sorry" and do not want to risk the possibility of status epilepticus if seizures recur when off anticonvulsants.

When a decision is reached to withdraw anticonvulsants, one drug at a time should be withdrawn. Anticonvulsants should be withdrawn slowly, at a rate of no more than one dose every five half-lives.

Compliance

1. Simple is best. A complex schema of drug administration may be clinicopharmacologically optimal but will be difficult for a patient to follow. A minimal number of daily doses should be used; for phenobarbital, a single daily dose is often effective, and phenytoin can usually be given in no more than two daily doses (once daily may be adequate). Adverse side effects resulting from large initial doses will lead to poor compliance later.

2. The physician must encourage prescription renewal when at least 1 to

2 weeks supply remains so that the patient will not run out of medications.

3. The patient should be encouraged always to carry on his or her person an extra full day's supply of anticonvulsant in order not to be stranded without medication.

4. When traveling, the patient should carry a letter or card from the physician stating diagnosis and medications in order to obtain an emergency supply of medicines or treatment. This is particulary true when traveling in foreign countries, where strict drug enforcement laws may require confiscation of legitimate anticonvulsant medication if it is not identified and justified.

5. Compliance can be assessed with the aid of blood anticonvulsant levels.

6. *First impressions count*: The first several months after the diagnosis is made are the most important in establishing a pattern of patient compliance in both medication and follow-up treatment. *Physician availability* is important. When patients first begin taking anticonvulsants, compliance can be fostered by the physician being available for telephone calls, or short, more frequent visits (every 3 to 6 weeks) to allay the patient's fears about side or toxic effects, what to do if a seizure occurs, and generally to demystify epilepsy.

7. Appropriate patient, parent, and sibling education is necessary to insure compliance. Generally, the more a patient knows about epilepsy, and the more responsibility he or she takes for the management of this disorder, the more likely compliance will occur (see following paragraphs on Patient Education).

Patient Education

1. When a patient receives the diagnosis of ''seizure disorder'' or ''epilepsy,'' there is usually initial denial, followed by anger and perhaps depression, before final acceptance. Therefore, the patient and physician should discuss the diagnosis in terms the patient can understand. No information should be released to employers or outside agencies without the patient's consent.

2. Automobile driver's license: The patient should be seizure-free for a period of time determined by law, which varies from state to state, with usually a minimum of 12 months. *With the patient's permission*, the physician may send a letter to the state bureau of motor vehicles, but only the state can decide when the individual will be allowed to drive.

3. School

   a. If seizures are frequent, a telephone discussion or a personal meeting between the physician and teacher or school nurse is helpful.

   b. The Epilepsy Foundation of America provides information useful for both the patient and family in dealing with the community and school and will sponsor in-service training for teachers and school officials on how to manage individuals with seizures.

c. If seizures are rare, it is not necessary to inform the school.

d. Learning disabilities and behavior problems can also occur in patients with seizures. These can relate to the seizures, the medications, or may coexist independently.

e. The physician must encourage vocational planning for patients with frequent seizures *early* in high school or even in junior high school.

4. Employment

a. If seizures are rare, it may not be necessary to inform the employer. Unfortunately, discrimination against individuals with seizures still occurs.

b. State agencies (generally in divisions of vocational rehabilitation) may be helpful in assisting the individual with seizures in finding employment or minimizing discrimination.

c. Individuals with seizures should be encouraged to avoid occupations in which a seizure would be hazardous to himself or fellow workers.

5. Alcoholic beverages

a. Consumption of alcoholic beverages in moderation will rarely increase the incidence of seizures, but alcohol and anticonvulsants have additive effects, usually resulting in lowered alcohol tolerance.

b. An alcoholic with seizures who continues to consume alcoholic beverages should probably not be given anticonvulsants, since compliance is often poor and seizures from medication withdrawal alone may occur. Drinking must stop before anticonvulsant prophylaxis can be effective.

6. Other drugs: Reassure patients that they do not become addicted to anticonvulsant drugs. Warn about drug interactions (see Table 11.4), although most commonly used over-the-counter medications, such as aspirin, have no significant drug interactions. Warn that drug abuse, with "speed," "uppers," or "downers" will result in significant drug interactions and probably exacerbate the epilepsy.

7. Birth control pills: Although it is commonly believed that seizures are exacerbated by oral contraceptives, in reality this is unpredictable in any single patient. Other methods of birth control are available if seizures are exacerbated. Generally, the higher-progesterone lower-estrogen containing oral contraceptives are less likely to exacerbate seizures.

8. Pregnancy: The risks of teratogenic effects of anticonvulsants on the fetus must be weighed against the risk of seizures occurring during pregnancy, with attendant effects on the pregnancy. Cleft lip, cleft palate, congenital heart defects, spinal dysraphism and mental retardation have been reported to result in babies born of mothers taking anticonvulsants dur-

Table 11.4.
Antiepileptic Drug Interactions

Drug	Serum Level Increased by	Serum Level Decreased by
Phenytoin	Chloramphenicol Disulfiram Isoniazid Dicumarol Salicylates Ethosuximide	Carbamazepine
Carbamazepine	Erythromycin	Phenytoin Phenobarbital Primidone
Valproic acid		Carbamazepine
Phenobarbital	Valproic acid Phenytoin	
Primidone	Valproic acid	Phenytoin

ing pregnancy. If at all possible, attempts should be made to keep mothers off anticonvulsants at least in the first trimester of the pregnancy. The usual problem clinically, however, is that the mother has already been pregnant for 6 to 8 weeks when the diagnosis of pregnancy has been made, and if there are teratogenic effects, the damage has already been done. There is a risk for a bleeding tendency in babies born of mothers taking phenytoin. Giving vitamin K orally to the mother in the last month of pregnancy prevents this.

9. Genetics: The primary generalized epilepsies (petit mal and grand mal) are the most hereditary of the epilepsies. The risk of a child having epilepsy when one parent has either petit mal or grand mal is estimated to be as high as 12%. The genetics of the primary partial epilepsies is unclear. Although the secondary partial epilepsies, simple or complex, are due to acquired lesions, whether these be demonstrable or not, there is some relationship to previous family history of epilepsy. Patients with severe head injury, for example, are more likely to develop posttraumatic epilepsy if there is a previous family history of epilepsy; however, it is not possible to predict the likelihood of epilepsy developing in offspring of parents, one of whom has an acquired partial epilepsy.

10. Safety: Anticonvulsants should always be stored in locked cabinets to prevent the possibility of theft or accidental ingestion by children.

11. Dentists and dental hygiene: Reassure dentists that there is no great danger of exacerbating seizures in the dentist's chair by giving local anesthetics

and that there is no great danger of anesthetics interacting with anti-convulsant drugs. Do instruct patients receiving phenytoin to visit their dentist at least twice a year and to brush their teeth at least twice daily. In addition, they should floss their teeth at least once daily.

12. Surgical operations: Phenobarbital and phenytoin can be given paren-terally at equivalent doses during preoperative and postoperative phases when the patient is NPO. Phenytoin should *not* be given IM, since it is poorly absorbed through that route. Because the period of NPO fol-lowing surgery is usually not more than 24 hours, parenteral admini-stration of other anticonvulsants is not necessary.

13. Physical limitations: Patients should be allowed to participate in phys-ical and recreational activities that maintain physical fitness. Perhaps the only activities that require some limitation are swimming (where the cau-tion of never swimming alone should be scrupulously observed) and con-tact sports, such as American football and ice hockey, in which serious injury could be sustained should a seizure occur on the field or rink (al-though there is wide room for individual physician judgment here).

14. Resources

   a. For information regarding services to epileptics, low-cost prescrip-tion services, and group life insurance, as well as general programs, the patient should contact the Epilepsy Foundation of America, 4351 Garden City Drive, Suite 406, Landover, MD 20785 (telephone: 301-459-3700 or 800-332-1000).

   b. Some reading materials that can be suggested for the individual with seizures include:

      Lagos JC: *Seizures, Epilepsy and Your Child*, New York, Harper & Row, 1974.

      Middleton AH, Altwed A, Walsh G: *Epilepsy*, Boston, Little Brown & Co, 1981.

      Svoboda WB: *Learning About Epilepsy*, Baltimore, University Park Press, 1979.

      Wright GN: *Epilepsy Rehabilitation*, Boston, Little Brown & Co, 1975.

Treatment of Convulsive Status Epilepticus (see also Chapter 20)

Convulsive status epilepticus is the state of continual seizures, or more com-monly, recurrent seizures in which the patient does not fully regain conscious-ness between seizures. Status epilepticus most commonly occurs in known epileptics who stop medication. Rarely, status epilepticus is the first presenta-tion of a seizure disorder, CNS infection (abscess or cerebral meningitis), meta-bolic disorders (hypoglycemia, hyponatremia, or hypocalcemia), or cerebrovascular disease (acute infantile hemiplegia).

1. *Do not panic*. The patient should be treated promptly, but carefully.

2. Establish an adequate airway:

   a. Remove false teeth.

   b. Turn patient or head to one side in order that secretions can drain out of the mouth.

   c. Extend neck (see Figure 11.1).

   d. Loosen tight clothing.

   e. Suction mouth as necessary.

   f. Place a padded object between teeth if the mouth is open (*do not force an object into a tonic, clenched jaw*).

   g. Oxygen is not necessary immediately, as long as the airway is adequate.

3. Insert needle into vein and draw syringe of blood for glucose, electrolytes, calcium determinations; through the same needle instill 50% glucose 1 to 2 mL/kg (50 mL in the adult) and then begin continuous IV-infusion with a 5% dextrose in water solution. Add thiamine 100 mg to the IV bottle.

4. Initially give diazepam 1 mg every 30 seconds up to a dose of 0.3 mg/kg (maximum dose 10 mg) or lorazepam 0.5 mg every 30 seconds up to a total dose of 0.1 mg/kg (maximum dose 8 mg). **THE PHYSICIAN MUST BE PREPARED TO SUPPORT RESPIRATION WITH AN**

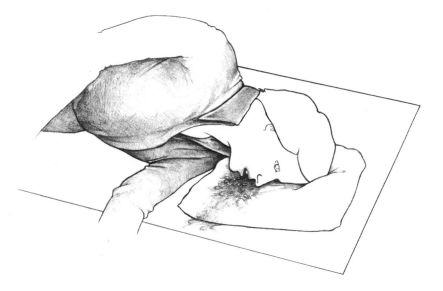

Figure 11.1. Positioning the patient in convulsive status epilepticus.

AMBU BAG, SINCE BRIEF RESPIRATORY ARREST MAY OCCUR AFTER BENZODIAZEPINE (DIAZEPAM OR LORAZEPAM) ADMINISTRATION. IF UNABLE OR UNPREPARED TO PROVIDE RESPIRATORY SUPPORT, DO NOT GIVE A BENZODIAZEPINE.

5. After diazepam or lorazepam administration, whether or not seizures stop, or if a benzodiazepine is not administered, administer phenytoin 20 mg/kg, up to 1000 mg. For proper IV injection of phenytoin see above section on phenytoin.

6. If seizures do not stop within 15 to 20 minutes after administration of phenytoin (the drug takes about ten minutes to reach a sufficient level in the brain to stop seizures), administer phenobarbital IV at a dose of 20 mg/kg. **AT THIS POINT THE PATIENT SHOULD BE INTUBATED.**

7. Continued seizures despite the previous medications are usually the result of a metabolic disturbance (such as hyponatremia or hypocalcemia) or a serious intracranial lesion (such as abscess or meningoencephalitis), and the seizures will not stop until the underlying disorder is treated. General anesthesia, such as pentobarbital coma, is a last resort and should be administered by an anesthesiologist under EEG monitoring.

8. Maintenance doses of the anticonvulsants should be started immediately and administered *intravenously* until oral doses can be started (NEVER INTRAMUSCULARLY). These are:

   a. Phenytoin 5 to 7 mg/kg/day (300-400 mg/day in adults) IV divided q6h, or

   b. Phenobarbital 3 to 5 mg/kg/day (120 mg/day in adults) IV q6h.

Treatment of Nonconvulsive Status Epilepticus

Seizures other than generalized convulsions can occur continuously, and although not life-threatening (because they do not derange respiratory function), they are disabling and must be recognized and treated.

1. *Absence status*: Absence seizures occur either continuously or with only a few seconds break between seizures. The patient appears dazed, blank, or confused, and may intermittently answer questions, usually slowly and irrelevantly. The EEG shows continual 3 Hz spike-and-wave complexes.

2. *Psychomotor (complex partial) status*: The patient may appear similar to the patient with absence status, except that there may be automatisms continuously. The EEG concomitant is continual 5 to 6 Hz theta waves.

3. These are *not* medical emergencies. However IV diazepam or lorazepam should immediately stop the seizures and confirm the diagnosis.

The loading dose of the appropriate long-term anticonvulsant should then be started.

BIBLIOGRAPHY

Aicardi J: *Epilepsy in Children.* New York, Raven Press, 1986.

Browne PR, Feldman RG: *Epilepsy Diagnosis and Management.* Boston, Little, Brown & Co, 1983.

Callahan N, Garrett A, Goggin T: Withdrawal of anticonvulsant drugs in patients free of seizures for two years. *N Engl J Med* 1988; 318:942-946.

Camfield PR, Camfield CS: Neonatal seizures: a commentary on selected aspects. *J Child Neurol* 1987; 2:244-251.

Dalessio DJ: Seizure disorders and pregnancy. *N Engl J Med* 1985; 312:559-563.

Delgado-Escueta AV, Wasterlain C, Treiman DM, et al: Current concepts in neurology: management of status epilepticus. *N Engl J Med* 1982; 306:1337-1340. [*Note:* There is an error in Table 1, procedure 4, line 4 of this article; it should corrrectly read: "An endotracheal tube should *now* be inserted."]

Dreifuss FE (ed): *Pediatric Epileptology. Classification and Management of Seizures in the Child.* Boston, John Wright-PSG, 1983.

Ferry P, Banner W Jr, Wolf R: *Seizure Disorders in Children.* Philadelphia, JB Lippincott Co, 1985.

Gastaut H, Zifkin BG: Classification of the epilepsies. *J Clin Neurophysiol* 1985; 2:313-326.

Green RC, Adler JR, Erba G: Epilepsy surgery in children. *J Child Neurol* 1988;3:155-166.

Kundt RS, Bickley SK, Shimp LA: Discontinuing antiepileptic therapy. *Am Fam Physician* 1985; 31(4):177-184.

Lee SK: Nonconvulsive status epilepticus. *Arch Neurol* 1985; 42:778-781.

Nelson K, Ellenberg JH: *Febrile Seizures.* New York, Raven Press, 1981.

Ogunyemi AO, Dreifuss FE: Syndromes of epilepsy in childhood and adolescence. *J Child Neurol* 1988;3:214-224.

Ojemann LM, Ojemann GA: Treatment of epilepsy. *Am Fam Physician* 1984; 30(2):113-128.

Porter RJ: *Epilepsy: 100 Elementary Principles.* Philadelphia, WB Saunders Co, 1984.

Rothner AD: Intractable seizure disorders of childhood. *Cleve Clin Q* 1984; 51:505-510.

Schomer DL: Partial epilepsy. *N Engl J Med* 1983; 309:536-539.

Shinnar S, Vining EP, Mellits ED, et al: Discontinuing antiepileptic medication in children with epilepsy after two years without seizures: A prospective study. *N Engl J Med* 1985; 313:976-980.

Wallace SJ: *The Child with Febrile Seizures.* London, John Wright, 1988.

Woody RC, Brodie M, Hampton DK, Fisher RH Jr: Corn oil ketogenic diet for children with intractable seizures. *J Child Neurol* 1988; 3:21-24.

XII

THE STROKE SYNDROME

A stroke is a sudden attack. In neurologic terms, it is a sudden focal deficit due to a central nervous system abnormality. Note that the term does *not* specifically imply cerebrovascular disease, atherosclerosis, hemorrhage, or any other etiology. It is true that the most common underlying cause is cerebrovascular disorder, but a significant number of stroke patients have curable or remediable causes such as subdural hematoma, tumor, seizures, postictal paralysis. For this reason, thorough evaluation is mandatory in nearly all patients. The task that faces the physician is as follows:

1. To localize the lesion by neurologic examination (cerebral hemispheres, brainstem, cerebellum)

2. To order the least invasive procedures most likely to reveal the cause of the lesion

3. To decide, on the basis of available knowledge, the best course of treatment

4. To provide supportive care while in the hospital

5. To initiate a program of rehabilitation

By casual inspection, even before taking a history, the physician can gain a general idea of the location of the lesion.

1. *Cerebral hemispheres*: Paralysis involves the contralateral face, arm, and leg. If the arm is more involved than the leg, suspect a lesion in the distribution of the middle cerebral artery. If arm and leg are equally involved, suspect a deep hemisphere lesion. If the leg is more severely

involved than the arm, suspect an anterior cerebral territory lesion. Aphasia and/or seizures suggest a hemispheric cortical lesion.

2. *Posterior fossa* (midbrain, pons, medulla, cerebellum) abnormalities are *crossed*, eg, ipsilateral paralysis of face or eye with paralysis of the opposite side of the body. Consciousness is often impaired. Speech is often slurred but not aphasic.

3. *Spinal cord*: Both legs are usually involved, bladder problems are common, and a sensory level exists.

The history taking should be guided by the physician's knowledge of the causes of stroke. The following anatomical classification may be helpful.

An Approach to Identifying the Cause of a Stroke

1. *Intravascular Causes*

   The physician must consider disease processes that result in hypercoagulable or hyperviscous states which increase the probability of infarction by thrombosis, while hypocoagulable states increase the probability of hemorrhage. Possible diagnostic considerations include leukemia, polycythemia, coagulation disorders, sickle cell anemia, and hemoconcentration from severe dehydration. Increased arterial pressure from hypertension increases the probability of hemorrhage.

2. *Causes Related to Blood Vessel Walls*

   These include congenital and mycotic aneurysms, infectious causes such as meningovascular syphilis, inflammatory disorders such as collagen vascular diseases, venous thromboses, and cranial arteritides. Cerebrovascular atherosclerotic disease may result in stroke syndrome either by arterial thromboses or embolism from an ulcerated plaque. Inflammatory diseases may also affect veins and cause venous thrombosis.

3. *Problems Related to the Great Vessels of the Neck*

   Disease of the great vessels of the neck (specifically the carotid arteries) may be surgically correctable. Included are stenosis of the carotid arteries and the subclavian steal syndrome. These are suspected when carotid bruits are heard in the neck but they can only be accurately diagnosed by four-vessel cerebral angiography. Palpation of carotid pulsation is an unreliable index of carotid artery stenosis or occlusion.

4. *Causes Related to the Heart*

   Patients with cerebral atherosclerosis often also have coronary artery disease. The frequency of heart disease (such as myocardial infarction or arrhythmias) in stroke patients is 2 to 3 times that of the age-adjusted general population without stroke. In other circumstances, such as bacterial endocarditis or postmyocardial infarction mural thrombus, there is a direct cause-and-effect between heart disease and stroke. Chronic or recurrent atrial fibrillation has been identified as a major risk factor for stroke. All patients with stroke syndrome need a thorough cardiac evaluation, which minimally would include an ECG, but may be extended to include rhythm monitoring procedures and echocardiography. Patients with transient ischemic attacks (TIAs) followed for 5 years die as often of heart disease as of stroke.

5. *Mass Lesions*

The neurologic deficits from mass lesions such as subdural hematoma or tumor are usually gradually progressive. Edema around a tumor or bleeding into a tumor from erosion of a blood vessel wall can make the clinical picture appear to be of sudden onset. Viral infections such as *Herpes simplex* encephalitis may present as a stroke syndrome.

6. *Hypotension*

In orthostatic or postural hypotension, a fall in systemic blood pressure may result in a focal neurologic deficit. Such deficits are usually transient, although in a patient with compromised cerebral circulation the deficit may become permanent. Recognition of hypotension as a contributory cause of cerebral injury is particularly important in the rehabilitation of the patient.

Caution: Prior to allowing a stroke victim to sit in a chair or ambulate, postural hypotension must be ruled out by measuring blood pressure in the lying, sitting, and standing position.

7. *Other causes*

Metabolic disorders such as hypoglycemia, hypoxia, and liver or renal disease can cause a preexisting subclinical cerebral deficit to become evident as a focal neurologic abnormality. It is important to emphasize the metabolic causes of stroke syndrome, since prompt intervention may reverse the clinical deficit. It is for this reason that, immediately following the onset of a stroke syndrome, the patient should have studies performed to assess blood sugar, liver and renal function, and arterial blood gases. Following focal seizures, paralysis may persist for 24 or more hours.

History

The history may be helpful in determining the etiology of the stroke syndrome. It is frequently important to corroborate the patient's story with a family member or a witness. In some cases, such as in comatose patients or patients with aphasia, family members may be the only source of history.

1. *Onset*

    a. Abrupt onset followed by gradual improvement suggests embolus ("While I was washing dishes, my right arm suddenly became paralyzed and I dropped a cup").

b. Acute onset with progression to maximal deficit over minutes to hours suggests thrombosis.

c. Stepwise development or onset during sleep usually suggests thrombosis.

d. Focal neurologic symptoms usually lasting minutes but no longer than 24 hours suggest a transient ischemic attack (TIA). Some of these TIAs represent small areas of damage that rapidly recover rather than true transient ischemia.

   Caution: The diagnosis of TIA is retrospective, made with certainty only after a thorough evaluation. Some TIAs may represent small areas of damage with rapid functional recovery rather than transient ischemia. Migraine, seizures, hypoglycemia, and cardiac arrhythmias may also present as TIAs.

e. Onset associated with headache or alterations of consciousness suggests intracerebral hemorrhage.

2. *Course*: In progressing stroke the patient displays increasing deficits during evaluation, and the differential diagnosis includes mass lesion and metabolic or infectious encephalopathy. In completed stroke the symptoms have stabilized and may improve.

   a. Rapid improvement suggests cerebral embolism.

   b. Gradual improvement over a day to a few weeks suggests thrombosis.

   c. Rapid deterioration over a period of several hours suggests intracerebral hemorrhage.

3. Questions should be directed to the following symptoms:

   a. Alteration of consciousness

   b. Headache

   c. Visual disturbances (*amaurosis fugax* -- monocular blindness of short duration -- usually indicates carotid artery disease with embolism to the ophthalmic artery, which is the first branch of the internal carotid artery) (see Figure 12.1)

   d. Disturbance of equilibrium (common in posterior fossa disorders)

   e. Motor or sensory disturbances

   f. Precipitating factors and risk factors:
      i. Hypertension
      ii. Atherosclerotic cardiovascular disease in patient or family members
      iii. Elevated low density lipoproteins
      iv. Cigarette smoking
      v. Obesity
      vi. Oral contraceptive use

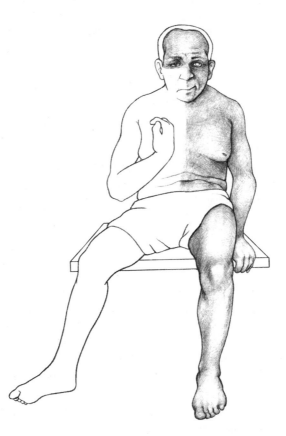

Figure 12.1. The combination of monocular blindness associated with contralateral hemiparesis strongly suggests carotid artery disease -- often medically or surgically treatable.

      vii. Age and sex -- middle-aged men and elderly individuals of both sexes are at higher risk

4. *Past medical history*: Especially of cardiovascular disease, hypertension, diabetes, head trauma, or recent infection.
5. *Family history*: Atherosclerotic cardiovascular disease or cerebral aneurysm.

Examination

In addition to the "routine" examination, the following are especially important:

1. Check for fever or stiff neck (often associated with intracranial hemorrhage or infections).

2. If possible, take the blood pressure in both arms, in lying and standing position (subclavian steal, postural hypotension).

3. Record level of consciousness using the Glasgow Coma Scale (see Chapter 13).

4. Check heart for arrhythmias, murmurs, and enlargement, and lungs for congestion and friction rubs.

5. Check all peripheral pulses (a mural thrombus may fragment and occlude arteries of the limbs).

6. Evaluate carotid artery blood flow by listening for carotid bruits. The classic bruit of carotid stenosis is harsh, systolic, emanates from the carotid bifurcation, and radiates to the angle of the jaw. A bruit on the same side as the brain lesion is especially important. Diminished carotid pulse is of no value because a completely occluded carotid may pulsate normally (pulsations are transmitted directly from the aorta). A bruit over the supraclavicular fossa suggests a stenosis of the vertebral or subclavian arteries. Observe, palpate, and compare the temporal, nasal, and supraorbital artery pulses; these branches of the external carotid artery are significant vessels used for collateral circulation to the brain following internal carotid occlusion (see Figure 12.2).

7. Examine optic fundi for:

   a. Early signs of papilledema (loss of venous pulsations and wet-appearing retina) indicating subarachnoid hemorrhage or mass lesion.

   b. Retinal infarction or cholesterol embolus (a small, bright yellow fragment in an artery) suggesting carotid artery ulceration.

8. Examine for signs of subacute bacterial endocarditis (SBE) such as petechial conjunctival hemorrhages or hemorrhages beneath the fingernails.

Laboratory Evaluation

The following laboratory studies are available in all hospitals and should be performed in every patient:

1. An ECG should be done immediately. Over one-third of stroke victims will show ECG abnormalities at some time during the first 24 hours.

2. Chest x-ray.

3. Complete blood count and platelet count.

4. Erythrocyte sedimentation rate (an elevated ESR may be related to infection or autoimmune process such as a temporal arteritis or lupus erythematosus).

5. Urinalysis (red cells in urine suggest emboli to the kidney as well as to the brain).

6. Blood glucose (before IV infusion is started).

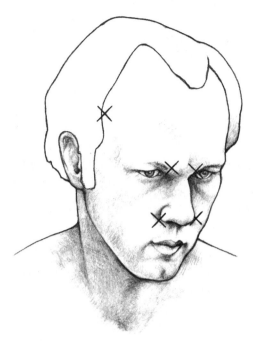

Figure 12.2. Palpation of temporal, nasal, and supraorbital pulses (*X* marks) may provide evidence of collateral circulation following a carotid occlusion.

7. Prothrombin time (PT or protime) and partial thromboplastin time (PTT).

8. Liver function and renal function tests such as determination of SGOT, alkaline phosphatase, BUN, and creatinine values.

9. Arterial blood gases if respiratory compromise is suspected.

10. Serologic test for syphilis (the vasculitis associated with syphilis is a treatable cause of the stroke syndrome).

11. If a myocardial infarction is suspected, appropriate serum enzymes should be drawn.

The following studies should be contemplated in every stroke victim. The decision as to whether they actually will be done or not will depend on availability and economics.

1. *CT (computed tomographic) scan:*

    a. A CT scan, ideally, should be done on every stroke victim *as soon as possible*. If the deficit is secondary to hemorrhage, this will immediately be apparent (and such patients should NOT be anticoagulated, even with low-dose aspirin or heparin). If the scan is normal or shows an infarct, the physician must immediately consider evaluation of the cerebral vasculature.

b. The CT scan findings must correlate with the patient's neurologic examination; patients may have old or clinically silent infarcts which are irrelevant to the acute situation. Obviously, the CT scan will identify most mass lesions. The physician with no access to a CT scan is indeed handicapped and should treat the patient with supportive measures only.

Caution: Never order a CT scan with contrast before knowing the patient's BUN and creatinine values, since contrast infusion in the patient with marginal renal function may precipitate acute renal failure.

2. *Four-vessel cerebral angiography via femoral catheter*: If the CT scan reveals a subarachnoid hemorrhage, this procedure is mandatory to identify an aneurysm or arteriovenous malformation. This test gives maximal information about the cerebral vasculature. This is also the procedure of choice if carotid endarterectomy is to be performed, since most vascular or neurosurgeons will not operate on the basis of Doppler studies or digital vascular angiography alone. The procedure should be ordered with caution, because it is associated with occasional morbidity and mortality. Ideally, it should be performed by an experienced radiologist trained in neuroradiology. Direct-puncture carotid angiography is almost never performed in the modern era.

3. *Digital vascular (subtraction) angiography*: This procedure avoids puncturing the femoral artery, but uses large amounts of contrast media. It is utilized primarily for identifying stenoses of the carotid artery, but it often misses carotid ulcerations.

4. *Doppler studies or other ultrasound studies of the carotid artery*: This type of study is safe and noninvasive. It is most useful for identifying carotid stenoses, but it often misses carotid ulcerations, and it gives no information about the intracerebral vasculature.

5. *Electroencephalography (EEG)*: This study is most useful in patients suspected of having a seizure disorder associated with their stroke or in identifying an underlying toxic-metabolic disorder. It is useful in confirming a diagnosis of a superficial hemispheric lesion.

6. *Magnetic resonance imaging (MRI)* is not essential for most stroke victims, but useful in providing more information about lesions already seen on CT scan and in diagnosing white matter lesions presenting as stroke (eg, multiple sclerosis) and lesions in the posterior fossa.

7. *Lumbar puncture*: Immediate lumbar puncture is indicated:

a. In suspected cases of CNS infection without evidence of increased intracranial pressure.

b. When a CT scan is not available and anticoagulants are anticipated; bloody or xanthochromic CSF would be a contraindication to anticoagulation. Normal lumbar puncture (often found with ischemic infarcts) decreases the probability that the deficit is caused by intracranial hemorrhage, tumor, or subdural hematoma.

Remember: If an infarct is present, cerebral edema will occur in 24 to 48 hours. This edema causes increased intracranial pressure and increases the risk of lumbar puncture.

8. *Skull radiographs*: Order only if a skull fracture is suspected or a CT scan is not available. The CT scan has largely replaced the skull radiograph.

9. *Radionuclide scan, pneumoencephalogram*: These are rarely performed in the modern era. Occasionally, a radionuclide scan is used to provide more information about a stroke due to *Herpes simplex* encephalitis.

Now That I've Made a Diagnosis, What Do I Do?

1. *Mass lesion*: Aneurysms, subdural hematomas, tumors, and abscesses should be referred to a neurosurgeon.

2. *Lacunar infarct*: The patient has a small infarct in the white matter and hypertension; these patients rarely need four-vessel angiography; treat hypertension and reduce the risk factors. Aspirin or anticoagulation therapy are not necessary.

3. *Carotid ulceration*: Patient may present with blindness in one eye and/or contralateral hemiparesis or have a cholesterol embolus in retina; the CT scan may be normal or show an infarct in the distribution of the middle cerebral artery. Treat with aspirin 325 mg/day. If attacks continue, consider carotid endarterectomy.

4. *Cardiac embolus*: Patient may have atrial fibrillation or mural thrombus; no hemorrhage is seen on the CT scan: Treat immediately with heparin, then later switch to warfarin sodium (Coumadin). Continue therapy for at least 6 months.

5. *Carotid stenosis*: The patient may have 80% stenosis of the internal carotid artery and symptoms on the opposite side of the body. Surgical treatment (endarterectomy) is controversial and is currently undergoing re-evaluation. The outcome depends in part on the experience and skill of the surgeon. The risk of endarterectomy in some communities is greater than the risk of conservative therapy and in such situations use warfarin sodium or aspirin 325 mg/day.

6. *Middle cerebral artery occlusion or arterial occlusion in the posterior fossa*: Extracranial-intracranial bypass operations have been shown to be of no value; treat with warfarin sodium or aspirin 325 mg/day.

7. *Seizure or migraine*: Treat specifically (see Chapter 11 or Chapter 3).

8. *Venous thromboses* are usually secondary to infection or to an underlying hypercoagulable state. Treat with antibiotics and anticoagulation.

9. *Carotid stenosis and no symptoms:* Endarterectomy is not recommended unless some other major surgical procedure is contemplated. Treat with aspirin 325 mg/day.

10. *Toxic-metabolic disorders* (eg, hypoglycemia or blood dyscrasia): Treat specifically.

Supportive Therapy for Stroke Victims

1. *Nursing orders to monitor neurologic status:* At least during the first 4 hours, the patient should be evaluated hourly. In addition to the Glasgow Coma Scale (see Chapter 13) and monitoring of blood pressure, pulse, temperature (rectal), and respirations, the nursing staff should be taught to evaluate pupillary size, equality, and reaction to light.

2. *Nursing management:* The following precautions may be beneficial:

    a. Above-knee elastic stockings may minimize the development of thrombophlebitis.

    b. Use dorsiflexion splints or a footboard and sandbags to maintain the foot of the paralyzed leg in dorsiflexion.

    c. Roll towels or other soft objects in the hand to maintain the hand in a position of function.

    d. The physician must be aware of and apprise the nursing staff of hemianopia and hemineglect and position the patient appropiately to accommodate these phenomena.

    e. Frequent turning of the patient prevents bedsores.

    f. If the patient cannot close the eyelids, instillation of artificial tears may prevent corneal ulcers.

    g. In the patient with diplopia, alternate patching of the eyes improves vision and is more comfortable.

    h. In the alert patient with difficult speech, a communication board with common requests may be helpful.

    i. Stool softeners should be instituted early to prevent fecal impaction.

    j. In the first few days after paralysis, the patient should be placed in an upright or sitting position intermittently to prevent development of postural hypotension.

    k. A simple explanation of the problem will relieve family anxiety. Especially in the case of the aphasic patient, explain to the family that speech difficulty is not associated with feeblemindedness.

3. *Blood pressure management:* Most stroke victims will have transient hypertension. A diastolic blood pressure of less than 120 torr is not cause for immediate concern. If the blood pressure is to be lowered, do so

gingerly over a time period of several days. A moderately elevated blood pressure may be the body's protective mechanism to insure adequate cerebral perfusion (even in hemorrhage, vasospasm is common).

4. *Nutritional Support*
   a. IV fluids should contain multivitamins (especially thiamine) to prevent Wernicke's encephalopathy.
   b. Syndrome of inappropriate antidiuretic hormone (SIADH) may occur with stroke; thus the patient should be kept on the "dry" side to treat both this and cerebral edema. Recording of fluid intake and output is important.
   c. Nitrogen and electrolyte balance is best accomplished with nasogastric feedings. The patient should receive nutrition via this route (rather than IV) as soon as possible.

5. *Bladder care*: Urinary retention in the acute phase is common, but an indwelling catheter should be used judiciously. If an indwelling catheter is used, intermittent clamping should be done to avoid loss of bladder tone. Bladder function returns more quickly in patients who have had intermittent catheterization. Patients with indwelling catheters tend to have severe urinary tract infections and bladder dysfunction due to chronic scarring.

6. *Pulmonary care*: Frequent suctioning of excess secretions, frequent turning, induced coughing, and deep breathing will help prevent atelectasis. Oxygen should be administered only when oxygen pressure is low.

7. *Cardiac care*: Because there is such a high correlation between cerebral infarction and cardiac abnormalities, continuous cardiac monitoring should, if possible, be instituted.

8. *Physical therapy*: Patients who remain bedridden for any length of time are at risk for developing serious complications such as pulmonary embolism or orthostatic hypotension. With the exception of patients with subarachnoid hemorrhage, stroke victims who are encouraged to sit or stand as soon as possible improve more rapidly and have fewer complications. If the patient is bedridden for any length of time, passive physical therapy may reduce the risk of pulmonary embolism. Physical therapy is also important in preventing contractures, since significant contractures may develop in the shoulder girdle rapidly.

9. *Anticoagulation*: Anticoagulation should be instituted only after establishing that the stroke syndrome was not the result of hemorrhage and that there is no gross bleeding into the area of infarction. Heparin and warfarin sodium are used for cardiac emboli and stenotic lesions; aspirin is used for platelet emboli (carotid ulceration).

a. In the acute phase, heparin is given IV by continuous infusion, preferably using an infusion pump. The effects of heparin must be monitored by frequent determinations of the activated partial thromboplastin time (PTT), which should be maintained at 1.5 to 2.5 times the normal value.

b. A coumarin compound such as warfarin sodium (Coumadin) may be of value for a period of 6 months or more in those individuals who have carotid stenosis or emboli from the heart. This drug reduces the hepatic production of vitamin K-dependent blood clotting factors (factors II, VII, IX, and X). Oral dosage should be individualized to maintain the prothrombin time (PT) at 20 to 25 seconds (twice normal). Initially, one dose of 20 to 60 mg is given followed by maintenance at a dosage of 2 to 10 mg daily. The prothrombin time must be determined at least once per week while the patient is receiving warfarin sodium. Once warfarin sodium is started, it probably cannot be stopped without a rebound increased risk of thrombosis. Therapy is complicated by the risk of major hemorrhage.

c. Aspirin, one tablet (325 mg) per day, inhibits platelet aggregation. Complications include gastric erosion from the aspirin (less likely if buffered) and hemorrhage after surgical procedures.

10. *Speech and language therapy*: If communication is disturbed by the stroke, speech and language therapy may be helpful. The language pathologist specifically evaluates auditory processing and retention, reading and writing abilities, and speaking abilities. From this evaluation, a treatment program is designed, utilizing the patient's strengths to improve weakness. The therapist identifies the specific problems in communication, consults with the physician and hospital staff, and counsels and advises the family members. The speech therapist assists the physician in educating the family regarding difficulties, such as those of aphasic patients, and works with the family and patient on a home program. Thorough explanation of the patient's communication difficulties to the family alleviates embarrassment stemming from misunderstanding. The patient should be encouraged to participate in social situations as much as possible. Follow-up treatment is usually arranged to reevaluate and update. Speech therapists may note minor changes in speech patterns, which may be subtle signs of recurring disease.

11. *Occupational therapy*: In the rehabilitation of stroke patients, the aims of occupational therapy overlaps speech and physical therapy with strong emphasis on functional skills for the activities of daily living. In cooperation with physical therapy, occupational therapy includes improving or maintaining the range of motion, strength, coordination, and balance

and reduction of spasticity. Therapists provide splints to prevent contracture, and slings to prevent subluxation of the shoulder. Evaluation and training is available for patients with perceptual dysfunctions. In conjunction with speech therapy, occupational therapists improve coordination for speech and fine coordination for writing. Special attention is given to retraining or assistance in the activities of daily living, such as dressing and feeding. Adaptive equipment is provided, and patients are taught how to use it most effectively.

12. *The rehabilitation hospital*: There is increasing pressure on the physician to discharge patients from the acute care hospital as soon as possible. Rehabilitation hospitals offer an environment where physical therapists, speech therapists, occupational therapists, and physicians specializing in physical medicine and rehabilitation work as a team to help the patient reach maximal functional capacity. A stroke victim will continue to improve for approximately 6 months. This alternative should be considered if the patient is moderately to severely disabled and rehabilitation efforts cannot be accomplished on an outpatient basis.

13. Educational materials and other information for patients and families may be obtained from the National Stroke Association, 300 East Hampden, Suite 240, Englewood, CO 80110-2622 (telephone: 303-762-9922).

Some Controversies Regarding Stroke

1. *Use of cerebral vasodilators*: At one time inhaled carbon dioxide was administered in the acute phase. This practice probably made the patient worse, since the undamaged vessels would dilate and shunt blood away from damaged areas which desperately need more oxygen and glucose.

2. *Treatment of cerebral edema*

    a. 48 hours after infarction, cerebral edema may develop and the patient will deteriorate. Steroids probably have little effect on this type of edema (as opposed to the dramatic effect on edema surrounding a tumor). If used, dexamethasone is recommended, 4 to 20 mg q4h. The steroid should be rapidly tapered and continued for no longer than seven to ten days.

    b. Keeping the patient moderately dehydrated by restricting IV fluids is probably most effective. As an adjunct to this, mannitol (in a 10%-20% solution), at a dose of 1 g/kg in extreme cases will aid in this dehydration. Daily weighting of the patient and monitoring of electrolytes is mandatory with this type of therapy.

3. *Surgical intervention for pathology of extracranial vessels*: A massive literature has developed regarding carotid endarterectomy and still no definitive advice can be given. The essential question is this: Do the risks of surgery outweigh the risks of medical treatment? The decision is an

individual one. It depends on the severity of the patient's symptoms and the skill of the surgeon. Both neurosurgeons and vascular surgeons perform this procedure; the choice depends on the training and skill of the surgeon, not his specialty.

4. *Transient ischemic attacks (TIAs)*

   a. *All temporary neurologic deficits should be evaluated.* A TIA is a neurologic deficit which lasts less than 24 hours. The most common cause is platelet emboli from an arterial ulceration in an older patient, but small emboli from the heart, collagen vascular disease, lacunar infarcts from hypertension, partial seizures, hemiplegic migraines, and small hemorrhages into a tumor may also cause transient deficits. Thus, a TIA may in reality involve the death of brain tissue and indeed not be transient ischemia at all.

   b. If the TIA is secondary to cerebrovascular atherosclerosis, 25% to 40% of these patients will have a stroke if followed for 5 years. Certainly, as a minimum, TIA patients should take a single aspirin tablet (325 mg) daily, and in selected cases the physician should consider warfarin sodium or surgical intervention. Therapeutic considerations are the same as those discussed earlier in this chapter.

Aphasia

Aphasia is considered in this chapter because it so commonly occurs in stroke victims, but it must be remembered that aphasia is a *symptom* (like a hemiparesis) and can occur in any disease process that injures the perisylvian dominant hemisphere. It is defined as an acquired disorder of language, and in the absence of other obvious neurologic symptoms, it can easily be confused with dementia and psychiatric disorders.

Aphasia is a disturbance of *language* only and must be differentiated from the myriad disorders of *speech*. For example, a patient with cerebellar dysfunction may have a loss of speech melody with an explosive irregular type of vocalization; a patient with vocal cord or tongue paralysis will have a normal speech cadence but a marked change in clarity and/or tone; and a patient with bilateral upper motor neuron lesions will have slow arduous speech. None of these patients would have any difficulty thinking of words or expressing thoughts appropriately. In addition, schizophrenic patients on occasion may have a senseless word salad in which there is apparently no connection between one word and the next; speech melody is normal, and when listened to closely, the patient's thought processes will fit into the patient's own private code. Aphasia is a disturbance of language only, whereas dementia is a disturbance of all cognitive processes including language.

It must be stressed that the diagnosis of aphasia should not be a casual diagnosis, but requires the physician to examine the patient specifically for an

Table 12.1.
Simplified Summary of Language Problems in Aphasia

	Type of Aphasia			
	Broca's	Wernicke's	Global	Anomic
Fluency	0	+	0	+
Comprehension	+	0	0	+
Naming	+	0	0	0

aphasic syndrome. In general, the physician should be able to differentiate four basic types of aphasic phenomena (see Table 12.1):

1. The patient understands language well but produces little spontaneous speech (*nonfluent* or *Broca's* aphasia).
2. The patient is unable to understand language, but produces voluminous verbalization with meaningless content (*fluent* or *Wernicke's* aphasia).
3. The patient with nonfluent speech and poor comprehension (*global* aphasia).
4. The patient who has good verbal output (fluent), good understanding of language, difficulty with word finding in spontaneous speech, and difficulty naming objects (*anomic* aphasia).

A. Nonfluent patient who understands well (commonly referred to as a motor aphasia, anterior aphasia, nonfluent aphasia, expressive aphasia, or *Broca's aphasia*):

1. In right-handed individuals, this is almost always associated with damage to the left frontal cortex and is usually associated with some degree of paralysis of the right side of the body.
2. The patient is aware of the speech difficulty and often becomes extremely frustrated and angry; secondary depression may frequently complicate the clinical picture.
3. Speech is effortful and ungrammatic with short telegraphic phrases poorly articulated. Speech melody and rhythm are abnormal and perseveration (repeating the same word) is common.
4. Auditory comprehension is well preserved, and the patient can follow most directions.
5. In the severe form, the patient may only be able to utter automatic speech such as obscenities and social amenities ("hello"). In the milder form or during recovery, more complicated automatic speech may be observed, such as singing "Happy Birthday" or reciting the Lord's Prayer.

6. Reading silently for meaning is relatively preserved but slow; reading aloud is impaired, and writing is large, messy, and effortful, paralleling the verbal expression.

Caveat: The diagnosis of aphasia cannot be made if the patient has absolutely no speech production.

B. Patient does not understand well, but has a voluminous verbal production (commonly called sensory aphasia, *Wernicke's aphasia*, posterior aphasia, receptive aphasia):

1. In right-handed persons, damage is almost always confined to the left posterior-superior temporal area. This aphasia is usually not associated with a paralysis, although some patients may have a homonymous right visual field defect.

2. In its pure form, the patient is unaware of the difficulty; usually the patient is pleasant and jovial but may become angry with the examiner's inability to understand his speech.

3. Speech rhythm and melody are normal, but the content is incomprehensible (true in all languages; eg, the aphasic German appears to be speaking German and the aphasic Frenchman appears to be speaking French, but the language is incomprehensible).

4. In mild form or during recovery, paraphasias are common; for example, "Resident pea gun staked on the telegram." = "President Reagan talked on the television." Speech with frequent paraphasias is also called jargon speech.

5. Patient has very poor auditory comprehension but may respond to whole-body commands such as "stand up," "walk backward," or "open your mouth."

6. Both reading aloud and reading silently for comprehension are defective; writing is well formed, but contains the same errors and lack of meaning as the verbal expression.

C. Patient who has nonfluent speech and poor comprehension (commonly called *global aphasia*):

1. As ordinarily used, global aphasia refers to the patient who has both frontal lobe and temporoparietal lobe damage; this is basically a combination of the fluent and nonfluent aphasias involving all aspects of language.

2. The patient is awake and alert but for the most part sits silently and is unresponsive.

3. Global aphasia is almost always associated with right hemiparesis in the right-handed patients; there is often a right homonymous hemianopia.

D. Patient with good verbal output and sound understanding, but word finding and naming difficulties (*anomic aphasia*):

Anomic Aphasia

1. In right-handed individuals this is usually due to a lesion of the left angular gyrus (at the junction of the parietal, occipital, and temporal lobes).

2. Speech is fluent, but may be hesitant because of word-finding difficulties (usually nouns).

3. As in fluent or Wernicke's aphasia, paraphasias (sound or word substitutions) are common in spontaneous speech.

4. Because of the word-finding difficulties, this syndrome is often confused with nonfluent or Broca's aphasia but can be differentiated from it because the anomic aphasic has fluent, nondysarthric, effortless speech, and in the pure form there is no accompanying hemiparesis.

5. Verbal comprehension is intact.

6. When presented with objects, the patient misnames them (often with paraphasic errors) or cannot produce the name, although the patient will select the correct name when given a multiple choice format.

7. Often accompanied by Gerstmann's syndrome (right-left disorientation, finger agnosia, acalculia, agraphia).

The aphasic syndromes can be more discretely defined and subcategorized, but familiarity with and identification of these four basic types by the physician will describe most aphasic patients.

Treatment:

1. Specific language therapy may accelerate a patient's recovery. Treatment should also be directed at the underlying lesion.

2. Rehabilitation of the patient with aphasia is necessary. For patients with intact understanding, it is important to find mechanisms to assist the patient with communication. The speech and language therapist may be of help in this regard. Simple signboards, letter boards, and other signaling devices are sometimes helpful, but new advances in computer technology in some areas have superseded these devices. The family must be educated to the patient's expressive difficulties and provide a nonstressful environment for the patient's expression. Appropriate reading materials and/or talking books should be provided for the patient. In the patient with abnormal understanding, supervised care may be necessary.

BIBLIOGRAPHY

Brodal A: Self-observations and neuro-anatomical considerations after a stroke. *Brain* 1973;96:675-694.

Chyatte D, Sundt TM: Cerebral vasospasm after subarachnoid hemorrhage. *Mayo Clin Proc* 1984;59:498-505.

EC/IC Bypass Study Group: Failure of extracranial intracranial arterial bypass to reduce the risk of ischemic stroke. *N Engl J Med* 1985;313:1191-1200.

Easton JD, Sherman DE: Carotid endarterectomy. *Mayo Clin Proc* 1983; 58:205-207.

Hurwitz BJ, Heyman A, Wilkinson WE, et al: Comparison of amaurosis fugax and transient cerebral ischemia: a prospective clinical and arteriographic study. *Ann Neurol* 1985; 18:698-704.

Kistler JP, Ropper AH, Heros RC: Therapy of ischemic cerebral vascular disease due to atherothrombosis. *N Engl J Med* 1984;311:27-34.

Ropper AH, et al: Carotid bruit and the risk of stroke in elective surgery. *N Engl J Med* 1982;307:1388-1390.

Sherokman BJ, Hallenbeck JM: Management of acute stroke. *Am Fam Physician* 1985;31:190-199.

Till JS, Toole JF, Howard VJ: Management of carotid artery plaques, murmurs, and transient ischemic attacks. *Arch Neurol* 1985;42:1198-1201.

XIII

THE COMATOSE PATIENT

Coma is a medical emergency. The purposes of this chapter are to:

1. Outline immediate measures to care for the comatose patient.
2. Establish criteria for deciding whether coma is secondary to a toxic-metabolic disorder (80% are) or a structural CNS disorder.
3. Provide guidelines for the management of coma secondary to a CNS disorder.

Immediate Measures

1. Establish and maintain a clear airway. In many cases this requires insertion of an endotracheal tube with ventilatory assistance.
2. Check pulse, blood pressure, and temperature. Apply ECG monitor. If profound hypotension is present, or if there are gross cardiac abnormalities, the cause of coma is evident and should be treated appropriately.
3. Insert an IV line and draw blood for glucose, electrolytes (Na, K, Cl, CO_2, Ca), CBC, BUN, and creatinine determinations. Arterial blood gases, toxic screening, and thyroid and liver function tests are often also drawn at this time.
4. Administer IV 50 mL of 50% glucose and 500 mg thiamine. Many authorities also suggest administration of naloxone hydrochloride (Narcan) 2 mg, especially if the patient has small pupils; however, if the patient does not respond to a total dose of 10 mg, the diagnosis of narcotic overdose is unlikely.
5. Catheterize the patient's bladder and monitor urinary output.

6. Determine the depth of coma:

   a. The Glasgow Coma Scale (Table 13.1) is commonly used to quantitate the severity of coma; it can be repeated at intervals to monitor the clinical course and effect of therapy.

   Note: This scale is especially useful in determining the prognosis in coma from head injuries and cardiorespiratory arrest. Thus 87% of patients who have a coma score of 4 or less at 24 hours after a head injury die or remain in a vegetative state. Of those with a score greater than 11, 87% show good recovery with mild to moderate disability.

   b. To evaluate the patient's response to noxious stimuli press the styloid processes (see Figure 13.1). This is an extremely painful stimulus that should be performed with caution; however, it is preferable to rubbing the sternum, twisting the nipples, or squeezing the testicles, which give less information, may leave unsightly marks that the family later questions, and are downright uncivilized. Note the type of response (arousal, decerebrate posturing, decorticate posturing, asymmetric response).

TABLE 13.1
GLASGOW COMA SCALE

(Add together to compute the total)

Eyes Open	
Never	1
To pain	2
To verbal stimuli	3
Spontaneously	4

Best Verbal Response	
No response	1
Incomprehensible sounds	2
Inappropriate words	3
Disoriented and converses	4
Oriented and converses	5

Best Motor Response	
No response	1
Extension (decerebrate rigidity)	2
Flexion abnormal (decorticate rigidity)	3
Flexion withdrawal	4
Localizes pain	5
Obeys	6

TOTAL SCORE	3-15

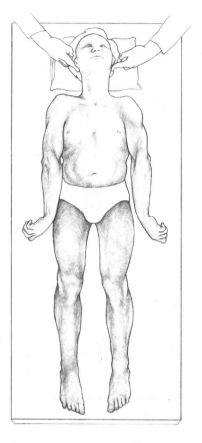

Figure 13-1 The examiner is applying pressure on the styloid processes in the comatose patient and producing decerebrate posturing. This posture is seen in patients with brainstem dysfunction.

    c. *Confused* patients respond to verbal stimuli, but are drowsy, slow, and often disoriented.
    d. *Stuporous* patients respond transiently only to vigorous stimuli.
    e. *Comatose* patients are unarousable and unresponsive, but may exhibit abnormal postures.

Examination of the Comatose Patient

Table 13.2 lists the mandatory examinations, which can be completed in a few minutes, and which allow the physician to make a tentative decision as to whether the coma is due to a toxic-metabolic cause or to a CNS lesion. Wasting time obtaining a CT scan on a patient dying from a metabolic disorder is inappropriate.

TABLE 13.2
Differentiation of CNS Lesion from Metabolic Coma

EXAMINATION	SUGGESTIVE OF STRUCTURAL CNS COMA	SUGGESTIVE OF METABOLIC COMA
Blood pressure	Increased	Decreased
Respiration	Ataxic	Regular or rhythmic
Temperature	Increased	Normal or decreased
Pupils	Asymmetric	Normal, usually reactive, even when brainstem function is suppressed
Oculocephalic and oculovestibular responses	Asymmetric or absent	Usually intact
Posture	Asymmetric	Symmetric
Fundi	Papilledema	Usually normal
Reflexes	Asymmetric	Symmetric
Neck suppleness	Stiff or normal	Normal
Myoclonus	Rare	Frequent

CNS Versus Metabolic Coma

This examination may reveal the following types of information:

1. *Blood pressure and pulse*: If the blood pressure is high and the pulse is low, severe increased intracranial pressure should be suspected. This finding is much more common in children than it is in adults. Most metabolic causes of coma cause hypotension.

2. *Breathing patterns* that may be seen in coma are:
   a. Normal respiration.

Inspiration

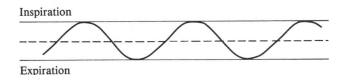

Expiration

b. Central neurogenic hyperventilation -- sustained, regular, rapid, deep hyperpnea (overbreathing); seen in midbrain lesions.

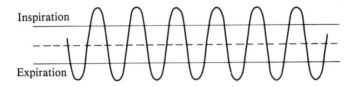

Inspiration

Expiration

c. Hypoventilation -- respiratory depression seen both with medullary lesion or in drug overdose.

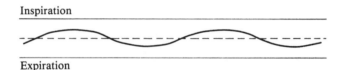

Inspiration

Expiration

d. Cheyne-Stokes respiration -- periodic smooth increase and decrease in respirations from apnea to hyperpnea; occurs both in bilateral lesions deep in the cerebral hemispheres and in metabolic coma.

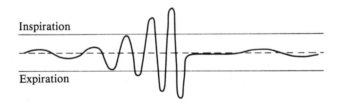

Inspiration

Expiration

e. Ataxic respiration -- completely irregular pattern due to a low brain-stem lesion, but may also occur in severe meningitis, cerebellar or pontine hemorrhage, direct medullary infarction, or trauma.

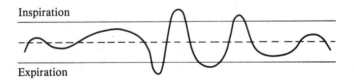

Inspiration

Expiration

Caution: Use of sedatives in a patient with ataxic breathing may cause respiratory arrest.

3. *Temperature*: A significantly elevated temperature in the presence of an altered state of consciousness strongly suggests CNS infection. Unless signs of imminent cerebral herniation or gross papilledema are present, the CSF must be examined and cultured before antibiotics are started. Subarachnoid hemorrhage may give a mildly elevated temperature, heat stroke a markedly increased temperature.

4. *Pupils*:
   a. Metabolic coma: Symmetric pupils that react to light suggest a metabolic disorder. Bilaterally fixed and dilated pupils are found in anoxia and in glutethimide, scopolamine, and atropine poisoning. Pinpoint pupils may occur in narcotic overdose but dilate and become reactive with a small dose of a narcotic antagonist.
   b. CNS coma is suggested by asymmetric pupils.

   Caution: Asymmetric pupils are occasionally seen in metabolic coma if there has been previous eye surgery or trauma.

5. *Oculocephalic response (doll's eye movement)* and *oculovestibular (caloric) test*:

   Caution: Do not perform in a patient with trauma.

   a. *Oculocephalic response*: Holding the patient's eyelids open, passively rotate the head rapidly to both sides. In the comatose patient, the eyes remain as if fixed on an object in the foreground (see Figure 13.2). Awake patients have no oculocephalic response. A unilateral response suggests a brainstem lesion. Presence of a normal doll's eye response in both directions indicates that the brainstem between cranial nerve III and cranial nerve VIII is intact, and this suggests that the cause of coma is not destruction of the brainstem. Absence of the response suggests a metabolic depression of the brainstem or severe brainstem dysfunction.
   b. *Caloric test*: If the doll's eye response is equivocal or if there is some reason the neck should not be rotated (as in head trauma or cervical spine injury), caloric testing (oculovestibular reflex) may provide the same type of information. Check to see that the tympanic membrane is intact and that the external auditory canal is not blocked by wax or blood. Slowly inject at least 10 mL of ice water through a small polyethylene catheter into the external auditory canal. The head should be elevated or flexed to approximately 30 degrees. In patients with suspected cervical spine fracture, instead of bending the neck, the head of the bed should be elevated. Deviation of the eyes toward the ear being stimulated suggests an intact brainstem and a metabolic cause of the coma (see Figure 13.3).

6. *Pressure on the styloid process*:
   a. Decerebrate posture (see Figure 13.1): This posture is character-

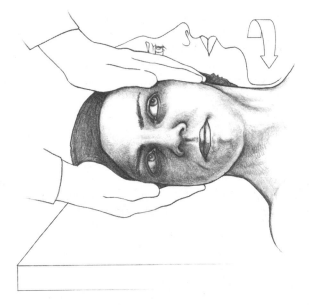

Figure 13-2 Doll's eye movements. The eyes remain relatively stationary when the head is rapidly turned to one side.

ized by extended and internally rotated arms and extended legs with plantar flexion of the feet. Asymmetric posturing (eg, one side moves, the other does not; or one side is decerebrate, the other decorticate) suggests structural CNS coma. Symmetric posturing is seen in brainstem and metabolic coma.

b. Decorticate posture (see Figure 13.4). This posture is characterized by flexion of the upper extremities, extension of the legs, and plantar flexion of the feet. Asymmetric posturing suggests structural CNS coma; symmetric posturing is seen in bilateral hemisphere lesions.

7. *Fundoscopy*: Look for early signs of papilledema including loss of venous pulsations, enlargement of veins, a wet appearing retina, and blurring of margins of optic discs. This may be seen in both CNS mass lesions and in metabolic disturbances causing cerebral edema.

8. *Reflexes*: Asymmetric reflexes suggest structural CNS coma; symmetric reflexes and bilateral Babinski reflexes are seen in both CNS and metabolic disturbances. Suggested techniques for eliciting the patellar and Achilles reflexes are shown in Figures 13.5 and 13.6.

9. *Neck suppleness*: A stiff neck suggests subarachnoid hemorrhage or infection.

Caution: The neck should not be manipulated in the case of head trauma in which there is a possibility of cervical spine fracture.

10. *Myoclonus*: This is manifested as uncoordinated generalized twitches and is more often seen in metabolic coma. Asterixis with flap tremor is another common finding in metabolic encephalopathy.

Note: Rarely, patients with metabolic coma may show focal CNS abnormalities. Asymmetric pupils may be congenital or a result of trauma. Fixed, pinpoint pupils may be secondary to treatment of glaucoma.

History of the Comatose Patient

The history, when obtainable, often eliminates the need for a number of diagnostic tests and points to a specific cause of the coma. The history may sometimes be obtained from relatives, friends, a family physician, or the police. It should include the following:

1. Onset: Abrupt onset indicates intracranial hemorrhage or infarction; gradual onset suggests a toxic or metabolic cause.
2. Preceding neurologic complaints: convulsions, confusion, hallucinations, headache, diplopia, vertigo, numbness, weakness, ataxia.
3. Recent trauma is suggestive of structural damage.
4. Past medical history: psychiatric disturbances, diabetes, heart disease, hypertension, renal disease, epilepsy, alcoholism.
5. Drug history: Both prescribed and illicit drugs are important.
6. Social history: Pay particular attention to any traumatic event that might be linked to depression and suicide attempt.

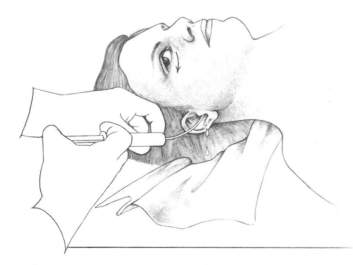

Figure 13-3 Caloric test. In a patient with intact brainstem (cranial nerves III through VIII), cold water in the auditory canal will cause the eyes to deviate toward the cold ear.

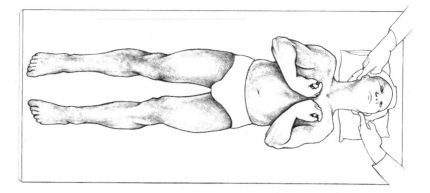

Figure 13-4 Decorticate posturing seen in patients with bilateral hemisphere dysfunction. This may be spontaneous or produced by painful stimulus.

Structural CNS Lesions Causing Coma

Hemispheric Lesions

A *unilateral* cerebral hemisphere lesion does not produce coma unless the lesion for some reason (eg, edema) causes damage to the other hemisphere as well. For coma to occur secondary to a CNS lesion either both hemispheres must be severely damaged or the reticular activating system in the brainstem must be damaged directly or indirectly because of a shift (usually laterally) in the hemispheres. When both hemispheres are involved, the neurologic ex-

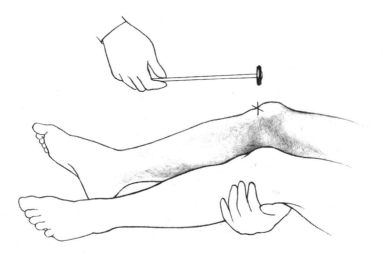

Figure 13-5 Patellar reflex testing in a comatose patient. Place arm under the knees so that they are slightly flexed as illustrated; pay close attention to asymmetries.

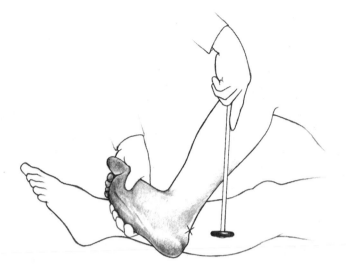

Figure 13-6 Achilles reflex. Cross legs as illustrated and slightly dorsiflex the foot before tapping the Achilles tendon.

amination almost always shows asymmetries; in this situation the CT scan should readily lead the physician to the correct diagnosis (massive intracerebral hemorrhage, subdural hematoma large enough to cause herniation, multiple infarcts from emboli, unilateral edema causing shifts in intracerebral contents).

Cerebral Herniation

The cerebral falx and the tentorium of the cerebellum are relatively rigid structures, which separate the cranial contents into three major compartments. Displacement of brain tissue by mass lesions (blood, edema, tumor) from one compartment to another is termed herniation (see Figure 13.7). The process is ominous because blood vessels may be compressed, causing additional damage by ischemia. Secondary hemorrhages in the brainstem are also common.

1. Herniation of a mass in the temporal lobe.
   a. Stretching of the third cranial nerve causes ipsilateral pupillary dilation.
   b. Pressure on the frontal lobe causes contralateral hemiplegia.
   c. As the process progresses, the cerebral peduncle is pressed against the sharp edge of the tentorium of the cerebellum, causing a severe ipsilateral paralysis.
2. Herniation of basal parts of both hemispheres through the incisura of the tentorium of the cerebellum (central herniation). The clinical picture is not particularly distinctive.

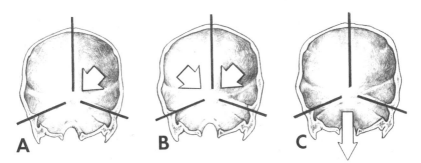

Figure 13-7 Herniation: A. Beneath the cerebral falx. B. Through the incisura of the tentorium of the cerebellum. C. Through the foramen magnum.

    a. Early: progressive loss of consciousness, small but reactive pupils, Cheyne-Stokes respirations, bilateral motor signs with decorticate posturing

    b. Late: central hyperventilation, hyperthermia, pupils unreactive to light and in midposition, loss of oculovestibular reflexes, decerebrate posturing

Treatment:

Herniation may temporarily be halted or reversed by the following agents:

  1. Mannitol 1 g/kg up to 50 g in a 25% solution IV administered over 20 minutes.

  2. Dexamethasone 0.3 mg/kg IV up to 12 mg IV followed by 0.06 mg/kg up to 6 mg q4h.

Posterior Fossa Mass (Cerebellar Hematoma, Posterior Fossa Subdural Hematoma, Rapidly Expanding Posterior Fossa Tumor)

  1. Subacute onset of symptoms

  2. Usually a past history of hypertension or occipital trauma

    Note: Cerebellar hematomas are a complication of chronic hypertension; symptoms are rapidly accelerating hypertension, headache, weakness, and confusion.

  3. Rapid progression of symptoms and signs, which may include the following:

    a. Early — occipital headache, repeated vomiting, dizziness, confusion, marked "malignant" hypertension

    b. Midstage — inability to stand or walk, bilateral extensor plantar responses, urinary incontinence, dysarthria, tonic deviation of eyes away from the side of the lesion, miosis, irregular respirations

    c. Late — coma, absent doll's eye responses and caloric responses, respiratory failure, flaccid limbs with diminished deep tendon reflexes

Caution: Lumbar puncture in the presence of a posterior fossa mass carries an especially high risk of cerebellar herniation and death.

Treatment:

This is a neurosurgical emergency. Immediate surgical decompression can be lifesaving. A definitive diagnosis is best established by CT scan; four-vessel cerebral angiography may be confirmatory, but is usually unnecessary.

Brainstem Infarction

1. Acute onset of symptoms with coma and other findings maximal at onset.
2. Often preceded by transient episodes consisting of diplopia, vertigo, dysarthria, dysphagia, motor weakness, and episodic loss of consciousness.
3. Respiratory disturbance prominent from onset (periodic breathing, central hyperventilation, or ataxic breathing).
4. Variable abnormality of pupils, which often are small and react sluggishly to light in a pontine lesion.
5. Dysconjugate position of the eyes or dysconjugate eye movements (seen in doll's eye or caloric tests) which suggest lesions of cranial nerves III, IV, or VI; absent or asymmetric doll's eye or caloric tests; facial paralysis is noted by asymmetric movement of the cheek during respirations.
6. Quadriparesis with extensor plantar responses (Babinski reflexes) and decerebrate posturing is often present. Cranial nerve abnormalities on one side with paralysis on the opposite side strongly suggest a brainstem lesion.

Treatment: Evaluation and treatment is discussed in Chapter 12.

Caution: Certain patients with upper pontine lesions may develop the locked-in syndrome (also referred to as pseudocoma or deafferented state) and have "a mind...clogged by a body rendered utterly incapable of obeying its impulses." Such an individual is awake but is unable to communicate except with eye movement ("a corpse with living eyes") such as the character M Noirtier de Villefort in *The Count of Monte Cristo*. These patients may be very much aware of their surroundings, and therefore the physician must be cautious in making comments in the presence of the patient. The locked-in syndrome must be distinguished from the persistent neurovegetative state (imprecisely referred to as coma vigil or akinetic mutism) in which the patient appears awake (and may even have a normal awake EEG) but is unable to communicate in any form (thought to be due to a high midbrain lesion).

Summary of Treatment of Patients with Coma Secondary to a CNS Lesion

1. Assure oxygenation with endotracheal suctioning, a cuffed endotracheal

tube, and assisted ventilation with oxygen.

2. Maintain the circulation by replacing blood volume losses, administering vasoconstrictors, and maintaining cardiac rhythm.

3. Insure adequate levels of blood glucose (the major substrate for brain metabolism) by administering 25 g of glucose IV in a 50% solution initially and by frequently monitoring blood glucose levels.

4. Lower intracranial pressure (optimally the intracranial pressure should be determined by direct measurement with a "bolt" installed by a neurosurgeon, but it is often treated based on clinical judgment alone).

   a. Hyperventilate to lower the carbon dioxide pressure to 25 to 30 torr (thereby decreasing cerebral blood flow).
   b. Mannitol 50 g in a 20% solution is given IV over ten to 30 minutes.
   c. Dexamethasone 10 mg IV, repeated with 4 to 6 mg q6h.
   d. If cerebral ventricular enlargement is evident on CT scan due to obstruction of CSF pathways, ventricular drainage may be lifesaving.

   Caveat: Hyperventilation should probably not be performed in patients with ischemia as a cause of coma. Mannitol is temporarily effective but may have a rebound. Steroids are most effective for edema due to brain tumors, but onset of action requires several hours. Steroids have a minor effect on edema secondary to ischemia. Thus the importance of combining the history, the neurological examinations, and the CT scan to obtain as accurate a diagnosis as possible.

5. Treat seizures, if present (see Chapter 11).

6. Treat infection, if present. A patient with fever, stiff neck, and coma should have an lumbar puncture *immediately*, even if a CT scan is not available. The risk from herniation in this situation is much less than the adverse effect of failure to identify the etiology of the meningitis, but the physician should be prepared to administer therapy to lower the intracranial pressure (see above).

7. Treat respiratory and metabolic alkalosis and acidosis; abnormalities may further depress respirations or worsen cardiovascular abnormalities.

8. Treat hyperthermia. An elevated body temperature may kill an already damaged brain and, if high enough, kill a normal brain. A cooling blanket is preferred.

Metabolic Coma

Approximately 80% of comas are caused by toxic-metabolic abnormalities; common causes include anoxia (cardiac arrest, pulmonary insufficiency), overdose (barbiturates or other sedatives, alcohol), diabetes (insulin overdose, ketoacidosis), uremia, hepatic failure, heat stroke, and meningitis.

Psychogenic Coma

Even astute physicians are sometimes fooled by a physiologically awake patient who does not respond to the environment and thus appears comatose. The following tests may be of value in confirming psychogenic coma:

1. The pupils and deep tendon reflexes are normal.

2. Caloric tests: 10 mL of cold water causes *nystagmus with the fast component away* from the irrigated side (in a truly comatose patient, the eyes will simply deviate toward the irrigated side).

3. Doll's eye movement: These are absent in an awake patient. Patients with absent doll's eye movement due to a brainstem infarct usually have other, obvious signs.

4. Hold the patient's hand over his face and drop it; the hand will hit the face of the comatose patient, but deviates to the side in an alert patient. (See Figure 9.3.)

5. Press the styloid processes; this very painful stimulus will arouse most noncomatose patients.

BIBLIOGRAPHY

Brooks DN, Hosie J, Bond MR, et al: Cognitive sequelae of severe head injury in relation to the Glasgow outcome scale. *J Neurol Neurosurg Psychiatry* 1986; 49:549-553.

Fitzgerald FT, Tierney LM, Wall SD: The comatose patient: A systematic diagnostic approach for you to follow. *Postgrad Med* 1983; 74:207-215.

Fraser CL, Arieff AI: Hepatic encephalopathy. *N Engl J Med* 1985; 313:865-873.

Levy DE, Caronna JJ, Singer BH, et al: Predicting the outcome from hypoxic-ischemic coma. *JAMA* 1985; 253:1420-1426.

Plum F, Posner J: *The Diagnosis of Stupor and Coma*, ed. 3. Philadelphia, F.A. Davis Co, 1980.

Posner JB: The comatose patient. *JAMA* 1975; 233:1313-1314.

Ropper AH: Lateral displacement of the brain and level of consciousness in patients with acute hemispheral mass. *N Engl J Med* 1986; 314:953-958.

Ropper AH, Kennedy SK, Zervas N: *Neurobiological and Neurosurgical Intensive Care*. Baltimore, Univrsity Park Press, 1983.

Silver JK: *The Comatose Patient*, videotape, Chicago, Division of Marketing and Meeting Services, American Medical Association.

XIV

INFECTIONS OF THE CENTRAL NERVOUS SYSTEM

Most infections of the central nervous system are life-threatening, the exception being the so-called aseptic or viral meningoencephalitis. Immediate diagnosis and treatment may prevent death or brain damage. Signs and symptoms may mimic other neurologic disorders, so the clinician must have a high index of suspicion. After the initial history and examination, the clinician makes an educated guess as to the likely causative organisms and then selects appropriate antibiotics. Antibiotics and management are subsequently modified, depending on laboratory results.

History and Examination Suggesting Infection

HISTORY

Historical points that direct the physician to consider CNS infection in the patient with developing neurologic signs or symptoms include the following:

1. *Fever* may be 40° C (105° F) or greater in adults, whereas other infections seldom produce fever this high. Fever may be absent in neonates and elderly patients.
2. Severe *headache* is worsened by movement of the head or neck, particularly flexion of the neck
3. Known *blood-borne infection* (such as bacteremia or endocarditis).
4. *Debilitating condition from other disease* (such as chronic renal failure) or from reduced immunity (such as in leukemia or lymphoma, administration of immunosuppressant drugs, or in congenital or acquired immunodeficiency syndrome).
5. *Infection of superficial or deep structures adjoining the nervous system*

(such as paranasal sinuses, skin of face, vertebral bodies), especially if there has been recent manipulation in the area.

6. *Abnormality of the blood-brain* barrier (such as in a recent ischemic infarction or emboli from congenital heart disease).

7. *Exposure of CNS structures secondary to trauma or surgery* (such as in compound or basilar skull fractures) or evidence of fistula connecting with the CNS subarachnoid space (such as through the nose, producing CSF rhinorrhea, or through developmental anomalies).

PHYSICAL EXAMINATION

Following are some aspects of the physical examination that suggest the presence of CNS infection:

1. Fever (especially with decreased level of consciousness, or progressing or fluctuating neurologic signs and symptoms).

2. Nuchal rigidity, a preference for lying in bed with the head extended and the back arched. Kernig's and Brudzinski's signs may be present (see Figures 14.1 and 14.2).
   Caution: In infants and some elderly patients, none of these signs may be present.

3. Neurologic findings suggesting multiple levels of involvement of the nervous system, such as cranial nerve palsies, alterations of sensorium, convulsions, and papilledema.

4. Signs of chronic or acute middle ear infection, particularly in children.

CEREBROSPINAL FLUID EXAMINATION (See Chapter 2)

1. CSF studies should be done in all patients *without delay* whenever meningitis or encephalitis is suspected.
   Caution: If there are focal findings or papilledema a CT scan is strongly recommended before the LP.

2. Gram's stain of CSF sediment will show organisms in 70% of untreated bacterial meningitis cases. India ink preparations for cryptococcus and acid-fast stains for tubercle bacilli are rarely positive tests but nonetheless should be performed.

3. Normally, the CSF contains *no* polymorphonuclear leukocytes and no more than five lymphocytes per microliter (cubic millimeter). *More cells* than this suggest CNS inflammation of some type.

4. A CSF glucose value of less than 40 mg/dL suggests bacterial infection. Simultaneous blood sugars are of little practical value, since blood glucose takes several hours to equilibrate with CSF glucose.

5. CSF protein and pressure are commonly elevated.

6. CSF *culture* and sensitivity testing should always include bacteria (aerobic and anaerobic), tuberculosis, brucellosis, and fungi. Although the

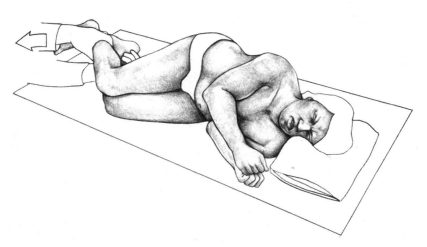

Figure 14.1. Kernig's sign: Patient with meningitis may lie in bed with knees and hips flexed. A positive sign (pain) is elicited when the legs are extended.

yield is very low, viral cultures should be obtained when viral meningoencephalitis is suspected and where facilities for viral culture are available.

7. Antigen-antibody studies:

    a. Cryptococcal antigen (latex particle agglutination test) determinations should be ordered when fungal meningitis is suspected and should be done routinely in all patients who are immunocompromised. Skin test antigen is of no value.

    b. CSF IgM may be elevated in *Herpes simplex* encephalitis.

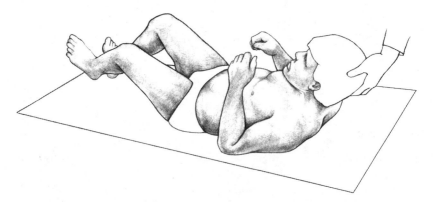

Figure 14.2. Brudzinski's sign: Passive flexion of the neck causes spontaneous flexion of the lower limbs.

   c. Routine countercurrent immunoelectrophoresis (CIE) may rapidly detect polysaccharide antigen associated with meningococcal, pneumococcal, and *Haemophilus influenzae* (type B) meningitis.

   d. Routine syphilis serology.

   e. CSF IgG and measles antibody titers must be obtained if subacute sclerosing panencephalitis is suspected.

8. Whenever possible, a 2 to 3 mL sample of CSF should be stored frozen to enable the physician to perform further studies if clinically indicated during the initial phase of the illness.

GENERAL PRINCIPLES OF ANTIBIOTIC TREATMENT

1. Antibiotics should be started empirically as soon as possible after the lumbar puncture is done. Choose antibiotics that are bactericidal against known or presumed causative organisms.

2. Combinations of drugs are to be avoided unless a synergistic effect is known to occur. Combinations of drugs may be necessary if:

   a. Sensitivities are initially unavailable.

   b. The organism is felt to be resistant (enteric gram-negative bacilli, fungal infection, tuberculosis, *Brucella*).

   c. The patient is immunosuppressed.

3. The antibiotics must be capable of penetrating into CSF in concentrations well above mean bactericidal concentration for the infective organism.

4. Intrathecal antibiotic administration is unnecessary in the initial treatment of the patient with acute meningitis and is only useful in certain circumstances (such as resistant fungal meningitis). Select the best antibiotic at the correct daily dosage (see Tables 14.1 through 14.3).

5. Be certain the patient is receiving what has been ordered. Serum level determinations can be done for chloramphenicol and the aminoglycosides, and the dosage may be adjusted accordingly.

BACTERIAL MENINGITIS IN NEONATES

Meningitis in the full-term and premature newborn has serious consequences.

1. Mortality rates are about 20 percent for *Escherichia coli* and group B streptococcal meningitis, which together account for 60% to 75% of cases.

2. Long-term sequelae range from blindness, deafness, seizures, or hydrocephalus, to cognitive disorders such as mental retardation, attention disorders, and learning disabilities.

Diagnosis

1. Early diagnosis is difficult because signs and symptoms may be non-

Table 14.1
ANTIBIOTIC DOSAGES FOR BACTERIAL MENINGITIS
(Birth to 2 Months)

Ampicillin	150-200 mg/kg/day, IV (q8h)
Penicillin G	
< 1 wk	150,000 units/kg/day, IV (q8h)
1 wk - 2 mo	150,000-250,000 units/kg/day, IV (q6h)
Group B *Streptococcus*	250,000-400,000 units/kg/day, IV (q6h)
Methicillin sodium	100 mg/kg/day, IV (q8h)
Nafcillin sodium	100 mg/kg/day, IV (q8h)
Carbenicillin	300 mg/kg/day, IV (q8h)
Ticarcillin	200-300 mg/kg/day, IV (q8h)
Piperacillin sodium	200 mg/kg/day, IV (q8h)
Kanamycin sulfate	
< 1 wk	20 mg/kg/day, IM or IV (q12h)
1 wk - 2 mo	30 mg/kg/day, IM or IV (q8h)
Gentamicin sulfate	
< 1 wk	5 mg/kg/day, IM or IV (q12h)
1 wk - 2 mo	7.5 mg/kg/day, IM or IV (q8h)
Tobramycin	
< 1 wk	5 mg/kg/day, IM or IV (q12h)
1 wk - 2 mo	7.5 mg/kg/day, IM or IV (q8h)
Amikacin	
< 1 wk	15 mg/kg/day, IM or IV (q12h)
1 wk - 2 mo	22.5 mg/kg/day, IM or IV (q8h)
Moxalactam disodium	100-150 mg/kg/day, IV (q8h)
Cefotaxime sodium	100-150 mg/kg/day, IV (q8h)
Vancomycin hydrochloride	
Birth to 1 wk	30 mg/kg/day, IV (q12h)
1 wk - 2 mo	45 mg/kg/day, IV (q8h)
Metronidazole	15 mg/kg/day, IV (q12h)
Chloramphenicol	
Premature (birth to 1 mo)	25 mg/kg/day, IV (q12h)
Full term (birth to 7 days)	25 mg/kg/day, IV (q12h)
Full term (7 - 30 days)	50 mg/kg/day, IV (q8h)
Full term (1 - 2 mo)	50-100 mg/kg/day, IV (q6h)

Table 14.2
ANTIBIOTIC DOSAGES FOR BACTERIAL MENINGITIS
(Over Age 2 Months up to 50 kg Body Weight)

Ampicillin	300-400 mg/kg/day, IV (q4)
Penicillin G	250,000 units/kg/day, IV (q4h)
Methicillin sodium	200-300 mg/kg/day, IV (q4h)
Nafcillin sodium	200 mg/kg/day, IV (q4h)
Carbenicillin	400-600 mg/kg/day, IV (q4h)
Ticarcillin	300-400 mg/kg/day, IV (q4h)
Piperacillin sodium	300-400 mg/kg/day, IV (q4h)
Chloramphenicol	75-100 mg/kg/day, PO or IV (q6h)
Gentamicin	4 mg/kg/day, IM (q8h)
Tobramycin	4 mg/kg/day, IM (q8h)
Amikacin	15 mg/kg/day, IM (q8h)
Moxalactam disodium	150 mg/kg/day, IV (q4h)
Cefotaxime sodium	150 mg/kg/day, IV (q4h)
Cefoperazone sodium	300 mg/kg/day, IV (q8h)
Ceftriaxone sodium	100 mg/kg/day, IV (q12h)
Rifampin	20 mg/kg/day, PO (q8h) (up to 600 mg)
Streptomycin sulfate	20-40 mg/kg/day, IM (q12h) (not over 1 g)
Vancomycin hydrochloride	60 mg/kg/day, IV (q6h)
Sulfadiazine	150 mg/kg/day, IV (q8h)
Metronidazole	40 mg/kg/day, PO (q8h) 30 mg/kg/day, IV (q6h)

specific or minor (irritability, poor feeding, jitteriness, lethargy).

2. CSF changes are delayed, especially in the premature infant, and the relatively poor defense mechanisms of newborns allows rapid progression of the disease.
3. Neonates require treatment based on suspicion alone.

Table 14.3
ANTIBIOTIC THERAPY FOR BACTERIAL MENINGITIS WITH A KNOWN ETIOLOGIC AGENT IN ADULTS

	ORGANISM	PREFERRED THERAPY (ANTIBIOTIC DOSAGE/24 HRS)	ALTERNATIVE THERAPY (ANTIBIOTIC DOSAGE/24 HRS)
G R A M	*Pneumococcus*	Penicillin G 24 million units IV	Chloramphenicol 4 gm IV
	multiply resistant	Vancomycin hydrochloride 2 g	IV Vancomycin 2 mg IV plus 2-5 mg intrathecally
P O S I T I V E	*Streptococcus*		
	Groups A and B	Penicillin G 24 million units IV	Chloramphenicol 4 gm IV
	Group D (enterococcus)	Penicillin G 24 million units IV + Gentamicin sulfate 5 mg/kg IM or IV	Vancomycin 2 gm IV plus 2-5 mg intrathecally
	Staphylococcus aureus	Nafcillin sodium 10-12 g IV	Vancomycin 2 gm IV plus 2-5 mg intrathecally
G R A M	*Listeria monocytogenes*	Ampicillin 12 g IV	Tetracycline 1.5 g IV
	Haemophilus influenzae	Chloramphenicol 4 g IV	Ampicillin 12-14 g IV
N E G A T I V E	*Meningococcus*	Penicillin G 24 million units IV	Chloramphenicol 4 g IV
	Escherichia coli, *Klebsiella,* *Proteus,* *Pseudomonas,* *Serratia,* and similar organisms	Carbenicillin 30-40 g IV + Aminoglycoside IV	Aminoglycoside 2-5 mg intrathecally

4. Pretreatment blood, urine, and CSF cultures are obtained and treatment is discontinued if these do not provide evidence of treatable infection.

5. Normal neonatal CSF protein may be as high as 150 mg/dL, the cell counts up to 25 WBCs/μL and 650 RBCs/μL, and peripheral WBC as high as 25,000/μL. By 1 month these values decrease to adult values.

6. CSF pressure is almost always greater than 180 mm water. Greater than 400 mm water indicates impending herniation.

Treatment:

1. Care of the neonate with meningitis may be complicated by respiratory insufficiency, hypoglycemia, dehydration, shock, or convulsions and is best undertaken in a neonatal intensive care unit. Unless the primary care practitioner has considerable experience with neonates, it is best to refer the patient to a pediatrician or neonatologist.

2. Recommendations for initial therapy are third generation cephalosporins combined with ampicillin. Cefotaxime sodium, 50 mg/kg IV q6h, or moxalactam disodium are preferred in combination with ampicillin until the pathogen is known. See Table 14.1 for other specific drug dosages.

3. Third-generation cephalosporins offer higher levels than the aminoglycosides; however hard data indicating therapeutic advantage over aminoglycosides are lacking.

4. All medication is given IV, and usually continued for 21 days after the CSF has been sterilized.

BACTERIAL MENINGITIS IN INFANTS AND CHILDREN

Bacterial meningitis is primarily a disease of early childhood.

1. Ninety percent of cases occur from age 1 month to 5 years.

2. The most common cause is *Haemophilus influenzae* type B, which accounts for 90% of cases from 3 months to 5 years of age, and 50% of all cases in childhood.

3. Pneumococci (*Streptococcus pneumoniae*) and meningococci (*Neisseria meningitidis*) account for most of the rest.

4. All three of these organisms colonize the nasopharynx of healthy children, and most children with meningitis have a preceding or concurrent nasopharyngitis.

Diagnosis

Signs and symptoms pointing to CNS invasion are more easily elicited in this group, compared to neonates.

1. Often, the main difficulty is distinguishing between acute viral and acute

bacterial meningitis, since the early symptoms are similar.

2. Antibiotics frequently have already been administered when the child presents, so that the differential diagnosis often is between partially treated bacterial meningitis and viral meningitis, both of which may show similar CSF profiles.

3. Appropriate smears and cultures are obtained anyway, countercurrent immunoelectrophoresis on the CSF performed, and if no evidence for bacterial infection is obtained, therapy can be discontinued.

Treatment:

1. *Initial therapy:* Ampicillin 300 to 400 mg/kg/day IV q4h, maximum daily dose 12 g to avoid cerebral irritability, plus chloramphenicol 75 mg/kg/day IV q6h.

2. A single antibiotic should be used whenever possible once sensitivity patterns have been determined. See Table 14.2 for drug dosage and regimens.

3. A second lumbar puncture should be obtained within 48 hours of starting antibiotic therapy. By this time no organisms should be detectable on stained CSF smears, or they should be greatly reduced; otherwise therapy must be re-evaluated.

4. CSF cells, glucose, and protein return to normal slowly, and so may still be abnormal at 48 hours. If the clinical course is satisfactory, it may not be necessary to perform a third lumbar puncture.

5. Duration of treatment is at least 14 days, but should be at least 21 days for gram-positive enterococci, and 28 days for gram-negative enteric bacilli.

Note: A new vaccine against *Haemophilus influenzae* type B is available and should be administered routinely to all children at 18 months of age. Its widespread use will potentially eliminate the majority of cases of this form of meningitis.

BACTERIAL MENINGITIS IN ADULTS

With treatment, fatality rates of adult bacterial meningitis are usually less than 10%, but severe neurologic sequelae are possible. The two leading causes in the adult are pneumococci (*Streptococcus pneumoniae*) and meningococci (*Neisseria meningitidis*).

1. Pneumococcal meningitis is usually preceded by pneumonia and often associated with alcoholism, debilitation, and old age, and usually occurs sporadically, except in developing countries. Confused elderly patients should be assumed to have meningitis until a clear and adequate diagnosis can be made.

2. Meningococcal meningitis occurs in epidemics (serogroups A or C) in

the pediatric age group, and may be acquired by susceptible adults.

3. Meningitis caused by gram-negative enteric bacteria is almost always a disease of the hospitalized or nursing home patient, and often follows bacteremia from other foci such as cellulitis or urinary tract infection.

Treatment:

1. *Initial therapy*: Penicillin G, aqueous, 2 million units IV q2h and chloramphenicol 1 g IV q6h. See Table 14.3 for other drug regimens.

2. Patients are customarily treated through five afebrile days, but not less than 1 week for meningococci, 10 days for *Haemophilus influenzae*, and 14 days for pneumococci.

COMPLICATIONS OF MENINGITIS

1. *Seizures*: Drug therapy is outlined in Chapter 11. These seizures may be transient and may not require prolonged anticonvulsant therapy or may persist for many years following brain destruction and scar formation. If a patient has a seizure during the acute episode, treat with anticonvulsants for 1 year. At that time, the drug may be discontinued, according to the guidelines in Chapter 11.

2. *Increased intracranial pressure*: This is usually a transient problem due to cerebral edema; if necessary, treat with fluid restriction, mannitol, or steroids (see Chapter 12).

3. *Subdural effusions*: These are especially common after *Haemophilus influenzae* meningitis in children; suspect with persistent fever and focal seizures. The effusions are usually treated by repeated subdural taps, but occasionally require neurosurgical intervention.

3. *Subdural empyema*: This is similar to a subdural effusion, except that the fluid contains live organisms and is consequently much more dangerous. Immediate surgical drainage and reassessment of antibiotic therapy are indicated.

4. *Infarction*: Venous infarcts may be caused by cortical thrombophlebitis, venous sinus thrombosis, or both. Cortical thrombophlebitis usually presents early with seizures that are difficult to control. Sagittal sinus thrombosis will manifest as increased intracranial pressure and stroke, predominantly with lower extremity findings. Arterial infarcts secondary to an inflammatory arteritis accompanying bacterial infection may not be evident until the recovery phase from the acute toxic illness, particularly in pneumococcal meningitis.

5. *Prolonged fever* may be due to local infection at the IV site, subdural effusion, inappropriate or inadequate antibiotic therapy, drug fever, and the presence of an unsuspected second organism.

6. *Inappropriate antidiuretic hormone (ADH) secretion*: The syndrome of

inappropriate ADH secretion (SIADH) is a frequent occurrence during the early phases of meningitis. Diagnosis is made by finding low serum osmolality and high urine osmolality. This is usually prevented by keeping on the low side of daily fluid maintenance requirements.

7. *Communicating hydrocephalus:* The infection may interfere with proper reabsorption of CSF, but more commonly, hydrocephalus is a late complication. The symptoms include deterioration of mental and behavioral function and bilateral corticospinal tract signs, especially increased reflexes in the lower extremities. The diagnosis is suggested by large ventricles on CT scan. If the condition does not spontaneously resolve, shunting of the CSF by a neurosurgeon may be necessary.

8. *Obstructive hydrocephalus*: This is suggested by an abnormal increase in head circumference and widening of sutures in infants or young children. In older children and adults, there will be progressive mental deterioration and ataxia, and the CT scan will show ventricular enlargement. Shunting by a neurosurgeon is often required. Acute obstruction results in coma and death if the pressure is not relieved promptly.

Prognosis

The prognosis of bacterial meningitis depends on the following:

1. The nature of the infectious agent and the severity of the initial process (convulsions and coma)
2. The age of the patient
3. The duration of symptoms before treatment
4. Appropriate and early antibiotic therapy

BRAIN ABSCESS

1. Presentation resembles that of any other mass lesion such as a tumor. Fever and leukocytosis may be minimal or absent, and thus do not rule out the diagnosis.
2. Abscesses are very irritating to brain tissue and cause edema, increased intracranial pressure, and seizures.
3. Predisposing factors include acute and chronic sinusitis and otitis, cyanotic congenital heart disease, and penetrating head wounds.
4. CSF culture is usually negative; cell count is normal or slightly elevated, and protein is slightly elevated.
5. All types of organisms cause abscesses; if neurosurgical intervention is undertaken, both aerobic and anaerobic cultures must be performed.
6. CT scan shows "doughnut sign" - an area of low density with a rim of higher density (capsule) and marked surrounding cerebral edema.
7. If CT scan demonstrates an abscess, lumbar puncture should be avoided due to risk of brain herniation.

8. Sinus and mastoid x-ray films should be performed to look for a source of infection in all cases.

Treatment:

1. Antibiotics against anaerobic *Streptococcus* and *Bacteroides* are given IV. Recommended are chloramphenicol 50 to 100 mg/kg/day in four doses (up to 4 g/day) and crystalline penicillin G, 100,000 to 400,000 units in four to six doses daily IV (up to 20 million units daily IV) if the organism is unknown.

2. Treatment of the cerebral edema usually requires dexamethasone 2 to 6 mg every four to six hours.

3. Neurosurgical excision or drainage of the abscess, with instillation of antibiotics locally, occasionally may be required, unless therapy is instituted very early at a "cerebritis" stage.

4. Duration of therapy remains empirical; however, 4 to 6 weeks is generally accepted as sufficient in most patients.

TUBERCULOUS MENINGITIS

Tuberculous meningitis is now rare in the United States, but should be suspected particularly in recent immigrants or in deprived populations.

1. The diagnosis is elusive because of the following factors:

   a. Onset is usually gradual without meningeal signs. Symptoms are nonspecific -- apathy, anorexia, malaise, low-grade fever. Later there may be drowsiness, seizures, cranial nerve palsies, and other focal (particularly brainstem) signs, and papilledema. The illness develops over weeks, not days.

   b. Tuberculous meningitis is seen in association with disseminated disease in young patients. In adults, the disease (secondary reactivation) usually manifests as CNS disease without dissemination.

   c. Only one-third of patients have evidence of active pulmonary disease, while one-third have a negative purified protein derivative (PPD) test.

   d. Stains for acid-fast bacilli in CSF sediment are frequently negative and cultures may take 4 to 6 weeks to become positive.

2. Strongly suspect the diagnosis under the following conditions:

   a. A history of recent exposure to tuberculosis.

   b. In any case where there is evidence of active tuberculosis, especially in young adults and children.

   c. In any patient with meningitis in whom the intermediate PPD is positive (especially if there is a recent conversion). CSF findings usually consist of increased lymphocytes with or without neutrophils, a decreased glucose, and increased protein.

Note: Tuberculoma does not present as a meningitis, but as a mass lesion.

3. For the above reasons, virtually all CSF with increased cells, even if the glucose is normal, should be cultured for acid-fast bacilli. Cultures and stains have a higher probability of being positive if the CSF is allowed to stand and the resulting proteinaceous precipitate is examined.

Treatment:

1. Once the diagnosis has been made on clinical grounds and adequate cultures have been obtained, treatment must be started immediately; delay of weeks until the culture is positive may lead to irreversible brain damage.

2. Treat routinely with triple therapy:

   Isoniazid (INH) 15 mg/kg/day PO to a maximum of 300 mg/day, for 12 months.

   Rifampin 600 mg/day PO, or 10 mg/kg/day, for 12 months.

   Ethambutol hydrochloride 25 mg/kg/day PO initially should be decreased to 15 mg/kg/day as soon as possible after treatment course is established, then maintained for 12 months.

   Note: Pyridoxine 10 to 20 mg/day should be given with isoniazid to prevent polyneuropathy.

3. Second-choice drugs that may be substituted for one or more of the above are:

   Pyrazinamide 20 to 40 mg/kg/day for a total of 3 g/day PO.

   Streptomycin 1 g/day IM.

Caution:

1. Antibiotic recommendations change from time to time, and consultation with an expert in infectious disease is recommended. Treatment must be monitored with repeated CSF examinations. The antibiotics listed here have a serious potential for toxicity with prolonged use; eg, ethambutol has been associated with optic neuropathy, and streptomycin may cause vestibular damage.

2. Rapid metabolizers (American Indians, Eskimos, Middle Easterners) do not tolerate doses higher than 300 mg INH combined with 600 mg rifampin: symptoms and signs of hepatic dysfunction usually appear within the first 2 months of treatment. Symptoms are dose-related and require only cessation of treatment for 1 to 2 weeks, then reinstitution at lower doses.

MENINGITIS DUE TO FUNGAL DISEASE

1. The diagnosis is often elusive.
2. Onset is often gradual.

3. Systemic symptoms initially may be mild.
4. CSF may show nonspecific findings of normal or low sugar, increased cells, and increased protein. These findings evoke a large differential diagnosis: herpes encephalitis, tuberculous meningitis, leptospiral meningitis, secondary neurosyphilis, partially treated pyogenic meningitis, sarcoidosis, cerebral abscess, and subdural empyema.
5. India ink preparations of CSF for *Cryptococcus* are not a reliable method of diagnosis, but nonetheless should be performed. In suspicious cases obtain cryptococcal antigen and antibody tests in the blood and CSF, as well as cultures of blood and CSF for *Cryptococcus*.
6. The index of suspicion should be especially high in *immunocompromised* or *debilitated* patients. Patients with Hodgkin's disease or acquired immunodeficiency syndrome (AIDS) are particularly susceptible.
7. The most common organisms are *Cryptococcus neoformans* (low-grade fever, cough, mental disturbance, eye abnormalities) and *Coccidioides immitis* (prolonged respiratory symptoms, subacute meningitis).

Treatment:

1. Amphotericin B 0.6 mg/kg/day IV in conjunction with flucytosine 150 mg/kg/day are lifesaving in most fungal infections. Because of their potential toxicity, the drugs should be administered by a clinician experienced in their use.
2. The course of treatment is determined by clinical response and CNS response documented by repeated CSF evaluation.
3. Occasionally intraventricular administration of amphotericin B is necessary to control the meningitis.

NEUROSYPHILIS

1. The clinical presentations of symptomatic neurosyphilis are protean ("stroke," "dementia," CNS mass lesion, meningitis, hydrocephalus); for this reason the CSF test for syphilis must be done on every patient undergoing a lumbar puncture; the diagnosis is most often made in this serendipitous manner.
2. The serologic tests for syphilis are:
   VDRL, rapid plasma reagin test (RPR), ART - nontreponemal tests
   FTA-ABS - fluorescent treponemal antibody absorption test
   MHA-TP - Microhemagglutination-*Treponema pallidum* test
   TPI - *Treponema pallidum* immobilization test
   a. Nontreponemal cardiolipin antibody tests (VDRL, RPR) are useful for screening.
   b. Treponemal tests confirm the diagnosis

   c. A decrease in nontreponemal titers documents adequate therapy

3. Patients with a past history of syphilis or who have a positive serum test for syphilis should have a lumbar puncture to rule out asymptomatic neurosyphilis.

4. In active neurosyphilis there is a high CSF IgM.

Treatment:

1. Neurosyphilis is a treatable disease; progression may be stopped in all cases, and most patients will show improvement.

2. There are several acceptable choices of antibiotic therapy:

   a. Aqueous penicillin G 2 to 4 million units IV q4h for 10 days, followed by penicillin G benzathine 2.4 million units IM weekly, for three doses.

   b. Amoxicillin 3 g/day PO plus probenicid 1g/day for ten days or aqueous procaine penicillin G IM 2.4 million units/day plus probenicid 500 mg qid for ten days, followed by penicillin G benzathine 2.4 million units IM weekly for three doses.

   c. For penicillin allergy, chloramphenicol 2 g/day for 15 to 30 days.

3. Patients with neurosyphilis must be followed with periodic serologic testing and repeat CSF exams for 3 years.

ASEPTIC MENINGOENCEPHALITIS

1. This is the diagnosis given to a patient who shows evidence of inflammation of the meninges and brain tissue, but without evidence of bacteria, fungi, spirochetes, or parasites. The CSF shows a slight increase in cells, usually lymphocytes, with normal glucose and protein.

   Caution: Although laboratory tests do not find the organism, this is not conclusive evidence that organisms are indeed not present.

2. Aseptic meningitis is most commonly caused by viruses. The differential diagnosis, however, is wide and includes:

   a. Parameningeal infections.

   b. Carcinomatous or lymphomatous meningitis. Careful examination of the CSF by a cytopathologist should identify this.

   c. Rarer conditions include Behet's disease, Vogt-Koyanagi syndrome, Mollaret's meningitis, and Lyme disease.

3. In cases where the CSF has an increased cell count, normal sugar, and moderately increased protein, the following laboratory tests should be performed:

   a. An acute serum should be drawn and frozen; 3 weeks later a second serum should be drawn and both should be sent to a laboratory where serum responses to specific infectious processes can be detected. The ability to make a diagnosis of a specific agent is of value for epidemiologic purposes (such as elimination of an arthropod vector) as well as care of the patient. If no rise in antibody is found, there should be a higher index of suspicion that the aseptic meningitis was caused by something other than a viral infection. Laboratories require that the physician specify which titers are to be checked; this should be done on the basis of a clinical picture of meningitis or encephalitis, season of year, and assorted factors (see Table 14.4).

    b. CSF tests for syphilis should be performed in all cases.

    c. A serum test for mononucleosis should be performed.

    d. Viral cultures of the CSF, pharynx, and stool are helpful in selected cases.

4. Presumptive diagnosis may be made during epidemics (arboviruses) or when there is a concurrent recognizable illness (such as mumps, measles, or infectious mononucleosis).

Treatment:

1. Supportive therapy, maintenance of fluid and nutrition (see Chapter 12).

2. Control of cerebral edema (see Chapter 13).

3. Control of seizures (see Chapter 11).

VIRAL DISEASES OF PARTICULAR IMPORTANCE

Acute Encephalitis

A. *Herpes simplex* encephalitis

This is the most common sporadic viral encephalitis. It affects primarily the temporal lobes (a focal encephalitis) although brainstem encephalitides do occur.

1. Presentation is of early personality and behavioral changes, followed by lateralizing and localizing neurologic signs such as hemiparesis or a visual field defect with increased intracranial pressure.

2. A CT scan of the brain may be normal very early in the course, while a radionuclide brain scan may show earlier signs of breakdown of the blood-brain barrier, but after 48 hours usually there are decreased densities in the temporal lobe(s).

3. The EEG characteristically shows early in the course periodic focal spikes from the temporal area with focal slowing or periodic lateralizing epileptiform discharges (PLEDS).

4. Brain biopsy with culture of infected brain establishes the diagno-

Table 14.4
Common Viruses

VIRUS	ASSOCIATED FACTORS	SEASON	PROMINENT MENINGITIC SYMPTOMS	PROMINENT ENCEPHALITIC SYMPTOMS
Enteroviruses				
Poliovirus types 1,2,3 Coxsackie A9, B1-5 Echovirus types 3,4,6 9, 11, 18, 30	Appear in epidemics of gastrointestinal illness	Summer, early Fall	X	
Arboviruses				
Eastern equine	Atlantic Gulf Coast (mosquito vector)			
Western equine	Western U.S. (2/3) (mosquito vector)			
Venezuelan equine	Florida, S.W. states (mosquito vector)	Summer, early Fall		X
St. Louis	All U.S., urban areas (mosquito vector)			
Powassan	Northern U.S., tick vector			
California	All U.S., primarily children (mosquito vector)			
Herpes virus				
H. Simplex, type 1	Adult (mimics temporal lobe tumor)	Sporadic, Winter		X
H. Simple , type 2	Neonatal			
Varicella-zoster	Shingles, chickenpox	Winter, Spring		
Epstein-Barr	Associated with infectious mononucleosis			
Cytomegalovirus	Infants, immunosuppressed adults			
Myxovirus and paramyxovirus				
Influenza	Rare	Winter		
Parainfluenza	Croup and/or bronchitis in young children	Winter		
Mumps	Parotitis, common cause of aseptic meningitis	Spring	X	X
Measles (rubeola)	Encephalomyelitis 1-14 days after rash	Peak in April		X
Adenoviruses	Primarily in neonates			X
Lymphocytic choriomeningitis	Contact with excreta of house mouse	Winter	X	X
Rabies	Animal bites			X

sis. There are characteristic electron microscopic findings. Positive antibody tests (immunocytochemistry) on the biopsy tissue give an early presumptive diagnosis.

5. There is a reduction in mortality and neurologic sequelae if the diagnosis is established early and treatment with specific antiviral agents started, particularly if started before coma ensues.

Treatment:

1. The efficacy of acyclovir (acycloguanosine) is established and its relative freedom from side effects proven, making it now the treatment of choice. Acyclovir 10 mg/kg IV q8h should be administered for a full ten-day course; stabilization or improvement of the patient's clinical symptomatology should be evident within 48 hours of beginning therapy.

2. Steroids (dexamethasone 10 mg IV initially followed by 4 mg IV q6h) may be used to reduce cerebral edema.

3. For *Herpes simplex* encephalitis, cultures of CSF, throat swabs, and stools are of no use in revealing the organism, but should be performed to rule out other pathogens.

4. A brain biopsy can be performed for definitive diagnosis, but in most centers now, if the diagnosis is probable on clinical grounds, treatment is immediately begun with acyclovir and biopsy is only performed if the patient does not become stable or improve within 48 hours.

5. Since *Herpes simplex* infection is ubiquitous in the population and infections outside the nervous system so common, acute and convalescent titers are usually not helpful.

B. Summer Encephalitides

1. These occur in epidemics and are usually secondary to arboviruses:

a. Equine encephalitis should be suspected anywhere in the United States when the horse population first becomes affected; with eastern equine encephalitis, 80% of cases will have neurologic sequelae, whereas western equine encephalitis is milder, with 5% to 10% of cases having neurologic sequelae.

b. St. Louis encephalitis occurs primarily in the far western United States.

c. Venezuelan encephalitis occurs primarily in southwestern United States.

d. California encephalitis occurs primarily in the midwestern United States.

2. Acute and convalescent viral titers need to be obtained, but treatment is symptomatic and supportive.

C. Poliomyelitis

    1. Poliomyelitis is now a rare disease in developed countries with compulsory immunization programs. Presentation is with a febrile illness followed by asymmetric weakness often involving only one limb (except for bulbar polio) associated with loss of deep tendon reflexes (see Chapter 15).

    2. There is a postpolio syndrome in which years after a stable deficit the patient apparently becomes progressively weaker. In the majority of cases, reduced muscle function is secondary to arthritic changes in long-stressed joints, improperly fitting prosthetic devices, and disuse atrophy of muscles from lack of exercise. Only rarely is this an ALS (amyotrophic lateral sclerosis)-like syndrome.

D. Rabies

    1. The presentation is of a brainstem encephalitis.

    2. Transmitted by animal bites, domestic or wild; particularly worrisome are unprovoked attacks by wild animals or bites from bats.

    3. Most dangerous are multiple bites or bites around the face.

Note: In the case of an animal bite, the animal should be impounded and observed. Vaccination should be instituted with vaccine produced in cultured human diploid cells. Passive immunization with human antirabies antiserum may be used adjunctively. In all suspected cases consult local or state health authorities and an infectious disease specialist.

Chronic Encephalitis

A. Acquired Immunodeficiency Syndrome (AIDS)

    1. The human immunodeficiency virus (HIV [formerly termed HTLV-3 or LAV-1]) responsible for AIDS resides chronically in the CNS long before clinical signs of systemic AIDS appear. Viral antibody titers are often positive.

    2. The neurologic complications of AIDS present as a wide spectrum of disorders from encephalitis to myelitis to neuritis to myositis. Neurologic signs and symptoms in an AIDS patient may be due to one or more of:

        a. Opportunistic infections in an immunocompromised host; eg, toxoplasmosis, progressive multifocal leukoencephalopathy, cryptococcal meningitis, disseminated *Mycobacterium avium intracellulare*

        b. Unusual primary or metastatic malignancies; eg, primary CNS lymphoma (reticulum cell sarcoma) or metastatic Kaposi's sarcoma.

c. The direct effect of the AIDS virus itself which seems to have a propensity for causing damage to the deep cerebral white matter.

3. Every patient with unusual or unexplained neurologic signs or symptoms should have serologic evaluation for the AIDS virus.

4. Biopsy of the brain, peripheral nerve, and/or muscle is necessary for characterization of the process. Material for cultures and other studies for opportunistic infections must be obtained at the time of biopsy.

Treatment:

No specific treatment for infection by the AIDS virus is yet available. Treatment specific for any documented opportunistic infection should be offered.

B. Progressive multifocal leukoencephalopathy (PML)

1. This is a rare condition, occurring in immune-compromised or debilitated patients, presenting as sequential multifocal neurologic signs.

2. CT scan shows multiple decreased white matter densities.

3. The disease is caused by a papovavirus.

Treatment: There is no effective treatment.

C. Jakob's disease (Jakob-Creutzfeldt disease or subacute spongiform encephalopathy)

A presenile dementia associated with either myoclonus or extrapyramidal movement disorder caused by a slow virus. No treatment is available. (See Chapter 6).

Caution: The nervous system tissue of patients is highly infective, even after being fixed in formalin. Fluids and tissues of demented patients should therefore be handled with care, unless the cause of dementia is certain. Tissue from these patients should never be used for transplantation.

D. Subacute sclerosing panencephalitis (SSPE)

1. Subacute sclerosing parencephalitis is a slowly progressive dementing and degenerative disease occurring primarily in children, caused by reactivation of a latent form of an altered measles virus, years after clinical measles; its incidence has decreased since widespread compulsory measles immunization in North America, but is still prevalent in underdeveloped countries.

2. Four clinical stages are identified:
   a. Stage I - Personality, behavioral, and cognitive changes often with apraxia and agnosia

    b. Stage II - Onset of characteristic slow myoclonus that is periodic, often involving the trunk and axial structures

    c. Stage III - Progression of focal neurologic signs

    d. Stage IV - A neurovegetative state followed by death

3. Characteristic EEG change of periodic complexes (usually generalized) in a relatively normal background occurs in late stage I or early stage II.

4. Markedly elevated measles antibody titers are identifiable in the CSF.

Treatment:

No curative treatment is available. Recent reports suggest that isoprinosine (Inosiplex) arrests the disease for a while in some cases. All cases in the United States should be reported to the SSPE Registry in Birmingham, Alabama (telephone 205-471-2159).

E. Progressive rubella encephalitis

Progressive rubella encephalitis occurs in children with congenital rubella (see Chapter 16) after 8 to 19 years and is characterized by progressive dementia, seizures, ataxia, and spasticity. CSF shows increased lymphocytosis, mildly increased protein, and markedly increased gammaglobulin. Serum and CSF show markedly increased rubella antibody titers.

Treatment: There is no effective treatment.

Postinfectious Encephalopathies

There are a number of uncommon acute toxic encephalopathies and acute and subacute hemorrhagic and nonhemorrhagic leukoencephalopathies which are best managed at a specialized center. However, prompt recognition and initial management of Reye's syndrome is imperative prior to referral.

A. Reye-Johnson Syndrome

1. Presents with vomiting then rapid decrease in consciousness in children with preceding viral infection (usually influenza B).

2. Differential clinical staging criteria have been proposed, but generally, if the patient reaches the state of coma, the point of irreversibility may have been passed.

3. Massive cerebral edema may be evident as papilledema or on CT scan of the brain. Lumbar puncture and measurement of CSF pressure should *not* be done without preparation for medical (by mannitol) or surgical decompression. Management usually requires an intensive care unit with ability to do continuous intracranial pressure monitoring.

4. Treatment is aimed primarily at decreasing intracranial pressure, supporting vital functions, and preventing complications of a co-

matose patient (see Chapter 13).

5. The role of aspirin or salicylates in causing this disease is still controversial. Recent data indicate a stronger association, and the present recommendation is that no salicylates be given to children with fever.

Herpes zoster (Shingles)

1. The varicella (chickenpox) virus resides asymptomatically in dorsal root ganglia, and for unknown reasons may occasionally migrate along sensory roots causing pain and later vesicular skin eruption in root distribution.
2. Pain may precede eruption of skin vesicles by several days, making the diagnosis obscure until eruption occurs.
3. Patients should be evaluated for underlying immune deficiency, especially lymphomas.
4. Acyclovir is useful treatment, decreasing pain and new vesicle formation. The dose is acyclovir 15 mg/kg IV in three divided doses daily for five to ten days. In otherwise healthy patients, prednisone 60 to 80 mg daily PO for 2 to 3 weeks may reduce the risk of postherpetic neuralgia.
5. Complications:
   a. Postherpetic neuralgia occurs in about 15% of patients with shingles. Treatment is symptomatic: amitriptyline hydrochloride 25 to 50 mg at bedtime in combination with carbamazepine 200 mg 3 or 4 times daily after meals.
   b. Ophthalmic zoster carries the danger of corneal scarring. Treatment is with local steroids and antibiotics; patients should be referred to an experienced ophthalmologist for care.
   c. Geniculate zoster will present with a peripheral facial palsy. Management is the same as with Bell's palsy (see Chapter 15).

BIBLIOGRAPHY

Bell WE, McCormick WF: *Neurologic Infections in Children.* ed.2. Philadelphia, WB Saunders Co, 1981.

Bell WE, McGuinness GA: Current therapy of acute bacterial meningitis in children, Part II. *Pediatr Neurol* 1985; 1:201-209.

Booss J, Thornton GF (eds): Infectious diseases of the central nervous system. *Neurol Clin* 1986; 4;1-325.

Johnson GM, Scurletis D, Carole NB: A study of 16 fatal cases of encephalitis like disease in North Carolina children. *NC Med J* 1963; 29:464-473.

Johnson RT: *Viral Infections of the Nervous System.* New York, Raven Press, 1982.

Johnson RT: *Current Therapy in Neurologic Disease 1985-1986.* Philadelphia, BC Decker, 1985.

Kaplan SL, Fishman MA: Update on bacterial meningitis. *J Child Neurol* 1988; 3:82-93.

Seay AR: Bacterial meningitis: future directions. *J Child Neurol* 1988; 3:80-81.

XV

FOCAL AND DIFFUSE WEAKNESS OF PERIPHERAL ORIGIN

Although generalized weakness may be due to a variety of medical problems (such as anemia or cardiac failure) or to psychiatric disturbances, in this chapter weakness is assumed to be due to disease of the peripheral nervous system (PNS) (muscle or nerve) or the CNS. Sometimes it is difficult to differentiate PNS disease from CNS disease. The following guidelines may be helpful:

1. Increased reflexes and extensor plantar responses (Babinski reflexes) are associated with CNS disorders.
2. Decreased reflexes generally indicate weakness of peripheral nervous system origin, except in the acute phase of CNS disease or in long-standing, extremely severe CNS disease.
3. Involvement of an arm and a leg on the same side is suggestive of CNS disease.
4. Multiple cranial nerve involvement suggests CNS disease, especially when there is motor weakness or sensory disturbance in the contralateral leg and/or arm.
5. Changes in muscle bulk (such as atrophy or hypertrophy) suggest PNS disease.
6. Trophic changes in skin and hair, especially if associated with changes in muscle bulk, suggest PNS disease.

Once the clinician has determined that the weakness is of PNS origin, Tables 15.1 and 15.2 may be helpful for determining whether the problem primarily involves the muscle or the nerve.

Table 15.1.
DIFFERENTIATION OF MUSCLE AND NERVE DISEASE ON CLINICAL EXAMINATION

SIGN	NERVE	EXCEPTIONS	MUSCLE	EXCEPTIONS
Reflexes	Absent early	Anterior horn cell disease, reflexes preserved	Usually present	In end-stage muscle disease and in polymyositis, reflexes are diminished or absent
Distribution of weakness	Distal	Occasionally in anterior horn cell disease and lead poisoning; weakness is proximal	Proximal	Myotonic dystrophy has distal weakness
Sensory disturbance	Usually present	Anterior horn cell disease	Absent	In inflammatory myopathy, nerve terminal branches can be involved
Atrophy	Early	Anterior horn cell disease	Late	Muscular dystrophy, "congenital myopathies"
Hypertrophy	Rare	Plexiform neurofibroma	Common in Duchenne's dystrophy	
Cramps	With initia- tion of exercise		After exercise	

Characteristic findings are:
1. Myotonia - Found in myotonic dystrophy, myotonia congenita, and periodic paralysis;

2. Fasciculations - indicate anterior horn cell disease but may be benign in situations such as excess caffeine intake.

Table 15.2
LABORATORY FEATURES THAT MAY BE HELPFUL IN CORROBORATING CLINICAL DIFFERENTIATION OF MUSCLE OR NERVE INVOLVEMENT

TEST	NERVE	EXCEPTIONS	MUSCLE	EXCEPTIONS
Creatine phosphokinase (CPK)	Normal	Elevated factitiously after injections and trauma; elevated 2-3 times normal in anterior horn cell disease	Markedly elevated 8-200 times normal	End-stage muscle disease, rare cases of inflammatory muscle disease and "congenital" myopathies
Needle EMG	Fibrillations and fasciculations (large amplitude units)	May be normal less than 3 wk from onset; in severe disease electrical activity not detectable	Small motor units	Fibrillations may occur in inflammatory disease
Nerve conduction velocity	Usually a decrease	Usually normal in anterior horn cell disease and selective axonal disorders	Normal	
Muscle biopsy	Small atrophic fibers and grouping of fiber types	Normal less than 3 wk from onset or sampling error	Necrotic muscle fibers and abnormal fiber architecture are common	Sampling error

DIFFUSE WEAKNESS OF PERIPHERAL ORIGIN

Polyneuropathy

Diabetic Neuropathy

There are three types of neuropathies associated with diabetes, and an individual may have one or any combination of all three neuropathies:

1. Diabetic peripheral neuropathy is also called diabetic sensory neuropathy because motor symptoms tend to be mild.

   a. Some degree of peripheral neuropathy is evident in almost all diabetics.

   b. Usual presentation is painless foot trauma or paresthesias or hyperesthesias of feet; suspect neuropathy when either exaggerated withdrawal response to plantar stimulation or summation are present (see Chapter 1).

   c. Significant peripheral neuropathies are almost always associated with absent ankle reflexes.

   d. Severity of neuropathy often is not directly correlated with control of blood sugar.

   e. Very severe diabetic peripheral neuropathy (pseudotabes) may be characterized by recurrent spontaneous pain (described as "deep in the bones"), loss of pain sensation in joints, sensory ataxia, and development of perforating ulcers.

   Note: It is sometimes necessary to differentiate peripheral polyneuropathy (symmetric involvement of all peripheral nerves, usually the result of metabolic disturbance and affecting the distal portions of extremities more than the proximal) from mononeuritis multiplex (involvement of multiple individual nerves, often asymmetric and proximal and usually the result of traumatic or vascular injury). Both types of peripheral neuropathy may occur in diabetics. The "stocking" component of the symmetric peripheral neuropathy is always clinically more evident than the "glove" component. When the upper limbs are equally or more affected than the lower limbs, mononeuritis multiplex is the more likely diagnosis.

2. Diabetic autonomic peripheral neuropathy.

   a. Commonly the patient complains of excessive sweating on the upper portion of the body (which is due to decreased sweating on the lower portion of body) and symptoms due to postural hypotension.

   b. Other symptoms may include impotence, atonic bladder, and abnormalities of gastrointestinal motility.

   c. Individuals with diabetic autonomic peripheral neuropathy are very susceptible to heat stroke.

3. Diabetic amyotrophy.
   a. Characterized by proximal weakness and atrophy, nocturnal pain in thigh, back, and perineum, and presence of fasciculations. Called "amyotrophy" (meaning without muscle nourishment) because of prominent motor involvement.
   b. Sensory loss is minimal; knee reflex may be absent while ankle reflex is present.
   c. Important to diagnose because improvement is often noted with better blood sugar control.

Treatment:

1. Diabetic control is important, but may not alter the course except in diabetic amyotrophy.
2. Pain should NOT be treated with narcotics. Amitriptyline hydrochloride 100 to 150 mg/day or a combination of fluphenazine 2 to 4 mg/day and amitriptyline offer the best pain control. Phenytoin 200 mg bid or carbamazepine 200 mg qid may also be used to relieve symptoms.
3. Thiamine 50 to 100 mg/day may be helpful.
4. Underlying etiology is hypoxia due to altered peripheral nerve-blood barrier; temporary marked improvement with hyperbaric oxygenation has been noted. Another abnormality noted is the increase in sorbitol and fructose in the peripheral nerve; agents such as sorbinil (an aldose reductase inhibitor) are being evaluated as possible treatment.

Polyneuropathies Associated with Deficiency States and Metabolic Disorders

Polyneuropathies associated with deficiency states and metabolic disorders are extremely common, and in most instances, closely resemble the diabetic polyneuropathies, although there are some individual differences in presentation.

A. Vitamin B_{12} deficiency (pernicious anemia, subacute combined degeneration, combined systems disease)
   1. The clinical presentation is variable, because the patient may have only one or all of the following four disturbances:
      a. Peripheral neuropathy: moderate to severe involvement of sensation and, in later stages, distal muscle atrophy and weakness.
      b. Posterior-column symptoms: markedly diminished or absent vibratory and position sensation (particularly in the lower extremities); sensory ataxia; on examination, patient will fall from a standing position with eye closure (positive Romberg test).
      c. Spasticity: corticospinal tract involvement with paraparesis or quadriparesis (tetraparesis); on clinical examination, bilateral

extensor plantar responses (Babinski reflexes) usually will be present.

    d. Dementia: may be clinically indistinguishable from other forms of dementia (see Chapter 6).

Remember: It may be difficult to demonstrate spasticity or posterior column disturbance in the presence of severe peripheral neuropathy, and demonstrating sensory disturbance may be difficult in the presence of significant dementia.

2. Diagnosis is established by low serum vitamin B_{12} levels and positive Schilling test.

3. Anemia or disturbances of blood cell morphology may be absent and should not be used as criteria for excluding this diagnosis.

Treatment:

Only *after* the diagnosis is *definitely established* should treatment be started. Vitamin B_{12} 1000 g, parenterally every week for ten doses and then monthly should be administered.

Caution:

Administration of only folic acid to a patient with vitamin B_{12} deficiency will result in further worsening of neurologic symptoms, while any hematologic disturbance will revert to normal.

B. Folic acid deficiency

1. The clinical presentation is often indistinguishable from vitamin B_{12} deficiency, except that dementia is usually the most prominent neurologic symptom.

2. Diagnosis is established by low serum folate levels.

Treatment:

Before folic acid is administered, vitamin B_{12} deficiency must be definitely excluded. Folic acid 5.0 mg should be administered daily.

C. Thiamine deficiency-alcoholic polyneuropathy

Thiamine deficiency most commonly presents in alcoholic patients (see Chapter 8) with absent ankle reflexes and paresthesias, although it may occasionally occur in nonalcoholic patients who suffer nutritional deprivation. Motor symptoms are minimal.

D. Other metabolic causes

1. Chronic renal disease

2. Chronic liver failure

3. Remote effect of carcinoma, particularly bronchogenic carcinoma

4. Drug-induced, particularly vincristine, cisplatin, nitrofurantoin, dapsone, isoniazid (INH), disulfiram

Polyneuropathies Associated with Heavy Metal Poisoning

Arsenic, lead, mercury, and thallium are the most common metal poisonings associated with peripheral neuropathy. Specific features of these polyneuropathies are summarized in Table 15.3. Bismuth, manganese, gold, antimony, barium, zinc, and copper in large doses have also been associated with neuropathy, but other systemic symptoms usually dominate the clinical picture.

Guillian-Barré Syndrome (Landry-Guillian-Barré-Strohl Syndrome, Inflammatory Polyradiculoneuropathy, "French Polio," Ascending Polyradiculoneuropathy)

1. Symmetric progressive weakness is greater distally than proximally and in the legs more than in the arms; an ascending paralysis that affects motor nerves more than sensory nerves.
2. Reflexes in the lower extremities are absent early in the disease.
3. The facial nerve may be involved.

   Caveat: Bilateral facial weakness of rapid onset with motor polyneuropathy is most often due to Guillian-Barré syndrome.
4. Sensory loss is variable, but usually mild; when present, position and vibration sense are more affected than pain.
5. Onset subacute (usually over one to two days); afebrile unless complications occur. One half of patients have a history of antecedent acute infection (usually influenza like or dysenteric) which has resolved by the time of onset of polyradiculoneuropathy; 10% of patients have had surgery 1 to 4 weeks previously; postimmunization occurrence has been reported.
6. Autonomic function is usually abnormal, but manifestations are variable and include bladder disturbance, fluctuating blood pressure with postural hypotension, anal sphincter weakness, gastrointestinal motility disturbances (including dysphagia), and sluggishly reactive pupils; abnormalities of cardiac rhythm may occur; loss of sweating in lower extremities may result in increased sweating in upper extremities.
7. After the first two or three days of paralysis, the CSF protein is elevated, and only a few lymphocytes are present, usually less than 10 cells/μL (so-called albuminocytologic dissociation). Peak levels of CSF protein (may be greater than 2000 mg/dL) occur 4 to 6 weeks after onset of illness and may continue to rise as clinical improvement occurs.
8. Maximum deficit occurs over three days to 6 weeks; spontaneous recovery occurs in a "descending fashion," over 6 weeks to 6 months, and is usually complete.

Table 15.3
PRINCIPAL METAL TOXINS

	Arsenic	Lead	Mercury	Thallium
Clinical tip-off	Red hands and burning feet with hyperhydrosis	Peripheral neuropathy which may appear to be single nerve involvement (such as wrist drop or foot drop)	Severe spontaneous arm and leg pain	Alopecia
Exposure	Homicide attempt, insecticides, medicinal arsenic, Paris green, accidental contamination, Fowler's solution (potassium arsenate)	Industrial ingestion; tetraethyl gasoline; lead paint; burning lead batteries; eating from pewter or dishware with glaze containing lead; melting for purposes of molding.	Ingestion, methyl mercury (Minamata disease), especially fish in polluted areas, industrial exposure, antifungal treatment of grain	Homicide, insecticide rodent poison
Clinical syndrome	"Stocking-glove" mainly sensory neuropathy; severe pain and paresthesias, especially of feet, "burning feet and hands", red hands with hyperhydrosis and subsequent motor neuropathy involving distal muscles of hands and feet	Primarily a motor neuropathy, which frequently may appear as though single nerves are involved such as radial nerve ("wrist drop"), median nerve (thenar atrophy), peroneal nerve ("foot drop"); painful joints; in children causes cerebral edema	Dementia with primarily motor neuropathy; occasional sensory "stocking-glove" neuropathy; acrodynia (Pink disease) in infants and young children	Distal sensorimotor neuropathy of "stocking-glove" type with alopecia
Diagnosis	24-hour urine analysis, hair analysis, blood arsenic level	Blood lead level, 24 hour urine analysis	24 hour urine analysis	24 hour urine analysis
Treatment	Penicillamine 250 mg qid (may also use BAL or EDTA)	Penicillamine 250 mg q.i.d. (may also use BAL or EDTA)	Penicillamine 250 mg q.i.d. (may also use BAL or EDTA)	Diphenyl thiocarbazone or sodium dicarbamate

9. Routine nerve conduction velocities are normal in up to 10% of patients; tests of F wave latency and the H reflex are usually abnormal.

10. Neurologic complications of arsenic poisoning or of acquired immunodeficiency syndrome (AIDS) may closely mimic Guillian-Barré syndrome and should be excluded by appropriate tests.

Note: Sometimes the first presentation of chronic relapsing polyneuropathy may mimic Guillian-Barré syndrome. However, such patients have multiple relapsing episodes at varying intervals and of varying duration, often without complete recovery between exacerbations.

Treatment:

1. The availability of an intensive care nursing unit is vital for managing the acute life-threatening complications of Guillian-Barré syndrome (see also Chapter 20).

2. Respiratory function initially must be closely monitored with frequent (at least hourly) bedside measurements of forced vital capacity (FVC) and inspiratory force (a direct pulmonary reflection of muscular strength). Respiratory function must be closely monitored even in patients with no apparent respiratory involvement, since rapid progression of weakness over several hours may produce respiratory failure. If FVC falls below 1400 mL in the 70-kg individual, tracheostomy must be very seriously considered. An inspiratory force of less than 25 cm also indicates probable need for tracheostomy. Tracheostomy is preferred over endotracheal tube placement. The frequency of monitoring of respiratory function may be reduced as the patient shows signs of clinical improvement.

3. Ventilatory assistance must be provided at the first sign of dyspnea or decreased blood oxygen saturation. Dysphagia may result in aspiration of food, and nasogastric feeding may be necessary. Paroxysmal hypertension, cardiac arrhythmias, and abnormal thermoregulation can occur and must be individually treated. Intercurrent infections must be treated vigorously. Pulmonary embolism can occur secondary to venous stasis in paralyzed limbs; thigh-length elastic stockings are recommended.

4. Treatment of the precipitating illness may be necessary; about 5% of cases have a preceding mycoplasma infection requiring antibiotic therapy. Also, the syndrome of inappropriate antidiuretic hormone may occur in some patients and should be treated with careful fluid restriction.

5. Nursing care and physical therapy are important adjuncts. Frequent turning is important to avoid pressure sores. Pressure on peripheral nerves (especially ulnar nerve at the elbow and peroneal nerve at the fibular head) can destroy the still intact nerve axons and the del-

icate regenerating myelin, resulting in permanent nerve palsies; this should be avoided by appropriate patient positioning and cushioning. Passive range of motion is important to prevent contractures. Early mobilization of the extremities is necessary to avoid the development of thrombophlebitis with subsequent pulmonary embolization; low-dose heparin therapy may also be useful in preventing this complication.

6. Corticosteroids have not definitely been shown to benefit Guillian-Barré syndrome, although in chronic relapsing polyneuropathy, there is definite benefit with corticosteroid therapy.

7. If available, plasmapheresis *early* in the course of the disease (during the first week) may decrease severity and hasten recovery.

Diseases of the Anterior Horn Cell

Amyotrophic Lateral Sclerosis (ALS)

1. Gradually progressive muscle weakness is characterized by fasciculations of arms, legs, and tongue. The initial weakness may be proximal and resemble a muscle disease.

2. Signs of upper motor neuron disease (hyperactive reflexes and extensor plantar responses) may be present initially, but are later masked by severe loss of anterior horn cells.

3. There are no significant sensory abnormalities.

4. Occasionally minor elevations of creatine phosphokinase (CPK) up to 3 times normal and elevation of CSF protein to 70 to 80 mg/dL may be noted.

5. Since the disease is fatal within several years in 80% of patients, ALS must be very carefully differentiated from the following potentially treatable conditions:

   a. Diseases of the cervical spinal cord (see Chapter 18), such as syringomyelia, spondylitic myelopathy, tumors (fasciculations only in upper extremities and upper motor neuron signs in the lower extremities)

   b. Parathyroid disease (elevated serum calcium)

   c. Diabetic amyotrophy (improved with blood sugar control)

   d. Benign fasciculations (often seen in patients with excessive caffeine intake)

   Treatment:

   1. The intellect in ALS is preserved; careful counseling of the patient and family concerning prognosis and death are mandatory.

2. If severe dysphagia is present, a feeding gastrostomy or pyriform sinus feeding tube may make the patient more comfortable.

3. Most physicians will not use ventilatory assistance, since this results in a totally paralyzed patient (eventually even eye movements become paralyzed) who suffers a prolonged and agonizing death.

4. Further information on services available to patients with ALS can be obtained from the Muscular Dystrophy Association, 810 Seventh Ave, New York, NY 10019 (telephone: 212-586-0808) or from the ALS Association, 21021 Ventura Boulevard, Suite 321, Woodland Hills, CA 91364 (telephone: 818-340-7500 or 800-782-4747).

Inherited Anterior Horn Cell Disease (Spinal Muscular Atrophies)

1. Infancy (*Werdnig-Hoffmann disease*)

    a. Presents as a floppy baby (see Figure 15.1) with progressive weakness and feeding difficulties.

    b. Fasciculations are more readily seen in the tongue and are difficult to see in the extremities because of baby fat.

    c. Death usually occurs in the first several years of life due to respiratory insufficiency.

    d. This disorder results from an autosomal recessive gene.

2. Childhood or adolescence (*Kugelberg-Welander disease*)

    a. Presents as progressive, proximal weakness sometimes associated with large calves.

    b. Fasciculations may be visible in the extremities and tongue. Upper motor neuron signs are absent.

    c. This disorder may result from an autosomal recessive or autosomal dominant gene.

3. The diagnosis is made on the basis of the clinical presentation, evidence of denervation on EMG studies, and characteristic pathology in histochemically stained muscle biopsies.

Treatment:

1. There is no specific treatment, but physical and occupational therapy should be directed toward maintaining limb function and preventing deformity.

2. Genetic counseling is necessary.

3. Emotional support for the family should be provided.

4. Further information on services available to patients can be obtained from the Muscular Dystrophy Association (address above).

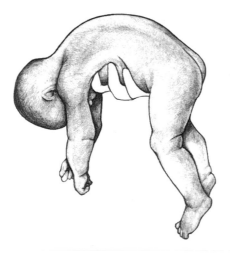

Figure 15.1. A 1-year-old "floppy baby" with infantile spinal muscular atrophy (Werdnig-Hoffmann disease). Note that there is a marked lack of muscle tone.

Peroneal Muscular Atrophy Syndrome (Charcot-Marie-Tooth Disease, Idiopathic Dominantly Inherited Hypertrophic Polyneuropathy, Hereditary Motor and Sensory Neuropathy)

1. This autosomal dominant disorder is associated with slowly progressive foot deformity (pes cavus and hammer toes) and atrophy of lower legs resulting in "stork legs" or "inverted champagne bottle legs" (see Figure 15.2).
2. Diagnosis is suggested by appropriate clinical findings, family history, and abnormal nerve conduction studies and EMG.
3. Clinical presentation of this disorder varies from family to family, but within a single family the symptomatology of affected individuals tends to be similar.
4. In some families other neurologic signs may be present such as sensory loss, enlarged nerves, or cerebellar ataxia.

Treatment:

There is no specific treatment for this disorder, although disability is usually mild and compatible with long life. Genetic counseling is necessary. Prevention of injuries to limbs that have reduced sensibility is imperative. Supportive physical and occupational therapy can often be provided through the Muscular Dystrophy Association (address above).

Poliomyelitis

1. Poliomyelitis is an acute viral infection of the anterior horn cells. The

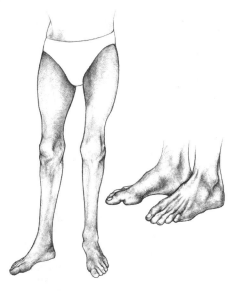

Figure 15.2. Patients with the peroneal muscular atrophy syndrome (Charcot-Marie-Tooth disease) have a ''stork-legs'' appearance due to atrophy of the lower leg and distal one-third of thigh musculature. Hammer toes and pes cavus may also be an early sign of this disorder.

weakness is often preceded by gastroenteritis.

2. The disease is usually asymmetric, with flaccid weakness.
3. There may be paralysis of the bulbar muscles.
4. Poliomyelitis is associated with aseptic meningitis.
5. The diagnosis is confirmed by acute and convalescent serologic titers.
6. Many years after the acute paralysis with varying degrees of subsequent recovery, occasional patients may experience apparent progressive weakness, sometimes accompanied by pain. Most often this weakness is not due to any new anterior horn cell loss, but is the result of:
   a. Normal age-related loss of muscle power (which compromises already marginal muscle function).
   b. Degenerative arthritis (developing in joints subjected to abnormal stresses from the long-standing muscle pareses) limiting joint and muscle function and resulting in pressure neuropathies or radiculopathies
   c. Bracing and prostheses, which are currently inappropriate (often not having been re-evaluated since the time of the initial polio episode).

Only very rare patients develop the ''postpolio syndrome'' of further progressive unexplained anterior horn cell loss.

Treatment:

1. There is no specific treatment for the infection.
2. Respiratory function may need to be supported.
3. The disease is now rare in North America due to prevention with appropriate vaccination. Contacts should be vaccinated if not previously done.

Diseases of the Neuromuscular Junction

Myasthenia Gravis

This is a disease of the neuromuscular junction in which weakness develops after repetitive muscle contraction (''fatigable weakness''); it usually presents with some degree of ophthalmoplegia.

1. Myasthenia gravis should be strongly suspected in any patient who reports excessive weakness at the end of the day. The complaints of weakness are frequently bizarre and are often interpreted as a psychiatric disturbance, especially since the routine neurologic examination is normal in most patients.
2. When the physician entertains the diagnosis of myasthenia, the following examinations should be performed:
   a. Since the eyes are most frequently involved, have the patient maintain a sustained upward gaze for at least three minutes without interruption. In the myasthenic patient, one or both eyelids will often begin to droop and/or the gaze will cease to be conjugate (see Figure 15.3).
   b. Have the patient perform repetitive muscle contractions related to the complaint, and observe for evidence of developing weakness. For example, if the patient complains of weakness in climbing stairs, repetitive deep knee bends will become progressively more difficult to perform. If the patient complains of weakness in the hands, repetitive squeezing of a manometer cuff will show a progressive decrease in power. If the patient complains of difficulty in swallowing, repeated sips from a large glass of water will be normal at first but subsequently result in choking.
3. Involvement of respiratory and/or pharyngeal muscles may occur with variable severity in the disease, and can lead to fatal respiratory failure or aspiration.
4. Definitive diagnosis:
   a. Tensilon (edrophonium chloride) test
      i. Establish parameters for success or failure of this test; for example, the disappearance of ptosis or restoration of strength after weakness had been produced by repetitive action.

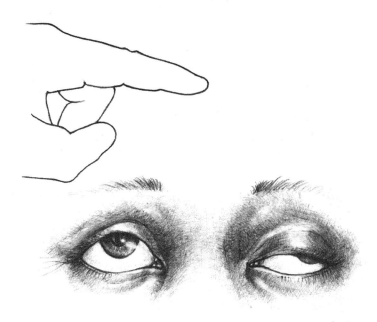

Figure 15.3. In myasthenia gravis fatigable weakness is evident on examination of eye movements. There is usually ptosis which becomes more evident as the patient attempts to sustain upward gaze.

    ii. Be sure that there is adequate preparation to deal with complications, which may include respiratory arrest and cardiac arrhythmias.

   iii. Establish an IV line in the patient and prepare the following solutions:

      (a) An IV bottle of either normal saline or 5% dextrose in water.

      (b) Normal saline is drawn up into a 2 mL syringe and labeled "A."

      (c) Tensilon (as 5 mg/mL-ampule) is drawn up into a 2 mL syringe and labeled "B."

   iv. The physician should be positive in statements about the effectiveness of each injection. First, inject syringe "A" (saline placebo) in 0.5 mL increments and appear very disappointed when there is no effect.

    v. Then syringe "B" (Tensilon) should be injected in 0.5 mL increments; often an effect will be evident with as little as 5 mg.

   vi. A dramatic improvement in the selected parameter should occur within 30 seconds after the injection of the Tensilon and revert to its original state after two minutes. Effects occurring with saline placebo or before 30 seconds and after two minutes with Tensilon injection should be suspect.

   b. Repetitive motor nerve stimulation (Jolly test) results in a characteristic pattern in myasthenia gravis; single-fiber EMG is abnormal.

   c. Tests of stapedial reflex fatigue may also be used to establish the diagnosis.

   d. Provocative tests for myasthenia (such as curare tests) are rarely essential for diagnosis and may be extremely dangerous if not carried out under carefully controlled in-hospital circumstances.

   e. Anti-acetylcholine receptor antibody (AChR-Ab) titers are elevated in 75% to 90% of myasthenic patients.

5. In certain circumstances myasthenic crisis (acute or subacute onset of respiratory failure) may be induced by drugs or infection, and treatment of this constitutes a neurologic emergency (see Chapter 20). Some of the drugs that can produce a myasthenic crisis are curare, succinylcholine, streptomycin, dihydrostreptomycin, kanamycin, polymyxin, lincomycin, tetracycline, oxytetracycline, gentamicin, viomycin, and quinine (tonic water).

Note: Agents which are safe in myasthenia gravis include penicillin, cephalothin, rifampin, vancomycin, amphotericin, and nystatin.

6. Thymic abnormalities (hyperplasia or thymoma) occur in about 80% of myasthenic patients.

7. During the neonatal period, 20% of infants born to myasthenic mothers have transient feeding difficulties, weak cry, breathing difficulties, floppiness, and other myasthenic symptoms (neonatal myasthenia), and require only supportive treatment.

8. D-Penicillamine can occasionally induce myasthenia gravis, which usually resolves within 1 year of discontinuing the drug.

Treatment:

   1. Initial treatment is usually with anticholinesterases (such as pyridostigmine bromide) for a trial period, although nearly all myasthenic patients require treatment in a tertiary hospital setting where therapy includes thymectomy (sternal splitting approach), plasmapheresis, alternate-day corticosteroids, and immunosuppressive therapy.

   2. Respiratory failure may occur during a crisis and is a neurologic emergency requiring ventilatory support (see Chapter 20).

Lambert-Eaton (Myasthenic) Syndrome

1. The Lambert-Eaton syndrome resembles myasthenia gravis with complaints of tiredness and weakness, but unlike myasthenia gravis, ocular involvement is rare.

2. Strength may improve temporarily after voluntary contraction, but prolonged effort results in fatigue.

3. Muscle tendon reflexes are depressed, but may improve after exercise.

4. Response to Tensilon is usually equivocal, and the diagnosis is established by characteristic findings with repetitive motor nerve stimulation.

5. Often associated with an occult malignancy (particularly lung carcinoma) or with autoimmune disease.

6. An antibody directed against the nerve terminal has been identified in affected patients; rare patients also have antiacetylcholine receptor antibodies and may have signs and symptoms of both myasthenia gravis and the Lambert-Eaton syndrome.

Treatment:

1. For the non-neoplasm-related syndrome, treatment includes plasmapheresis, prednisone 30-60 mg qid, and/or azathioprine 1.5 to 2.0 mg/kg/day. For neoplasm-associated disease, antitumor therapy is required; plasmapheresis and/or prednisone may be used in addition, but immunosuppressive therapy should be avoided.

2. Symptomatic improvement of strength and exercise tolerance may be achieved with guanidine 10-35 mg/kg/day or 4-aminopyridine 40 to 200 mg/day; potential side effects of guanidine include ataxia, gastrointestinal distress, bone marrow depression, and renal failure; side effects of 4-aminopyridine include seizures and a confusional state.

Botulism

1. Botulism presents as subacute paralysis of extraocular muscles with subsequent involvement of pharyngeal muscles.

2. Respiratory compromise secondary to skeletal muscle weakness occurs 24 to 48 hours after onset.

3. Botulism is caused by ingestion of toxin produced by *Clostridium botulinum,* which may be found in improperly canned acidic foods such as green beans.

4. Diagnosis can be confirmed by characteristic findings on repetitive nerve stimulation.

Treatment:

1. Polyvalent botulinum antitoxin should be administered, and stomach and intestinal contents removed.

2. Respiratory failure is a major concern and should be monitored and treated in a manner similar to the respiratory problems of Guillian-Barré syndrome.

Diseases of Muscle

Myotonic Dystrophy (Steinert's Disease)

1. The patient will complain of muscular stiffness, which is relieved after repetitive activity.
2. Myotonia is a delayed relaxation of muscles, clinically recognized by:
   a. Having the patient make a tightly clenched fist for 30 seconds and observing the difficulty in opening the hand.
   b. Percussion of the thenar eminence with a reflex hammer will cause the thumb to oppose the little finger and remain so for several seconds.
   c. Percussion of the gastrocnemius produces a transient hard lump in the gastrocnemius.
   d. EMG shows a characteristic "dive-bomber" pattern.
3. The patient develops slowly progressive distal weakness, especially in the upper extremities; a foot drop may develop later.
4. Facial features are often characteristic (see Figure 15.4); other characteristics include pronounced frontal balding, ptosis, cataracts, cardiac

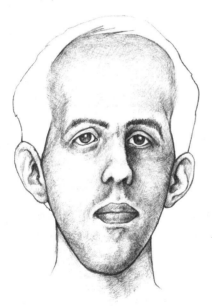

Figure 15.4. Patients with myotonic dystrophy have characteristic facial features of frontal baldness, depression of the temporal region (due to atrophy and loss of bulk of the temporalis muscle), and a long thin face with a pointed chin.

conduction defects, glucose intolerance, disturbed gastrointestinal motility, sleep problems (daytime somnolence), and psychological disturbances (depression).

5. The disorder is transmitted by an autosomal dominant gene.

6. Myotonic dystrophy may present in infancy as a floppy baby with respiratory distress and difficulty in feeding, usually in myotonic infants
born to myotonic mothers.

7. Some other diseases with myotonia include myotonia congenita and
hyperkalemic periodic paralysis.

Treatment:

1. Most patients do not require treatment of the myotonia, but in occasional patients with incapacitating myotonia, phenytoin 100 to 400
mg/day is the preferred drug for relief of symptoms, although alternate drugs are available on an experimental basis.

2. Genetic counseling should be provided.

3. Cardiac evaluations are mandatory and a pacemaker insertion may
be necessary to prevent fatal cardiac arrhythmias.

4. Depressive psychological (and possibly other personality) disturbances may be improved by imipramine hydrochloride 50 to 150
mg qhs.

5. Pregnant females with myotonic dystrophy should be warned that
there may be difficulty with the delivery and that the infant may
have respiratory and feeding difficulties (neonatal presentation of
myotonic dystrophy).

Duchenne's Dystrophy (X-Linked Pseudohypertrophic Muscular Dystrophy,
"Common Muscular Dystrophy")

1. This is a hereditary disorder that affects only boys and is first manifested around the age of 3 years by difficulty in climbing stairs.

2. On clinical examination, the following are seen:
   a. Calves that are larger than normal, and which have a rubbery feel
   on palpation.
   b. When the boy attempts to go from a lying to a standing position,
   he will attempt to climb up on his legs (Gowers' maneuver) (see
   Figure 15.5).

3. The diagnosis is confirmed by an extremely high serum CPK (8 to 200
times greater than normal) and by characteristic pathologic findings in
histochemically stained muscle biopsies.

4. Associated intellectual impairment is common.

Treatment:

Patients should be referred to the local Muscular Dystrophy Association

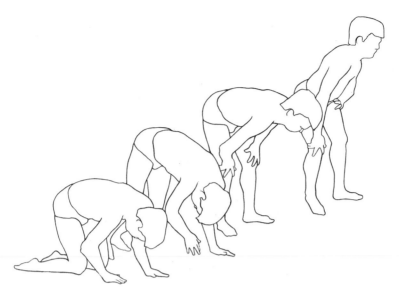

Figure 15.5. In Duchenne's muscular dystrophy, the patient will get up from the floor with the Gowers' maneuver. The boy will "walk up" his body with his hands as he arises.

clinic (national headquarters address above) which provides diagnostic facilities, genetic counseling, physical therapy, appliances such as braces and wheelchairs, and social services.

Polymyositis and Dermatomyositis

1. The patient (child or adult) presents with subacute onset of proximal weakness and muscle pain (a common complaint is difficulty in climbing stairs).

2. Neurologic examination is usually normal except for the presence of proximal weakness demonstrated by difficulty performing deep knee bends or arising from a chair (see Figure 15.6)

3. Skin lesions may be present and include malar flush, reddening at base of fingernails, a scaly rash over the extensor surface of the joints, and subcutaneous calcifications.

4. Diagnosis is established by elevated serum CPK, elevated ESR, and characteristic pathologic findings in histochemically stained muscle biopsies.

5. Occasionally associated with occult malignancy, autoimmune disorders, or AIDS.

Treatment:

Prednisone in a dose of 60 mg/M^2 (children) or 100 mg (adults) every other day will often result in a remission, but treatment with other ad-

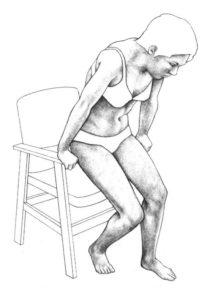

Figure 15.6. The proximal muscle weakness found in polymyositis results in difficulty arising from a chair. Note that the patient must use her arms to push off the chair to come to a standing position.

ditional immunosuppressive drugs may be necessary.

Muscle Weakness Associated with Systemic Disease (Type II Muscle Fiber Atrophy)

1. Patient presents with proximal weakness of subacute or chronic onset.
2. This is the most common cause of proximal muscle weakness.
3. Associated with disuse ("disuse atrophy") or with various chronic disorders such as cachexia, hypercorticism ("steroid myopathy"), hyperparathyroidism, cancer ("carcinomatous myopathy"), or hyperthyroidism ("thyroid myopathy").
4. EMG, nerve conduction studies, and serum CPK are usually normal.
5. Definitive diagnosis is by characteristic pathologic findings in histochemically stained muscle biopsies.

Treatment:

1. Weakness is generally reversible if the underlying cause can be corrected.
2. This potentially treatable cause of muscle weakness must be carefully differentiated from the untreatable causes of proximal muscle weakness.

Malignant Hyperthermia (Hyperpyrexia)

1. Malignant hyperthermia is characterized by sudden onset of marked hyperthermia (body temperature of 42° C or 107° F and higher) during general anesthesia with halogenated anesthetics (halothane, enflurane) or succinylcholine. Additional symptoms are extreme muscular rigidity, hyperkalemia, tachycardia, tachypnea, severe metabolic and respiratory acidosis, and myoglobinuria.

2. Frequently familial; occasionally associated with neuromuscular diseases including central core disease and myotonia congenita.

3. Susceptible patients often have elevated serum CPK in preoperative blood studies.

Treatment:

1. Death occurs in over 60% of patients in whom treatment is delayed. Immediate IV administration of dantrolene in a dose of 1 to 10 mg/kg will usually abort an episode, followed by oral dantrolene 1 to 2 mg/kg qid for one to three days to prevent recurrence.

2. Prevention is most important. If there is a family history of anesthetic-associated deaths, the known precipitating anesthetic agents should be avoided. If surgery in a known susceptible individual is indicated, preoperative treatment with dantrolene 1 to 2 mg/kg every six hours for one or two days before surgery with a last dose of 2 mg/kg three hours preoperatively may prevent development of the syndrome.

FOCAL WEAKNESS OF PERIPHERAL ORIGIN

Nerve Lesions

Localized weakness is frequently due to injury of the peripheral nerve, plexus, nerve root, or nerve cell body (see Figure 15.7). In most cases, there is both motor and sensory disturbance. The specific site of the nerve injury is recognized by the pattern of muscle weakness and by the distribution of the cutaneous sensory disturbance. Sometimes it is difficult to determine the exact muscle involvement by clinical examination, and in this instance, the EMG may determine the specific muscles involved. Most clinicians who do not frequently evaluate patients with peripheral nerve lesions will find help in the booklet: *Aids to the Examination of the Peripheral Nervous System* (London, Baillière Tindall, 1986). This thin, inexpensive paperback book can be readily carried in a physician's bag. Although specific etiologies of focal peripheral nerve weakness are not discussed in this chapter, the root lesion is most commonly caused by a herniated intervertebral disc, the plexus lesion by trauma or infection, and the peripheral nerve lesion by trauma, pressure, or vascular occlusion. Multiple individual nerve

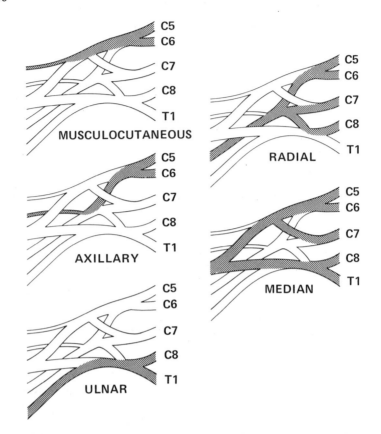

Figure 15.7. Diagram of the relationship between cervical nerve roots, brachial plexus, and peripheral nerves.

lesions may occur in a single extremity (as in trauma, vascular injury, or infection) or in multiple extremities (mononeuritis multiplex). The following is a description of common peripheral weakness patterns that should be recognized by the clinician:

Root Lesion

Common cervical root syndromes involve the C-6 and C-7 roots and are discussed in Chapter 18. The relationship of the cervical roots, brachial plexus, and peripheral nerves are shown in Figure 15.7. Common lumbar root syndromes involve the L-4, L-5, and S-1 roots and are discussed in Chapter 17.

Peripheral Nerve Lesions

 A. Radial nerve (see Figure 15.8)
     1. Weakness of extension of wrist and fingers (wrist drop)

2. Only small area of sensory loss along dorsum of base of thumb ("anatomical snuff-box")

3. Known as "Saturday night palsy" because paralysis commonly occurs from prolonged pressure on the nerve in the upper arm, such as might occur in an intoxicated person resting with an arm hanging over a park bench in a semistuporous state.

   Treatment:

   1. If injury is due to pressure, spontaneous recovery will usually occur over a 2 to 6 month period.

   2. A cock-up splint for the wrist may make the hand more functional.

B. Median nerve

1. *Carpal Tunnel Syndrome (median nerve lesion at wrist)*

   a. The patient will complain of pain and paresthesias in the hand, especially the thumb and index finger. The patient may also complain of pain more proximally in the forearm, upper arm, or shoulder. The pain is frequently worse at night, awakening the patient; pain relief is obtained by rubbing or shaking the hand and arm or letting the hand hang over the side of the bed.

   b. Although the patient may complain of reduced sensibility in the thumb and index finger, the actual sensory loss may be difficult to demonstrate on formal testing.

   c. Weakness and atrophy of the thenar muscles are usually late signs.

   d. Tinel's sign (see Figure 15.9) may be helpful. This is performed by lightly tapping the median nerve at the wrist, with such a

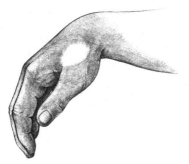

Figure 15.8. With a radial nerve palsy, there will be a wrist drop (due to weakness of the radial-innervated wrist extensor muscles) and a small patch of sensory disturbance in the area of the "anatomical snuff-box."

tap reproducing the symptoms. Hyperextension or hyperflexion of wrist may produce the same effect.

e. May be bilateral, but is usually worse in the dominant hand.

f. The definitive diagnosis may be made by nerve conduction velocity and EMG study.

g. Associated with rheumatoid arthritis (collagen vascular diseases), hypothyroidism, obesity, acromegaly, gout, and multiple myeloma; carpal tunnel syndrome initially presenting during a pregnancy usually resolves after delivery.

Treatment:

1. Treatment of any underlying disease is necessary.

2. Symptomatic relief may be obtained with a wrist splint.

3. Every patient with carpal tunnel syndrome does not necessarily need surgery, although sectioning of the carpal ligament may relieve pressure on the nerve.

2. *"Bridegroom's Palsy" (median nerve lesion in upper arm)*

a. Injury to median nerve along its course beside the brachial artery in the medial portion of the upper arm may occur from unsuccessful attempts to catheterize the brachial artery or from an abnormal sleeping position (the name is derived from the sleeping position of bridegroom's outstretched arm under bride's head).

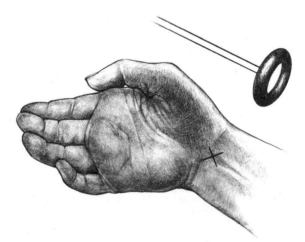

Figure 15.9. Tinel's sign is a burning-tingling sensation in the fingers, produced by tapping over the median nerve at the site of entrapment under the carpal ligament in the carpal tunnel syndrome.

b. Weakness of the prehensile abilities of the thumb is evident, including difficulty opposing the thumb to the little and index fingers; after many months atrophy of the thenar eminence may occur with recession of the thumb to form a "simian hand."

c. Sensory loss over the entire thumb, index and middle fingers, and the lateral half of the ring finger may be demonstrated.

C. Ulnar nerve

1. The commonest location of injury is at the condylar (ulnar) groove at the elbow; the commonest modes of injury are pressure and arthritis; previous fracture or a shallow condylar groove predispose to injury; "tardy ulnar palsy" refers to recurrent injuries to the ulnar nerve at the elbow, resulting in a slowly progressive loss of ulnar nerve function (frequently involving the dominant hand).

2. In mild or early injury there is:

   a. Weakness of finger extension (especially the ring and little fingers).

   b. Weakness of little finger abduction.

   c. Mild weakness of wrist flexion.

3. In severe or long-standing injury there is:

   a. Atrophy of the hypothenar eminence.

   b. Atrophy of the intrinsic hand muscles with hollowing between the metacarpal bones (especially evident in the space between the thumb and index finger; see Figure 15.10).

   c. Clawhand or "beer stein holder's hand" deformity.

4. Sensory loss of little finger and medial half of ring finger may be found.

   Treatment:

   1. Padding the elbow and educating the patient to avoid ulnar nerve injury at the elbow may result in return of ulnar nerve function.

   2. Anterior surgical transplantation of the nerve may be necessary to avoid repeated injury.

Caveat: The radial, ulnar, and median nerves all supply the muscles of the thumb. Extension is served by the radial nerve, adduction by the ulnar nerve, and opposition by the median nerve (see Figure 15.11).

D. Facial palsy (Bell's palsy)

1. In facial palsy, there is acute or subacute onset of complete or partial unilateral paralysis of the facial muscles including the forehead (see Figure 15.12). This paralysis may be associated with a pre-

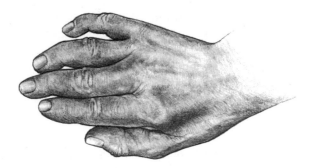

Figure 15.10. Lesions of the ulnar nerve produce atrophy of the interossei of the hand, which is evident as a ''guttering'' between the carpal bones.

vious nonspecific viral illness and is not associated with any other neurologic abnormalities.

2. Patient may complain of hypersensitivity to noise on the same side due to paralysis of the stapedius muscle.

3. If the injury to the facial nerve is proximal to the chorda tympani, examination of taste on the anterior two-thirds of the tongue on the same side as the paralysis will reveal loss; however, patients rarely complain of any change in taste.

4. Patient may complain that food accumulates in the paralyzed cheek

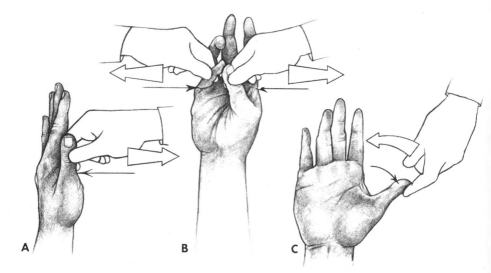

Figure 15.11. Functional integrity of the radial, median, and ulnar nerves can be tested by examining the strength of the thumb: A. Adduction — ulnar innervated muscles. B. Opposition — median-innervated muscles. C. Extension — radial-innervated muscles.

(due to buccinator muscle paralysis) resulting in difficulty in chewing; there is no true dysphagia.

5. *Caution*: Bell's palsy is an idiopathic disorder with a good prognosis for spontaneous recovery. However, it must be differentiated from other causes of facial paralysis, including the following:

   a. If there is decreased hearing or a decreased corneal reflex, suspect an acoustic neuroma.

   b. If there are vesicles in the external auditory canal then the Ramsey-Hunt syndrome (infection of the geniculate ganglion with herpes zoster) must be suspected. There may be an underlying lymphoma.

   c. Chronic otitis media or mastoiditis may damage the facial nerve.

   d. The facial nerve passes through the parotid gland and infection or inflammation (including sarcoidosis) of the parotid may cause facial nerve paralysis.

   Treatment:

   1. Spontaneous recovery usually occurs.

   2. Corticosteroids have not been shown to be of definite benefit, although it is common practice to administer prednisone 80 mg qd for five days if the patient is seen within

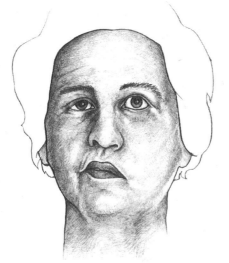

Figure 15.12. The patient with Bell's palsy (facial nerve palsy) will demonstrate an unwrinkled forehead, widely opened eye (with weakness of eyelid closure), flattening of the nasolabial fold, and a droop of the corner of the mouth.

three days of the onset or if pain in or behind the ear is prominent.

3. The eye is vulnerable because lid closure is impaired, and the cornea must be protected with ophthalmic ointments, patches, and/or goggles.

E. Femoral nerve

1. The patient presents with difficulty in climbing stairs due to weakness of one or both quadriceps muscles (sometimes incorrectly called "quadriceps myopathy"). The patient may compensate for this weakness by walking with the knee rigid. With a long standing or severe lesion there is wasting of the quadriceps and, in children, development of genu recurvatum.

2. The patellar (knee) reflex is reduced or absent.

3. Sensory loss may be detected over the anteromedial thigh.

4. Femoral neuropathy is often associated with diabetes mellitus or trauma. Femoral neuropathy must be differentiated from disuse atrophy (in which the knee reflex is preserved) and polymyositis (in which the serum CPK is elevated and/or the muscle biopsy is abnormal).

F. Peroneal nerve

1. The patient presents with foot drop ("slapping foot"). A peroneal nerve lesion causes weakness of extension of the foot and toes and weakness of eversion (turning out) of the foot. In long-standing or severe lesions, there is wasting of the anterolateral compartment of the lower leg (see Figure 15.13).

2. Sensory loss may sometimes be demonstrated over the lateral and anterior portions of the lower leg and dorsum of the foot

3. Common peroneal nerve injury in the lateral knee where the nerve courses around the head of the fibula often results from:

   a. Sitting with legs crossed

   b. Pressure during sleep, coma, or anesthesia.

   c. Pressure by casts, garters, boots, or braces.

   d. Trauma or laceration to the area of the fibular head (as in climbing over a barbed wire fence).

Caveat: A peroneal nerve injury resembles an L-5 root lesion; however, the internal hamstring reflex is diminished in an L-5 root lesion but not in a peroneal nerve lesion (see Chapter 17), and the posterior tibial muscle (which inverts a plantar-flexed foot) is weak in an L-5 root lesion but not in a peroneal nerve lesion.

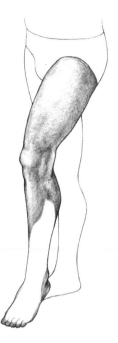

Figure 15.13. In long-standing or severe lesions of the peroneal nerve there is wasting of the anterolateral compartment of the lower leg.

G. Lateral femoral cutaneous nerve (meralgia paresthetica)

1. Patient presents with a sensory disturbance on the lateral aspect of the thigh (see Figure 15.14). This abnormal sensation may be reduced sensibility, a pins-and-needles feeling, or a burning discomfort. Abnormal sensations may be exacerbated by touching the skin (as from clothing or stockings) or by prolonged standing or walking.

2. Since this is a sensory nerve to the skin, weakness is never present.

3. Symptoms are due to compression of the lateral femoral cutaneous nerve in its passage under the inguinal ligament.

4. This condition is common in obesity, pregnancy, diabetes, trauma to the inguinal area, or after wearing tight-fitting corsets.

Brachial Plexus Lesions

Lesions of the brachial plexus are difficult to diagnose but should be suspected when there is more extensive involvement than would be produced by a lesion of a single nerve or root.

A. Upper trunk of brachial plexus (Erb-Duchenne palsy)

1. The patient presents with weakness about the shoulder and the el-

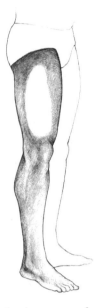

Figure 15.14. Meralgia paresthetica is an uncomfortable (burning) sensation in the distribution of the lateral femoral cutaneous nerve. Both the hypersensitivity to sensory stimulation and loss of normal sensibility can usually be demonstrated in this distribution.

bow. The arm may dangle at the side with the fingers slightly flexed and the palm facing backward (the so-called porter's tip position; see Figure 15.15). This is due to inability to abduct and externally rotate the shoulder and to supinate and flex the forearm.

2. Biceps and brachioradialis reflexes are absent.

3. Sensory loss is minimal but, if present, may be found over the lateral shoulder, thumb, and index finger.

4. The patient usually complains of a diffuse discomfort or pain in the shoulder.

5. Lesions are produced by sudden traction that pulls the shoulder downward and pulls the neck away in the direction opposite to the shoulder; may occur during anesthesia, motorcycle accidents, "rucksack paralysis," or as a birth injury.

Note: An upper trunk injury resembles a C-6 root lesion; external rotation and abduction of the shoulder are severely affected in the plexus lesion but not in the C-6 root lesion. Also, sensation is usually intact in the upper trunk lesion but a sensory disturbance is present in the C-6 root lesion (see Chapter 18).

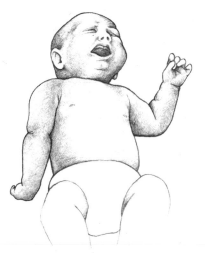

Figure 15.15. An Erb-Duchenne palsy (lesion of upper trunk of brachial plexus) will result in an inability to abduct and externally rotate the arm with weakness of wrist extension leading to the characteristic "porter's tip" posture. Such an injury is not uncommon in infants due to traction on the head and neck during delivery.

    B. Lower trunk of the brachial plexus (Klumpke-Dejerine palsy)

        1. The patient presents with weakness of forearm flexors and all intrinsic muscles of the hand; in long-standing or severe lesions, there will be atrophy of the intrinsic muscles of the hand, recession of the thumb into the plane of the hand, and extension of the wrist.

        2. Triceps reflex is absent.

        3. Often there is no sensory disturbance but, if present, may be found along the posteromedial aspect of the forearm and the ulnar side of the hand.

        4. Patient will frequently complain of a diffuse pain in the shoulder and axilla.

        5. May be associated with Horner's syndrome (ptosis, miosis, and facial anhidrosis on same side as the injury) due to damage to preganglionic sympathetic nerve fibers in the T-1 root.

        6. Results from sudden upward pull on the shoulder; for example, parent jerking upward on the arm of a falling child.

    C. Brachial plexus neuritis (brachial plexitis)

        1. Patient will present with the sudden onset of severe pain, usually at night, in the shoulder and/or arm, which is exacerbated by arm movement and elbow flexion.

2. Weakness develops progressively within 2 weeks of the onset of pain, usually involving the shoulder girdle musculature innervated by the upper trunk of the brachial plexus with lesser diffuse involvement of the musculature innervated by the rest of the plexus.

3. Reflexes will be variably reduced depending on the extent and degree of involvement.

4. Sensory loss is minimal or not detectable.

5. May involve both arms but is usually asymmetric with greater involvement in the dominant arm.

6. CSF is normal.

Treatment:

Spontaneous recovery usually occurs but may take up to 2 years. Contractures may develop unless physical therapy range-of-motion exercises are undertaken until strength returns.

Other Lesions Causing Focal Weakness

Cervical Bony Anomalies

The most common problem is the *thoracic outlet syndrome* (also see Chapter 18):

1. Thoracic outlet syndrome is characterized by weakness and atrophy of the thenar musculature with lesser weakness and atrophy of other intrinsic hand muscles and flexor muscles of the forearm.

2. The finger and wrist extensors and the proximal arm musculature are preserved.

3. Biceps and triceps reflexes are preserved.

4. Intermittent aching pain in the arm is often present for many years, particularly the ulnar side of the forearm and hand (frequently exacerbated at night) with numbness and tingling in the forearm.

5. Differentiation from the carpal tunnel syndrome is the presence of weakness in nearly all small hand muscles.

6. The EMG shows denervation in the hand musculature. Nerve conduction velocities are slightly, but uniformly, slow without localized delay at the wrist (as in carpal tunnel syndrome) or elbow (as in tardy ulnar palsy).

7. The diagnosis is based on correlating the clinical and electrophysiologic findings with radiographic evidence of a long down-curving transverse process of C-7 or a rudimentary cervical rib.

Treatment:

If symptoms are not relieved by physical therapy, surgical release of the dense fibrous band connecting the first rib to the transverse process of C-7 or to a rudimentary cervical rib may be necessary to free the C-8 and T-1 roots stretched and angulated over this band.

Focal Myositis

1. Muscle inflammation may occur secondary to bacterial infection (*Staphylococcus* or *Streptococcus* abscess), parasitic infestation (toxoplasmosis, trichinosis, *Toxocara*), or granulomatous disease (tuberculosis, histoplasmosis, actinomycosis, sarcoidosis).
2. The patient presents with swelling, weakness, pain, and tenderness in the affected muscles. This may be confused clinically with nerve, plexus, or root lesions, but may be differentiated by finding serum CPK elevation.
3. Definitive diagnosis may be made by muscle biopsy with histochemical staining, bacterial and fungal stains, and culture.

Treatment:

Treatment is of the basic disease process. Fasciotomy may be necessary to prevent ischemic necrosis if associated swelling is marked.

Dupuytren's Contracture

1. There is progressive flexion contracture of the proximal joints of the ring finger, little finger, and middle finger, frequently bilateral. Thickened bands of palmar fascia may be seen and palpated (see Figure 15.16).
2. May be confused with a carpal tunnel syndrome because of associated mild dull ache or tingling sensation in the palm.
3. Muscles and nerves are not involved, although secondary disuse atrophy of muscles may develop.

Treatment:

Orthopedic surgical fasciotomy or fasciectomy.

Volkmann's Ischemic Contracture

1. After acute trauma or embolism to the forearm, usually within six to 48 hours of the injury, swelling of injured tissue may occlude blood vessels causing acute ischemia and infarction of muscles and nerves.
2. Subsequent contracture may be confused with brachial plexus injury because of pronation of the forearm, flexion of the wrist, flattening of the hand (paralysis and atrophy of intrinsic hand muscles with loss of the thenar and hypothenar eminences), hyperextension of fingers at the proximal joints, flexion of the fingers at the middle joints (clawhand), and glove sensory loss (see Figure 15.17).

Treatment:

1. Acutely, surgical intervention may be necessary to relieve the forearm congestion and prevent ischemia and infarction.

260

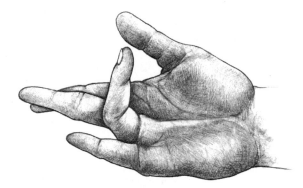

Figure 15.16. A bandlike thickening of the palmar fascia is evident in Dupuytren's contracture.

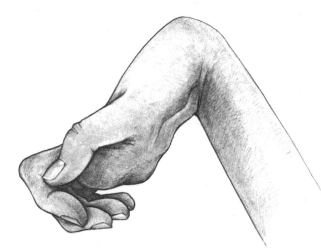

Figure 15.17. In Volkman's ischemic contracture there is atrophy and fibrosis of the forearm and hand resulting in a fixed posture.

2. Once the contracture develops, orthopedic procedures may be performed to provide some hand function.

BIBLIOGRAPHY

Asbury AK, Johnson PC: *Pathology of Peripheral Nerve*. Philadelphia, WB Saunders Co, 1978.
Brooke MH: *A Clinician's View of Neuromuscular Diseases*. ed.2. Baltimore, Williams & Wilkins Co, 1986.

Brumback RA, Gerst J (eds): *The Neuromuscular Junction*. Mount Kisco, NY, Futura Publishing Co, 1984.

Brumback RA, Leech RW: *Color Atlas of Muscle Histochemistry*. Littleton, Mass, PSG Publishing Co, 1984.

Carpenter S, Karpati G: *Pathology of Skeletal Muscle*. New York, Churchill Livingstone, 1984.

Dubowitz V: *Muscle Disorders in Childhood*. London, WB Saunders Co, 1978.

Dyck PJ, Thomas PK, Lambert EH, et al (eds): *Peripheral Neuropathy*, ed 2. Philadelphia, WB Saunders Co, 1984.

Engel AG, Banker BQ (eds): *Myology*. New York, McGraw-Hill Book Co, 1986.

Gamstorp I, Sarnat HB (eds): *Progressive Spinal Muscular Atrophies*. New York, Raven Press, 1984.

Lund H, Nilsson O, Rosen I: Treatment of Lambert-Eaton syndrome. *Neurology* 1984; 34:1324-1330.

Mulder DW (ed): *The Diagnosis and Treatment of Amyotrophic Lateral Sclerosis*. Boston, Houghton Mifflin, 1980.

Nakano KK: *Neurology of Musculoskeletal and Rheumatic Disorders*. Boston, Houghton Mifflin, 1979.

Vinken PJ, Bruyn GW, Ringel SP (eds): *Handbook of Clinical Neurology. Volume 40. Part 1-Diseases of Muscle*. Amsterdam, North Holland Publishing Co, 1979.

Vinken PJ, Bruyn GW, Ringel SP (eds): *Handbook of Clinical Neurology. Volume 41. Part II-Diseases of Muscle*. Amsterdam, North Holland Publishing Co.,1979.

Walton J: *Disorders of Voluntary Muscle*. ed 5. New York, Churchill Livingstone, 1988.

XVI

THE CHILD WHO IS NOT DEVELOPING OR LEARNING NORMALLY

Children are frequently brought to the physician for evaluation of neurologic problems. Apart from the focal neurologic symptoms described in other sections of this book, children may be referred for evaluation of deviation from the expected normal pattern of development. In this chapter, the problems are categorized according to the age at which the child is most likely to present to the physician for evaluation and treatment. For many of the disorders, a multidisciplinary approach to evaluation and treatment is required. For the child under 3 years of age, the physician usually needs to coordinate the services of these various disciplines, but for the child over 3 years of age school systems (as required by Public Law 94-142, Education for All Handicapped Act of 1975) may coordinate services with the physician acting as a member of the multidisciplinary team. Table 16.1 lists some of the kinds of problems.

Every child under the age of 3 years who visits a primary care physician should be screened for developmental delays, as part of the general physical examination or well-baby visit. This task can be simplified by providing a growth and developmental questionnaire for parents to fill out in the waiting room, by routinely plotting heights, weights, and head circumference measurements (see Appendix D) and by training an office assistant or nurse to administer the Denver Developmental Screening Test (see Appendix D). Observations by a sensitive receptionist or secretary of behavior in the waiting room are also helpful. Remember that during the first 2 years of life, the child's responses are limited and consist mainly of motor responses. After that period,

Table 16.1.
Developmental, Learning, and Behavioral Problems by Age

AGE OF CHILD	ASSESSABLE RESPONSES	TYPES OF ABNORMALITIES
Infants and toddlers (Birth to 3 yr)	Developmental screening Gross motor Speech Dysmorphic features Neurometabolic urine screening Denver Developmental Screening Test	"Cerebral palsies" Dysgenetic ("FLK") syndromes Inborn errors of metabolism Chromosomal disorders
Preschool years (3-6 yr)	Language Fine motor Adaptive and social development	Hearing loss Mental retardation syndromes

School age (6-12 yr)	Cognitive development
	Emotional/social development
	Moral development
	Behavioral development
	Minor neurologic signs
	  ("soft signs") through special
	  neurologic examinations
		Developmental language
		  disorders
		Hyperactivity-attentional
		  disorders
		Learning disability syndromes
		Childhood depression
		Behavioral disorders
		Petit mal epilepsy

Adolescence (12-18 yr)	Emotional health Neuropsychological assessments	Attentional disorders Written language disabilities Adolescent adjustment reactions Psychiatric disorders Alcohol and drug abuse

language develops and makes assessment of intellectual functioning easier. Once the child enters school, abnormalities of learning and various types of behavior disorders may also become evident.

One of the most important roles of the physician is to determine whether the child's deviation from normal is the result of slow development, developmental arrest, or developmental deterioration, since this will determine the types of disease processes considered and hence the evaluation undertaken (see Figure 16.1). The rate of acquisition of new milestones provides dynamic clues to developmental disabilities. By schematically graphing time against courses of abnormal development for any given series of developmental milestones, it is possible to show three different schematic graphs. Children with slow development (Figure 16.1A) require evaluation by psychosocial and educational services and referral to appropriate community resources. The presence of developmental arrest (Figure 16.1B) or deterioration of functioning (Figure 16.1C) will almost always require referral to a specialized diagnostic center.

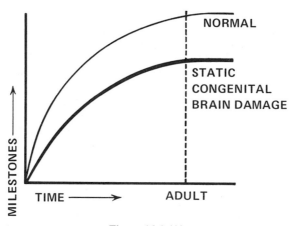

Figure 16.1 (A)

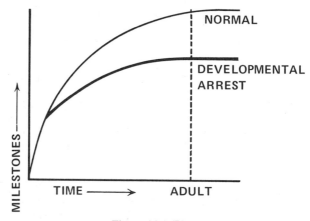

Figure 16.1 (B)

Figure 16.1. (A). In slow development the child starts slowly and gradually falls further behind his normal peers, because the rate of development is also slow. This type of developmental curve is seen in the child with a static congenital encephalopathy or with Down's syndrome. (B). Developmental arrest occurs in the child who has shown normal development from birth, but stops acquiring new skills. This type of developmental curve may be found in the child who has been successfully treated for bacterial meningitis or who has sustained significant head trauma. (*Caution*: This type of curve may also be seen in the early phases of a degenerative process when the natural acquisition of developmental milestones may balance the deterioration.) (C). Deterioration of functioning (the actual loss of previously acquired milestones) implies an ongoing destructive process in the brain. This type of curve may be found in hydrocephalus, untreated galactosemia or phenylketonuria, or rare CNS neurometabolic diseases.

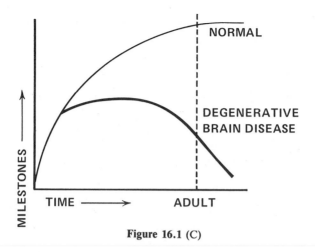

Figure 16.1 (C)

INFANTS AND TODDLERS

How to Identify an Infant Who is Not Developing Normally

Obtain the history to determine whether the child has any of the risk factors such as those listed in Table 16.2. The infant at risk for later developmental, learning, or behavioral problems is one:

1. Whose prenatal and perinatal history reveals certain risk factors (see Table 16.2).

Table 16.2
EXAMPLE OF SOME FACTORS THAT PLACE AN INFANT IN THE HIGH-RISK CATEGORY FOR FUTURE ABNORMAL DEVELOPMENT NECESSITATING CAREFUL PHYSICIAN FOLLOW-UP

1. Maternal diabetes
2. Maternal toxemia
3. Maternal viral infection (especially rubella)
4. Maternal alcoholism or drug ingestion
5. Teenage mother
6. Old mother (over 35 years old, especially if first pregnancy)
7. Fetal distress during delivery
8. Breech presentation
9. Prematurity
10. Infant small for gestational age (assessed by Dubowitz scale of newborn age and Lubchenko charts)
11. Neonatal respiratory distress
12. Neonatal seizures
13. Neonatal infection (especially meningitis)
14. Prolonged neonatal jaundice

2. Who acquires illnesses that may injure the brain, such as head trauma, meningitis, or malnutrition.

3. Whose rate of acquisition of developmental milestones deviates from normal expectancy.

Note: Risk factors are not only biological, but more importantly are often psychosocial, such as poor maternal-child interaction, inappropriate parenting by primary caregivers, and child abuse or neglect. Other risk factors are poverty, with its attendant cultural deprivation and accompanying emotional and nutritional deprivation, although wealth, with its tendency for overindulgence, can also inhibit emotional and behavioral development. The physician cannot alter the nonbiological risk factors but can exert great indirect influence by compassionate parent education and sensitive referral to psychological and social services. Any infant in the high-risk category should receive special attention.

Caveat: The majority of causes of mental retardation tend to fall into a few broad categories:

Perinatal hypoxia and ischemia
Infection - prenatal, perinatal, or neonatal
Down's syndrome
Fragile-X syndrome

Obtain *history* of developmental milestones in infancy, in particular looking for evidence of:

1. Absence of social smile after 8 weeks

2. Poor head control while sitting on mother's lap after 4 months

3. Inability to sit unsupported after 8 months

4. Inability to play games such as peek-a-boo, bye-bye, and pat-a-cake after 12 months

5. Inability to walk independently by 15 months

6. Persistent hand preference before 12 months

7. Delay in speech milestones (see Tables 16.3 and 16.4)

8. Peculiar postures or modes of crawling (lying frog-legged, crawling on one side, kicking of legs symmetrically after 4 months)

Physical Examination of the Infant

The essential parts of the pediatric neurologic examination include the following:

1. Head circumference: Measure frontal-to-occipital head circumference (see Figure 16.2) and plot on an appropriate growth chart (see Appendix D). Values less than the fifth or greater than the ninety-fifth percentiles are abnormal. Serial measurements are more reliable than single measurements. Growth should be along a percentile line, and deviation

Table 16.3.
Important Speech and Language Milestones (Ages 6-30 Months)

RECEPTIVE LANGUAGE	AGE (MONTHS)	EXPRESSIVE LANGUAGE
Turns to sound of bell	6	Cries, laughs, babbles
Waves "bye-bye" Knows meaning of "no" and "don't touch"	9	Imitates sounds and makes dental sounds during play ("da-da")
	12	1-2 words ("da-da," "mama," "bye")
Responds to "come here"	15	Jargon (speechlike babbling during play)
Points to nose, eyes, hair	18	8-10 words (1/3 are nouns), puts 2 words together ("more cookie"), repeats requests
Points to a few named objects and obeys simple commands	24	Asks 1- to 2-word questions ("Where kitty?")
Repeats 2 numbers and Can identify by name. "What barks?" and "What blows?"	30	Uses "I," "you," "me," names objects, uses 3-word simple sentences

Table 16.4.
Important Speech Milestones (Ages 3 to 6.5 Years)

RECEPTIVE LANGUAGE	AGE (YEARS)	EXPRESSIVE LANGUAGE
Responds to prepositions "on" and "under"	3	Masters consonants b, p, m
Responds to prepositions "in," "out," "behind," "in front of"	4	Speaks in 4- to 5-word sentences, uses future and past tenses, and masters consonants d, t, g, k
Can repeat a sentence of 7 words	5	Masters consonants f, s, v, and names red, yellow, blue, green
	6.5	Masters consonant th, uses sentences of 6-7 words length, and says numbers up to 30s

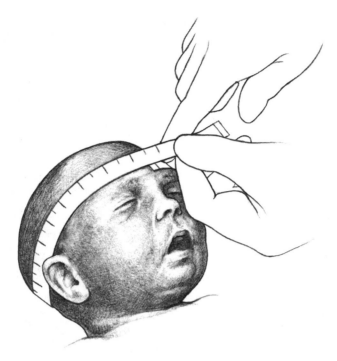

Figure 16.2. The occipital-frontal circumference (OFC) is measured by using a steel or paper centimeter tape measure, which is placed over the forehead and the occipital protuberance (see also Appendix D).

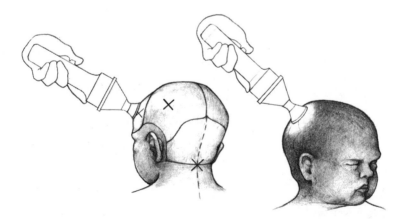

Figure 16.3. Transillumination of the head. The flashlight with rubber adaptor is placed over symmetric frontal and parietal skull areas. The rim of light around the edge of the rubber adaptor is usually no more than a few millimeters and should be symmetric (the illustrated rim is abnormal). The flashlight is placed in the midline below the occipital protuberance to inspect posterior fossa transillumination.

is abnormal. Head circumference growth should be correlated with growth in height and weight.

2. Transillumination of the head (see Figure 16.3) is performed in the newborn period and before age 1 year. A flashlight with an appropriate rubber adaptor should be used to perform this in a light-tight, darkened room after appropriate dark adaptation. A small rim of light on the scalp should surround the rubber adaptor symmetrically in similar positions on each side of the head and in the midline posteriorly at the base of skull. Excessive transillumination suggests absence of brain tissue, necessitating further evaluation. This procedure has generally been supplanted by sonograms and CT scans.

3. The skin is examined for café au lait spots, vitiliginous spots, and hairy patches over the midline (or other neurocutaneous stigmata). A Wood's lamp (ultraviolet lamp) may be helpful in detecting vitiliginous patches.

4. Observe for abnormal facial features in the eyes, ears, nose, and chin. Does the child look significantly different from the parents?

5. Observe for leg postures, particularly:
   a. Frog legs (suggests hypotonia; see Figure 16.4).
   b. Kicking legs symmetrically beyond 4 months of age (suggests spastic diplegia)

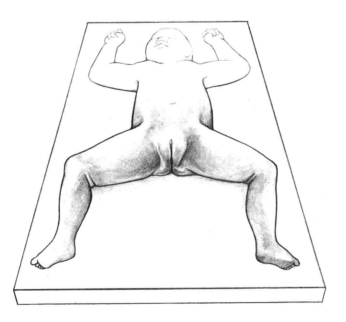

Figure 16.4. Frog-legged posture, suggesting hypotonia. Extremities are abducted proximally and flexed at elbows and knees.

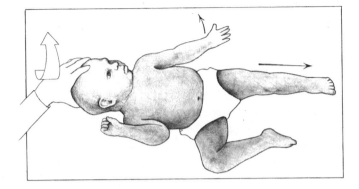

Figure 16.5. Tonic neck response: With the infant supine the arm (and leg) extend on the side toward which the head is turned while the other arm (and leg) flex ("fencing posture").

     c. Kicking only on one side (suggests spastic hemiplegia involving the less mobile side)

6. An asymmetric tonic neck response present from 2 to 6 months of age is normal; it is abnormal if the child is unable to move out of the posture (too obligatory) or if the response persists beyond age 6 months (see Figure 16.5).

7. The Moro (or startle) reflex (see Figure 16.6) in the waking state is normally present from birth to age 3 months. Persistence beyond this time is abnormal. Asymmetry in this reflex at any time is abnormal and may suggest hemiparesis, brachial plexus injury, or spinal cord defect.

8. Observe for excessive opisthotonic posturing, either spontaneously or upon being handled. This is an early sign of "cerebral palsy," which may be present before obvious diplegia or other major motor deficits.

9. In testing the child on the pull-to-sit (traction) test, the child's arm resistance, as well as head control, must be observed. By 5 months of age the head should come up with the body and not lag. The child should pull symmetrically against the examiner with both arms (see Figure 16.7). Persistent head lag is associated with hypotonic disorders. Asymmetrical arm pull suggests a hemiparesis.

10. Test for joint hyperextensibility - extending the knee beyond 180 degrees, extending the wrist back on the arm, and dorsiflexing the foot on the shin. Abnormalities are found in hypotonic children with a variety of neurologic defects.

11. Observe postural responses at 6 months in a sitting position (see Figure 16.8):

     a. When pushed to the side, the child should extend the arm to catch self.

b. When pushed backward, the child should extend the legs. Asymmetry suggests hemiparesis, and nonextension of the legs suggests a diparesis.

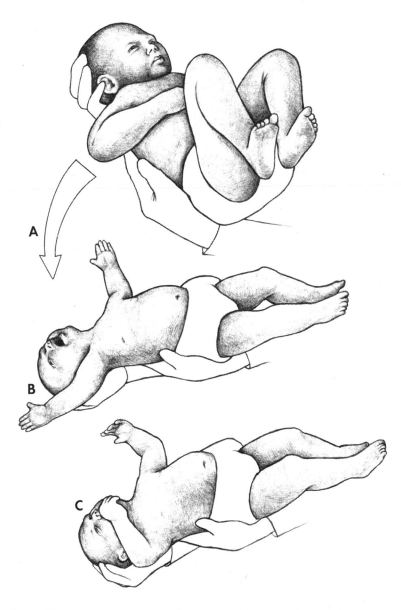

Figure 16.6. The Moro (startle) reflex is elicited by suddenly extending the baby's head (A). The normal response has two phases: first, sudden extension and abduction of the arms and extension of the legs (B); and second, slower adduction of the arms (C).

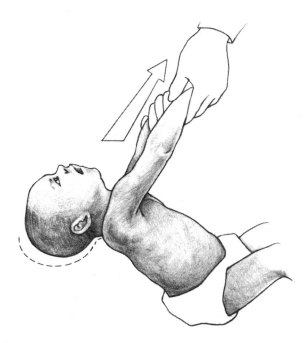

Figure 16.7. Pull-to-sit (traction) maneuver. This is tested from the newborn period to 6 months. The pull of the child's arms as well as the degree of head lag is observed.

12. Test for the parachute response (see Figure 16.9).
13. A Denver Developmental Screening Test should be done on initial contact and on the first few subsequent visits, if developmental delay is suspected. Serial developmental assessments are more predictive of later outcome than single assessments (See Appendix D).

Laboratory Studies

1. If there is *developmental delay*, the following screening procedures may be done:
   a. Urine neurometabolic screening (see Chapter 2).
   b. Neurosonography: This simple portable procedure (necessitating no radiation exposure or sedation) should be performed in all neonates with abnormal head circumference, dysmorphic features, or in whom any suspicious neurologic or behavioral signs are evident.
   c. Thyroid testing: Serum TSH, T_3, T_4
   d. If congential intrauterine infection is suspected, TORCHES (*Tox*-oplasmosis, *R*ubella, *C*ytomegalovirus, *H*erpes simplex, *S*yphilis) titers, hepatitis-B titers, and HIV (formerly known as HTLV-3 or LAV-1) titers for AIDS need to be done.

e. If dysmorphic features are prominent, chromosome studies are warranted. Chromosome breakage syndromes and the fragile-X syndrome require special media and methods, and the cytogenetics laboratory must be so alerted.

f. Skull x-rays (specifically for abnormal calcification, suture synostosis or splitting, and beaten copper appearance).

g. If developmental anomalies of the brain are suspected, CT scan or MRI of the brain is warranted.

2. If there is *developmental regression*, referral to a center with a pediatric neurologist is indicated.

3. Diseases in which there is *developmental arrest and then regression* tend to fall into only a few categories:

a. Previously diagnosed cerebral palsy, which turns out to be a misdiagnosis and is really a slowly progressive, rather than static, encephalopathy.

b. Complications of developmental brain anomalies, such as the development of hydrocephalus.

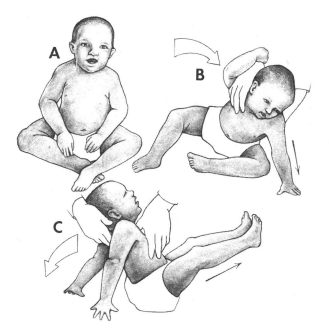

Figure 16.8. Responses to thrust in an infant in the sitting position (A). When pushed to the side, the baby extends outward the arm on that side, as if to catch the fall (B). At 6 months, when the infant is suddenly pushed backward, the legs should kick out symmetrically (C).

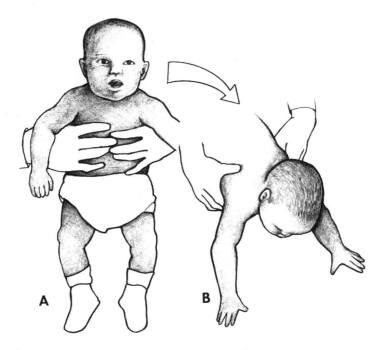

Figure 16.9. The parachute response appears at 8 months. It is elicited by suspending the baby in the upright position (A) and then rapidly propelling the head toward the examining table (but stopping short of hitting the table). The arms should thrust out symmetrically, as if to break the fall (B).

    c. Resistant seizure syndromes - infantile spasms and Lennox-Gastaut syndrome.

    d. Infectious disease, such a AIDS, SSPE (subacute sclerosing panencephalitis), or rare slow virus infections, such as progressive rubella encephalopathy or progressive multifocal leukoencephalopathy.

    e. Neurometabolic disease, such as certain aminoacidurias, lysosomal storage diseases, or peroxisomal diseases, involving primarily gray matter, or white matter, or both.

    f. Rare syndromes of episodic neurologic disturbance, associated with lactic acidosis, hyperammonemia, or progressive disorders of unknown cause such as spinocerebellar disorders or juvenile Huntington's disease.

IDENTIFIABLE CAUSES OF DEVELOPMENTAL DELAY

A. *Neonatal Hypothyroidism*

    1. Profound mental retardation will develop if treatment is delayed beyond the neonatal period. If treatment is instituted under age 3

months, 80% of infants may be normal; if treatment is delayed beyond 3 months, less than 30% will be normal.

2. Lethargic floppy infant with poor sucking.

3. Prolonged neonatal jaundice.

4. The presence of the triad of large tongue, abdominal distention, and constipation is rare and is usually found only in severe cretinism.

5. Diagnosis by heel-stick blood sample analysis for thyroxine; this is done as a routine neonatal screening in most states.

Treatment:

Immediate oral thyroxine supplementation, desiccated thyroid 15 mg qd. Patient should be followed closely with thyroid studies.

B. *Phenylketonuria (PKU)*

1. Usually a normal-appearing neonate who fails to gain weight and has feeding difficulties in the first weeks of life.

2. Seizures, poor growth, and profound mental retardation develop if untreated.

3. Autosomal recessive pattern of inheritance.

4. Diagnosis by heel-stick blood sample (drawn after milk feeding) analyzed for phenylalanine level (this screening procedure is done by law in all states) or by positive urine ferric chloride test (see Chapter 2).

Treatment:

A diet low in phenylalanine (formula such as Lofenalac) is necessary. Genetic counseling should be provided to the family.

C. *Galactosemia*

1. Normal-appearing infant who develops vomiting, diarrhea, and/or seizures of variable severity after several days or weeks of milk feeding, including breast feeding.

2. Prolonged neonatal jaundice is often present.

3. Blood glucose levels are in the hypoglycemic range only if assayed immediately after a milk feeding.

4. Autosomal recessive mode of inheritance.

5. Cataracts, hepatosplenomegaly, seizures, and profound mental retardation will develop if untreated.

6. Diagnosis after a feeding by finding low blood glucose, positive urine sugar (Clinitest tablets) but negative urine glucose (glucose oxidase urine dipsticks); quantitative galactose levels also can be obtained.

Treatment:

A galactose-free diet is necessary. Genetic counseling should be provided to the family.

D. *Down's Syndrome*

1. The clinical diagnosis of Down's syndrome is made by following criteria:
   a. Oblique palpebral fissures
   b. Epicanthal folds
   c. Brushfield's spots (light speckling) of the iris
   d. Flat nasal bridge
   e. Clinodactyly of the fifth fingers and bilateral transverse palmar creases
   f. Wide spacing of the first and second toes
   g. Hypotonia
2. Down's syndrome is more frequent in pregnancies of women over 40 years of age.
3. There is a high incidence of associated problems such as congenital heart disease, tracheoesophageal fistula, duodenal atresia, megacolon, and lymphoreticular malignancies.
4. The diagnosis is confirmed by chromosomal studies - 95% of cases have trisomy 21, the remainder have translocations or mosaicism.
5. Hip x-ray films showing a characteristic change in the acetabulum may be helpful.
6. Progressive upper cervical spine abnormalities may result in spinal cord symptomatology in late childhood or early adolescence.
7. Progressive personality changes and intellectual deterioration begin in the late twenties or early thirties with all patients having histopathologic Alzheimer's disease by age 40 years.

Treatment:

1. Although no specific medical treatment is available, there is evidence now that early intensive developmental stimulation programs and early special education programs, as well as psychosocial support result in achievement of higher functioning than what might have been predicted in the past. The degree of psychomotor retardation varies from mild to moderate, and allows placement into trainable or educable special education classes. Employment as adults in sheltered situations is possible, and independence in self-care the rule.
2. The recurrence risk after trisomy 21 is 1% to 2%; in translo-

cations, 0% if the parents are chromosomally normal. Referral to a pediatric geneticist is advisable.

3. Support groups for families are available.

4. Patient and physician information materials can be obtained from the National Down Syndrome Society, 141 Fifth Ave, New York, NY 10010 (telephone: 800-221-4602) or the National Down Syndrome Congress, 1800 Dempster St, Park Ridge, IL 60068-1146 (telephone: 800-232-NDSC).

E. *Fragile-X Syndrome*

1. Associated with moderate to severe mental retardation.

2. Dysmorphic features include large ears, prominent jaw and forehead, broad nose, high-pitched voice, macro-orchidism.

3. Often associated with seizures.

4. An X-linked disorder affecting only males, but females are carriers.

5. Chromosome studies show excessive breaks when cultured in special media.

Note: Because special culture media are required to demonstrate the chromosomal abnormality, it is imperative to alert the laboratory if this diagnosis is considered.

Treatment:

1. No specific treatment is available; seizures should be treated symptomatically (see Chapter 11); genetic counseling of the family is necessary.

2. Patient and physician information materials can be obtained from the Fragile X Foundation, PO Box 300233, Denver, Colorado 82203 (telephone: 303-861-6630).

F. *Congenital Intrauterine Infection*

1. Depending on the type and duration of the prenatal infection, the presentation of the child may vary from a small-for-dates, premature severely microcephalic infant with hepatosplenomegaly, purpura, and severe jaundice to a normal-appearing child, who does well in infancy but who develops poorly in late childhood.

2. Most common agents are in the TORCHES groups (*T*oxoplasmosis, *R*ubella, *C*ytomegalovirus, *H*erpes simplex, *S*yphilis), but other agents include the hepatitis-B virus, enterovirus, and, increasingly, HIV (the virus of AIDS).

3. Diagnosis is by determination during neonatal period of elevated (preferably from cord blood) serum IgM (and disease-specific IgM).

The agents can sometimes be cultured from the stool, urine, or throat. Serologic tests are available through state health laboratories.

4. Skull x-ray films and/or CT scans of the brain reveal punctate periventricular calcifications in cytomegalovirus infection and larger, scattered calcifications of toxoplasmosis.

5. The degree of neurologic impairment varies with the severity of infection:

   a. Seizures and severe retardation are more common with *Herpes simplex*, toxoplasmosis, and cytomegalovirus.

   b. Visual disturbances are more common with toxoplasmosis and rubella (cataracts), and hearing loss alone with cytomegalovirus.

   c. Hearing impairment together with autism is more common with rubella. A progressive rubella encephalitis continuing after the neonatal period and through the first year is now recognized.

   d. Cytomegalovirus is the most common infectious cause of mental retardation and also the most underdiagnosed.

   e. Almost any symptom can be associated with HIV infection.

Treatment

1. In congenital syphilis, procaine penicillin G 50,000 units/kg IM in single daily dose for 14 days must be administered.

2. Toxoplasmosis is treated in the child less than 1 year of age with pyrimethamine 1 mg/kg/day orally (with leucovorin calcium 5 mg twice weekly) and sulfadiazine 50 mg/kg/day orally in divided doses for 21 days. If there is evidence of active disease, additional corticosteroid (prednisone 1 to 2 mg/kg/day) may be necessary. Complicated cases requiring additional or other courses of treatment should be referred to an infectious disease center. Chorioretinitis should be managed by an ophthalmologist.

3. Since the child with any congenital infection is potentially contagious, contact with other infants and with pregnant women should be avoided (excretion of high titers of virus may continue for several months in congenital cytomegalovirus and rubella infections).

4. General supportive care only is available for rubella and cytomegalovirus, while acyclovir is available for neonatal *Herpes simplex* encephalitis (usually secondary to type 2, or genital herpes).

5. Currently there is no treatment for HIV infection, but the mother should be counseled about the risk of having further infected children.

G. *Static Congenital Encephalopathy with Predominant Motor Involvement (Cerebral Palsies)*

1. The static encephalopathies are defined as a group of disorders in which there is a major motor deficit secondary to a brain lesion acquired at or around the time of birth. Hypoxia and ischemia, infection, hemorrhage, and brain anomalies account for the majority of static encephalopathies.

2. Infant has delay in achieving motor milestones, while social and behavior development may be normal. The infant often has normal or above-normal intelligence, but 40% have varying degrees of mental retardation.

3. Some specific patterns of motor involvement can be recognized. Some children may display combinations of these patterns (mixed forms) and may show variation over time (note that the mixed forms have a worse prognosis):
   a. Hemiplegia or hemiparesis (arm and leg on same side involved; undergrowth and abnormal posturing of that side).
   b. Diplegia or diparesis (both legs involved, with minimal to absent involvement of the upper extremities) is the most common form. Usually there is delayed standing, early walking on tiptoes, and walking with scissoring or knees crossing, and in the first years of life hypotonia and decreased reflexes, but with later increased tone and hyperreflexia.

      Note: The term paraplegia refers to acquired leg paralysis secondary to spinal cord injury usually at the thoracolumbar level.

   c. Tetraplegia or tetraparesis (involvement of both legs and arms; very poor head control and trunk control on sitting) is better described as a bilateral hemiplegia, since the lesions responsible are usually bilateral hemispheric.

      Note: The term quadriplegia usually refers to paralysis of arms and legs secondary to cervical spinal cord injury.

   d. Ataxic/atonic (presentation of hypotonia in infancy, then marked unsteadiness and incoordination when the upright posture is attempted).
   e. Choreoathetosis (abnormal choreoathetoid posturing of arms and legs) is the least common form. Presentation in infancy is usually with hypotonia, which then evolves into rigidity and choreoathetoid movements.

4. Speech may be abnormal in tone, rate, and quality due to impairment of the motor aspects of articulation, while basic language expression and reception is normal. The most severe motor speech disorders,

sometimes to the point of anarthria, are seen in the choreoathetoid syndromes. Occasionally the speech disorder is disproportionately severe relative to the involvement of the extremities.

5. Epilepsy occurs in one-third or fewer of cases, primarily in those with spastic cerebral palsies (hemiplegic, diplegic, tetraplegic). When some combination of major motor defect, mental retardation, and epilepsy occurs, with or without deafness or blindness, the term *multiply handicapped* is often applied. These distinctions are important because they determine the kind of intervention programs that are appropriate.

6. Of importance in the neurologic examination is the observation of postures -- early excessive opisthotonos, obligatory spontaneous asymmetric tonic neck postures, and the persistence of developmental reflexes that should have been inhibited. The persistence of the asymmetric tonic neck reflex augurs for a poor prognosis for walking.

Caveat: "Minimal cerebral palsy" occurs in a number of children, and presents as a clumsy child, or one with "visual-perceptual" difficulties, or sometimes as an attentional-hyperactivity disorder. The diagnosis is made upon finding minimal, but definite neurologic signs, such as shortened Achilles tendons, with hyperactive lower extremity reflexes and Babinski reflexes, or mild but definite signs of congenital hemiparesis. Usually the children have no real functional handicap from the motor deficits.

Treatment:

1. Physical therapy, occupational therapy, and developmental stimulation programs must be established *early*, preferably in the first year of life, to permit maximum socialization and education of the child and to minimize the development of fixed skeletal deformities.

2. The infant that does best is the child with "pure" spastic diplegia or hemiplegia.

3. Many forms of neurodevelopmental therapies are available, which are usually administered along with routine physical-occupational therapy.

4. Follow-up care needs to be coordinated. Regional Crippled Children's Service clinics are available.

5. Information for physicians and patients may be obtained from United Cerebral Palsy Associations, 66 East 34th St, New York, NY 10016.

Caution: In patients with cerebral palsies in which there is a change in motor or mental functioning for the worse, or in which there is a family history of cerebral palsy or deaths from neurologic conditions, suspect hereditary neurometabolic disease, and refer to a pediatric neurologist.

THE PRESCHOOL YEARS (AGES 3 TO 6)

Identifying the Child Who Is Not Developing Normally

During the preschool period, the child develops language and behavioral patterns that indicate temperament or personality. Delay in speech and language is the most important disorder to assess during this period. Speech or language delay is the single most consistent predictor of later learning disabilities, particularly in reading and writing. Motor disabilities are less commonly noted for the first time during this period.

Parents may bring a child to the physician with a primary complaint of delayed speech or language. However, the astute physician must be able to recognize delayed or aberrant speech and language:

1. During routine physical examinations

2. During follow-up of children who have been identified earlier as high risk

3. During examination for another complaint such as a cold

In the preschool years physicians should become aware of risk factors that warn of academic or behavioral difficulties when first grade begins:

1. The presence of hyperactive and attentional disorders: These can be suspected by reports from nursery school or kindergarten teachers that a child is more ''immature'' than expected for his or her age. Parents will report discipline problems and problems that the child has playing with peers.

2. Delayed speech and language: If a language disorder is present, there is a high risk for delayed acquisition of reading and writing skills (possible dyslexia and dysgraphia). Speech disturbances alone (developmental articulation disorders, stuttering) do not presage learning disabilities.

3. Lack of achievement of academic readiness skills at the end of kindergarten (counting, reading and writing the alphabet, naming colors, etc) which are predictive of readiness for the first grade.

4. Poor drawing abilities for age, clumsiness, or incoordination do not necessarily presage academic learning disabilities, although they may lead to difficulties in handwriting and in art classes.

The physician has many therapeutic services open to patients at this age. Private or public community agencies, Headstart programs, preschool handicapped programs, and formal speech therapy are available in most communities even before the formal kindergarten period. Various nursery schools that provide more than baby-sitting by incorporating child development approaches are becoming more widely available. The special services of special education departments of the public school systems are mandated to provide educational services for preschool children, beginning at age 3 years, under the Education for All Handicapped Act (PL94-142), depending on state law.

IDENTIFIABLE DISORDERS

A. *Hearing Loss*

1. Deviation from the normal rate of development of sound reception and expression (see Tables 16.3 and 16.4) suggests possible hearing impairment.

2. There may be a delay in the development of speech and/or abnormal tone or quality of speech sounds. For example, with mild hearing loss words with high-frequency sounds will be misunderstood by the child, and the high-frequency sounds in words will be omitted from the child's speech ("stop" will be heard and spoken as "top").

3. The most common and frequently neglected cause of hearing loss is middle ear disease.

4. The child may display autistic features.

5. The child will be fascinated by loud sounds (especially vibrating bass sounds), and the parents may complain of the child's turning the radio or television on very loudly.

6. The child may develop lip reading, gestures, and pantomime to communicate.

7. Diagnosis necessitates detailed audiometry by an audiologist experienced with young children. Recording of brainstem auditory evoked potentials may be necessary in younger children.

   Caution: An apparent normal response to a bell in office testing is an inadequate assessment of the child with possible hearing loss. Screening audiograms in the school usually will not detect the child with anything less than profound hearing loss.

   Treatment:

   Thorough otologic and audiologic assessment is usually necessary. Amplification devices may be helpful in some children. Modification of the classroom environment or special schooling for the deaf may be necessary.

B. *Mental Subnormality (Mental Retardation)*

1. In the child with normal hearing (after thorough audiologic testing) who has delay in speech or language, the most common cause is

a global deficit in intellectual-cognitive skills termed mental retardation.

2. The important language milestone is a *two- to three-word sentence (must be a subject-verb sentence) by 24 to 30 months.*

3. Testing by a psychologist experienced in assessing children must be done in order to discriminate appropriately the presence of an intellectual-cognitive deficit. Such tests as the Bayley Scales of Infant Development, the Stanford-Binet Form L-M, the Wechsler Preschool and Primary Scale of Intelligence (WPPSI), and the Kaufmann Assessment Battery for Children (K-ABC) are the most useful. Extreme caution must be exercised in making prediction of future performance potential based on the test numbers alone.

4. Mental retardation is documented not only by intellectual cognitive testing, but by social-behavioral testing as well. Significant deficits in both areas must be present for the diagnosis to be accurately applied.

5. Mental retardation is actually only a description of a symptom complex (intellectual-cognitive and social-behavioral deficit that occurs before the age of 18 years) and may be the end result of multiple possible etiologies.

6. There are a number of conditions that may mimic mental retardation (pseudo-mental retardation):
   a. The most common is developmental language disorders (developmental dysphasias). These will give test results showing a low Wechsler Full-Scale IQ score, with the Verbal scale usually 15 to 20 points below the Performance scale.
   b. Multiple specific disabilities but normal intellectual potential, as indicated by normal adaptive behavior, age appropriate play, and social functioning, and average or better IQ subtest scores on subtests that are indicative of cognitive ability (Wechsler Similarities and Information subtests).
   c. Borderline intellectual potential, but complicated by specific developmental disabilities, attentional disorders, emotional disorders, or sensory impairments.
   d. Others include deafness or severe hearing impairment (presenting as speech and language delay), behavioral disorders (including childhood depression), attentional activity disorder, bilingualism (and ethnic-cultural differences), and pharmacologically induced cognitive dysfunction

7. Etiologic screening: Look for treatable causes (see Laboratory Studies above). Known genetic causes require genetic counseling of parents and siblings of childbearing age; referral to a pediatric geneticist is helpful. If any screening tests are positive, refer to an ap-

propriate specialist for further in-depth diagnostic assessment.

8. Psychoeducational management: Refer patients less than 3 years of age to community infant stimulation programs; after age 3 years refer children to the public school department of special education for preschool handicapped programs and development of individual education plans (IEPs) under the Education for All Handicapped Act (PL94-142). Physician and parent information may be obtained from the National Association for Retarded Citizens, 2709 Avenue E East, Arlington, TX 76011, and the Council for Exceptional Children, 1920 Association Drive, Reston, VA 22091.

C. *Infantile Autism*

1. Onset before age 18 months.

2. Abnormal interpersonal relationship ("doesn't relate to people as people but to people as objects"); the child avoids eye contact and tactile contact. He may, for example, use the mother's hand "as a tool" to grasp a doorknob. Does not cuddle as an infant.

3. Bizarre mannerisms (motor stereotypies): repetitive movements resembling tics, such as flapping arms at sides, rocking, or other self-stimulating maneuvers, whirling and spinning.

4. Abnormal play: child uses toys inappropriately in a stereotyped manner; eg, trucks are lined up (never rolled) while buildings are rolled.

5. Aberrant language
   a. Variable acquisition rates; eg, markedly delayed verbal comprehension and production but in later childhood "cocktail party chatter."
   b. Reading acquired before spoken language
   c. Pronoun inversion ("I" for "you")
   d. Echolalia and perseveration

6. On formal intellectual testing, child's scores are in the "retarded" range, but the child appears to be functioning at a much higher level.

7. Splinter skills may be present. These are precociously developed but isolated abilities such as calendar skills (eg, being able to tell what day of the week it was on September 25, 1896).

8. Compulsive need for sameness in environment and in routine.

9. Although this is a rare disorder, it is often misdiagnosed, in children who are retarded, aggressive, hyperactive, and nonverbal, as severe or profound mental retardation.

10. Similar disorders, with milder features (eg, less severe language disability), begin in children after age 18 months. These autistic-like disorders have been termed pervasive developmental disorders.

Treatment:

1. Neuropsychopharmacologic management is at present entirely symptomatic and empirical:
    a. Haloperidol may be used if there is much hyperactive aggression, self-mutilation, or marked motor stereotypies (the bizarre mannerisms). Starting dose: 1 mg bid to tid.
    b. Amitriptyline hydrochloride may be used, starting with 25 mg at bedtime, if there is much hyperactivity, trouble sleeping at night, or reversal of the diurnal cycle.
    c. Carbamazepine, beginning at 200 mg bid to tid, may be used if there is much aggressive behavior, and the child also has seizures.
    d. Lithium carbonate, beginning with 300 mg qd to tid, may be used for sustained hyperactive behavior akin to mania.
    e. The CNS stimulants, methylphenidate, dextroamphetamine, and pemoline hydrochloride, may also be used for prominent attentional hyperactivity disorders.
2. Psychoeducational management: Refer patients less than 3 years of age to community infant stimulation programs; after age 3 years they should be referred to the public school department of special education for preschool handicapped programs and development of IEPs under the Education for All Handicapped Act (PL94-142). Physician and parent information may be obtained from the National Society for Autistic Children, 306 31st St, Huntington, WV 25702.

D. *Developmental Hyperactivity (Attentional/Activity Disorder with Hyperactivity)*

1. Parents describe the child as "always on the go" from birth (may even have been more active in utero).
2. A child may never crawl but walks early enough and runs rather than walks.
3. The child characteristically is impulsive, distractible, immature, and clumsy, with a short attention span and difficulty in following directions, often racing from task to task without completing any one task.
4. Frequently parents and other caretakers have difficulty tolerating the child. Many behavior problems may develop. Peers have difficulty tolerating the child.
5. There is a "paradoxical reaction" to certain drugs - the barbiturates (sedative in normal individuals) markedly increase the hyperactivity, whereas stimulants such as amphetamines, methylphenidate,

and pemoline reduce the hyperactivity and increase the attention to tasks.

6. Boys are more frequently affected than girls.

7. Subtle neurologic signs on special extended neurologic examinations may be demonstrated (see *Psychopharmacology Bulletin* 1985;21:773-800 or Tupper, *Soft Neurological Signs*, Orlando, Grune & Stratton, 1987).

Treatment:

1. The physician's immediate task is parental education about the nature of the condition, and the appropriate place for the home, school, and medication in management of the attentional, behavioral, and academic problems. Parents should be referred to the appropriate literature on dealing with the hyperactive child (see Appendix D).

2. Pharmacologic management is effective, if given in conjunction with a comprehensive program of behavioral modification and environmental adjustment in the school and the home, along with appropriate pedagogical intervention, cognitive attentional training, and training in organizational skills. Modification of the school and home environment is necessary; ie, more structure, less distraction, short circumscribed tasks, a check list for developing self-monitoring abilities, and home chores to develop time management ability and responsibility.

3. Pharmacologic management utilizes primarily the CNS stimulants methylphenidate, dextroamphetamine, or pemoline. Dosage is clinically titrated to achieve a therapeutic effect. Hyperactivity may abate with a lower dose than that necessary to improve attentional or behavioral disturbance. Failure with one drug does not necessarily mean that the other drugs will also fail.

4. Before initiating treatment with the selected drug, the physician must establish a baseline assessment of motor, attentional, and behavioral parameters; a variety of standardized questionnaires and continuous performance tasks are available. The use of central auditory processing tests by an audiologist experienced with children is also a good method to establish a baseline for attentional tasks, and for follow-up monitoring. These measures will insure that data from a number of sources, other than the physician's own observation of the child in the examining room (which is often misleading), are available for an accurate view of the child's functioning.

a. Methylphenidate is the recommended first drug of choice. If treatment is unsuccessful, discontinue and treat with dextroamphetamine. Medication should be given in a twice-daily regimen, just after breakfast and lunch, to avoid anorexia and maximize absorption. Medication after 4 PM should be avoided to prevent insomnia. Suggested beginning doses are:

   Methylphenidate 5 mg bid

   Dextroamphetamine 5 mg bid

   Pemoline may be used as a single morning dose after breakfast, if successful treatment cannot be achieved with the other drugs. Starting with a dose of 37.5 mg every morning.

b. Medication should be given daily, although some children who display symptoms only during school need not be given the drug on weekends, school holidays, or during summer vacation.

c. The child should be carefully followed up on a weekly basis with upward adjustment of the dosage if necessary to achieve the desired therapeutic effect. After a maintenance regimen has been established, height and weight should be monitored and charted at least monthly to detect growth failure. A drug-free holiday is necessary if growth failure is documented. The child on a maintenance regimen must be followed regularly to monitor for undesirable side effects.

THE SCHOOL AGE YEARS (AGES 6 TO 18 YEARS)

Entry into school can be a traumatic period in which intellectual, motor, and emotional disorders may become more prominent. Disorders as previously described, such as hyperactivity-attentional syndromes, may become more obvious during this period. However, difficulty in school performance may be the first indication of a developmental or learning disability. Some specific behavioral and educational disorders may first become evident at this time.

This is a particularly trying time not only for the child but for the family as well. It is imperative that all professionals provide the family with accurate, comprehensive, and noncontradictory information. Because of the presence of a disabled child, family interactions may be tumultuous, affecting the psychosocial adjustment of siblings and parents, as well as family unity. A well-coordinated support system for the family may be as beneficial as any intervention prescribed for the child individually.

A. *Childhood Depression*

1. Endogenous major depression in a child may first present during school age (also see Chapter 9).

2. The family history is often strongly positive for depression, mania, nervous breakdown, mental illness, suicide, or alcoholism.

3. There is a history of recurrent episodes of change in behavior, including:
   a. Changed activity level, either hyperactivity (especially fluctuating) or reduced activity.
   b. School problems secondary to distractibility or decreased attention span or a new learning disability.
   c. Excessive moodiness or irritability.
   d. Appetite disturbance, sleep disturbance.
   e. Medically unexplained headaches, recurrent abdominal pain, or recurrent vomiting.
   f. Secondary enuresis (see Chapter 5) without demonstrable urologic or neurologic abnormality.
   g. Phobias or excessive fears.
   h. Preoccupation with death, suicide attempts, setting fires, running away.

4. Sadness and low self-esteem are encountered in long-standing learning disabilities, underachievement, or school failure, but in these cases are not associated with the variety of other symptoms characteristic of depression.

Treatment:

Antidepressant pharmacotherapy is usually necessary along with supportive psychotherapy and family therapy, and is generally best accomplished by referral to appropriate specialists.

B. *Educational Dysfunction*

There are many non-CNS factors that can account for below-expected academic performance. Some of these are:

1. Sensory deprivation (blindness or deafness)
2. Schools with deficient teaching programs
3. Belonging to a minority group with different values from those of the predominant culture
4. Bilingualism
5. Primary emotional or psychiatric disturbance

If non-CNS factors cannot be identified as the cause of poor achievement, then one or more of several kinds of educational dysfunction may account for poor academic performance.

1. *Mild to moderate mental retardation.* This child has global intellectual, cognitive, adaptive, and social-behavioral deficits. Formal psychological testing as well as serial developmental and neurologic assessments over time are required to make this diagnosis.

Caution: Skepticism must be used in evaluating intelligence test scores that report "characteristic of mental retardation." Psychological tests produce numerous false-negative and false positive results. Careful detailed neuropsychological testing is necessary for precise characterization of mental retardation.

Treatment:

Usually public schools have resource rooms or special classes for the educable or trainable retarded. An individual educational plan (IEP) is required for each child according to the Education for All Handicapped Act (PL94-142).

2. *Borderline intelligence*. The child with borderline intelligence shows cognitive potential below normal on formal psychological testing but which is above that of mental retardation. Although not mentally retarded this child will perform more slowly than normal, because his or her potential is lower than normal.

Treatment:

This child will require an IEP, usually incorporating more tutoring at a slower pace than that of the comparable regular classroom. This is the group correctly referred to as "slow learners." More information for parents may be obtained from the Center for Slower Learners, 5931 Buffridge Trail, Dallas, TX 75252 (telephone: 214-248-2984).

3. *Disorders of attention-activity* (attention deficit disorder [ADD], with or without hyperactivity): These are children with developmental hyperactivity in which the short attention span and distractibility, and not necessarily the motor hyperactivity, are the presenting features and the reason for academic underachievement. This group of disorders is one of the most common problems for which schools refer children to physicians. The referral information usually has terms such as "immaturity," "underachievement," "learning disability," or "behavior problem." Motor hyperactivity tends to abate with age, but the attentional disorder may persist through high school. The older the child, the more the physician must look for complicating secondary emotional complications, such as conduct disorder.

Treatment:

All management previously discussed in the section on developmental hyperactivity applies. In addition, continual and clear communication with school teachers and administrators is necessary for effective monitoring of the child's responses to pharmacologic intervention.

4. *Specific learning disabilities*: Children with specific learning disabilities have normal intellectual potential but greater than expected difficulty in acquiring one or more of the basic academic skills of reading, writing. arithmetic, or spelling. The incidence is about 3 % of the school population. Specific reading disabilities (sometimes termed developmental dyslexia), with later spelling and written language disabilities, are common. Arithmetic disability (sometimes called developmental dyscalculia) has been less well studied, and the actual incidence is not known.

   a. The classic neurologic examination is almost always normal, but usually subtle neurologic signs can be demonstrated. A neurodevelopmental evaluation may reveal aberrant or delayed functioning.
   b. Speech articulation can be tested by repetition of test phrases such as "la-la," "mi-mi," "go-go."
   c. Spoken language can be rapidly screened by repetition of sentences of varying length and syntax.
   d. Arithmetic ability can be screened in the early school age child by addition and subtraction of single digits, and in the older school age child by multiplication of two digit numbers by two digit numbers (written).
   e. Note whether errors in reading, writing, or arithmetic may be attentional errors, such as skipping lines, wrong lining up of columns, or impulsive errors, such as writing down the first things to come to mind, and frequent erasing. These are clues to the presence of an attentional disorder that may be presenting as a learning disability.
   f. Ascertain if there is a family history of reading or other learning disabilities, or of attentional-activity disorders.
   g. Screen for visual-motor problems by Draw-a-Person test, drawing a clock, or copying geometric figures.
   h. There are a number of specific learning disability syndromes such as the developmental Gerstmann's syndrome, developmental dyslexia, developmental dyscalculia, developmental clumsiness or apraxia, developmental dysgraphia, and developmental dysphasia (see also *Pediatric Clinics of North America* April 1984;31[3], and *Journal of Child Neurology* April 1986;1[2]).
   i. Although psychometric testing may be helpful in elucidating these disorders, many psychological tests produce false positive and false-negative results. Therefore detailed neuropsychologic testing is often necessary to characterize more precisely a clinically diagnosed learning disability.

j. Learning disability syndromes may occur alone or in combination, and also may coexist independently within attention deficit disorder, with or without hyperactivity.

k. Many neurobiological correlates of learning disabilities are now known, and may suggest techniques in the future for supplementary diagnosis.

l. Physician and parent information are available from the Association for Children with Learning Disabilities, 5225 Grace St, Pittsburgh, PA 15236, and The Orton Dyslexia Society, 724 York Rd, Baltimore, MD 21204 (telephone: 301-296-0232 or 800-ABCD123).

BIBLIOGRAPHY

Adams R, Lyon G: *Neurology of Hereditary Metabolic Disease of Children*. New York, McGraw-Hill Book Co, 1981.

American Psychiatric Association: *Diagnostic and Statistical Manual of Mental Disorders*, ed 3 [DSM-III]. Washington, American Psychiatric Association, 1980.

Bakwin H, Bakwin RM: *Clinical Management of Behavior Disorders in Children*. Philadelphia, WB Saunders Co, 1972.

Barlow CF: *Mental Retardation and Related Disorders*. Philadelphia, FA Davis Co, 1978.

Capute AJ, Accardo PJ: Linguistic and auditory milestones during the first two years of life. *Clin Pediatr* 1978; 17:847-853.

Fisher WF, Burd L, Kena DP, et al: Attention deficit disorders and the hyperactivities in multiply disabled children. *Rehabil Lit* 1985;46:250-254.

Golden G: Neurobiological correlates of learning disabilities. *Ann Neurol* 1982;12:409-418.

Herskowitz J, Rosman NP: *Pediatrics, Neurology, and Psychiatry - Common Ground*. New York, Macmillan, 1982.

Noshpitz JD (ed): *Basic Handbook of Child Psychiatry*. New York, Basic Books, 1979.

Palfrey JS, Mervis RC, Butler JA: New directions in the evaluation and education of handicapped children. *N Engl J Med* 1979;298:819-824.

Paine R, Oppe T: *Neurological Examination of Children. Clinics in Developmental Medicine. Volume 20/21*. Philadelphia, JB Lippincott Co, 1966.

Peters JE, Romine JD, Dykman RA: A special neurological examination of children with learning disabilities. *Dev Med Child Neurol* 1975;17:63-78.

Rapin I: *Children with Brain Dysfunction: Neurology, Cognition, Language, and Behavior*. New York, Raven Press, 1982.

Swaiman KF, Wright FS: *The Practice of Pediatric Neurology*, ed 2. St Louis, CV Mosby Co, 1982.

Touwen BC: *The Examination of the Child With Minor Nervous Dysfunction*, ed 2. Philadelphia, JB Lippincott Co, 1981.

Volpe J: *Neurology of the Newborn*, ed 2. Philadelphia, WB Saunders Co, 1987.

XVII

LOW BACK PAIN

Low back pain with or without leg pain, is one of the most common complaints seen in medical practice. It is estimated that up to 80% of the American population may suffer at least temporary disability from low back pain. Low back pain is only a **symptom** which can result from several conditions and hence the term should not be equated with herniated lumbar disc. Each patient must be evaluated with a detailed history, an adequate physical examination, and relevant investigations so that a correct diagnosis is reached and appropriate treatment initiated. The etiologic factors include:

1. Trauma:
   a. Acute lumbosacral sprain.
   b. Fracture of lumbar vertebrae.
2. Tumors:
   a. Metastases to the spine: Common sources are prostate, breast, and kidneys.
   b. Tumors compressing the cauda equina.
3. Metabolic: Osteoporosis (particularly in postmenopausal females), myeloma, and hyperparathyroidism.
4. Degenerative processes involving the intervertebral disc or the joints between the articular processes of adjacent vertebrae: A posterolateral herniation of the nucleus pulposus usually compresses a nerve root.
5. Other structural lesions of spine:
   a. Spinal stenosis.
   b. Spondylolisthesis.

6. Infections of the disc space or vertebrae.

7. Inflammatory disorders involving:

    a. Vertebrae, eg, ankylosing spondylitis.

    b. Meninges, eg, arachnoiditis.

8. Vascular:

    a. Abdominal aortic aneurysm eroding the vertebrae.

    b. Occlusive vascular disease causing radicular or plexus ischemia.

9. Direct involvement of lumbosacral plexus or sciatic nerve, eg, trauma, tumors, injections into or close to the sciatic nerve.

10. Psychogenic, especially when litigation is involved.

History

It is of utmost importance that the history be derived without using leading questions. Patients with pain problems are often overly susceptible to suggestion. Leading questions may only provide misinformation to the initial examiner and allow the patient to develop a symptom complex that will mislead subsequent examiners. For example, do not ask whether specific activities aggravate the pain, ask whether there are any known factors that aggravate the pain. Do not ask whether the pain goes into the leg; ask whether the pain extends into any other part of the body from the lower back. The answers to such questions may help to differentiate organic from functional problems. With experience, the examiner should (in approximately 15 minutes) be able to take a history regarding the back pain problem that will provide the following information:

1. The chronological sequence of the events involved in the pain problem leading up to the time of examination: "Tell me the whole story of your problem from the very beginning."

2. An exact description of the type of pain, its location, extent, and radiation, if any: "Tell me exactly what this pain is like."

3. Factors that precipitate the pain and activities that exacerbate or relieve the pain: "Does anything affect this pain?"

4. A description of any back injury (and whether there is litigation related to that injury): "Have you ever injured your back?"

5. Associated motor or sensory complaints-nature and extent: "Have you noticed any weakness or loss of feeling?"

6. Interference with bowel, bladder, or sexual function: "Do your bowels and bladder work all right?" "Have you had any problems with your sexual function?"

7. A detailed description of previous therapy for the pain and what effect it may have had: "Have you ever had any treatment for your back; if

so, describe.'' (Pay attention to the description of traction and its effect and to the use of medications, especially narcotics.)

Hypothesis Formation

From the history a hypothesis as to the possible source of pain should be formulated:

1. If the pain is localized to the low back, without radiation to the leg, it is unlikely that there is nerve root involvement. Osteoporosis, spinal metastasis, degenerative disc disease, disc space infections, all can present with low back pain alone.
2. If the pain radiates to the lower extremity take into consideration the following:
   a. Root pain:
      i. Worse with factors that increase intraspinal pressure (coughing, sneezing).
      ii. Distribution is usually in the L-4, L-5, or S-1 dermatome.
   b. Claudication:
      i. Related to exertion-especially with iliofemoral occlusive vascular disease.
      ii. Lumbar spinal canal stenosis: Pain is worse with exertion.
      Caveat: Stenosis commonly produces numbness and weakness; vascular disease does not.
   c. Posterior longitudinal ligament involvement (most often a bulging disc which does not stretch a nerve root):
      i. Seldom radiates below knee.
      ii. Pain is vague, not associated with paresthesia.
   d. Hip joint disease and pelvic pathology may also cause lower extremity pain.

Physical Examination

1. Examination of *gait* is a very important part of the physical examination of patients with back pain. The physician must pay particular attention to the following:
   a. Whether the patient is walking with a list of the spine; this is highly indicative of an organic back problem (see Figure 17.1).
   b. Whether the patient can support his weight on his toes and heels (motor weakness in muscles below the knee).
   c. Whether the patient can hop on one foot or the other (weakness of quadriceps or gluteus muscles).

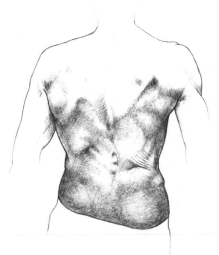

Figure 17.1. Patient with an organic back pain problem frequently walks with forward flexion of the trunk and with one iliac crest higher than the other. A lateral curve of the spine is often present.

2. Examination of the *back* should be carried out with the patient in the upright standing position. Conditions to be noted include the following:
   a. Muscle spasm (noted by prominence of paraspinal muscles on one side or flattening of lumbar lordosis) (see Figure 17.2).
   b. List or curvature. The patient often leans away from the site of his pain and the scoliosis becomes more prominent as the patient tries to bend forward.
   c. Any palpable mass or tenderness along the vertebral column (including percussion of the flanks looking for kidney disease and percussion over the spinous processes with a tendon hammer) (See Figure 17.3).
   d. Range of motion in flexion, extension, and sideways bending: Often the patient will keep the spine rigid and do the flexion at the hip.
   e. Dimples, birth marks, abnormal patches of hair (clues to congenital malformation or tumors).
3. Straight leg raising test is the **key to identifying nerve root irritation**. With the patient lying flat on his back, passively raise the extended leg until pain occurs (see Figure 17.4); normally an 80-degree movement can be made with little discomfort; if the pain is only in the back of the thigh, it is likely to be due to hamstring tightness and not due to nerve root tension, irritation, or compression. If the pain radiates to the back

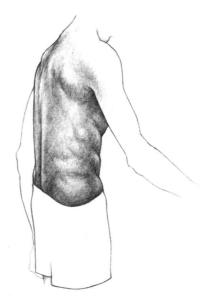

Figure 17-2. A patient with an organic back problem will often have the lower lumbar curve obliterated. Unilateral paravertebral muscle spasm on one side elevates the iliac crest. This is most commonly seen with a root lesion.

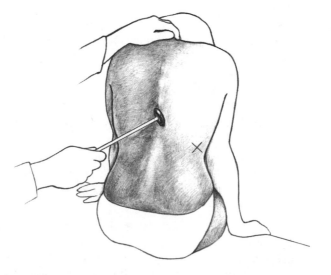

Figure 17-3. Percussion of the spinous processes will often cause more discomfort over the involved vertebrae. Be certain also to percuss the costovertebral angle in search of renal disease.

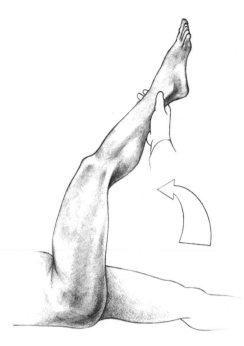

Figure 17-4. Straight leg raising: With disc disease, raising the affected leg will often cause pain in the distribution of the affected root. This pain is centered in the buttocks at the sciatic notch and radiates down the leg. Pain at the knee from tight hamstring muscles does not constitute a positive straight leg raising test.

as well as to the leg, it often indicates nerve root involvement. When in doubt, use one or more of the following maneuvers to confirm a positive straight leg raising test.

a. The straight leg is brought down until the pain just disappears when an attempt is made to suddenly dorsiflex the ankle; genuine root pain will be reproduced by this maneuver.

b. Have the patient sit up in bed with the legs extended at the knee or repeat the test with the patient in the sitting position with his legs dangling over the edge of the table (see Figure 17.5). When the leg is extended at the knee, the patient should complain of pain and lean backward to produce the same angle as for the straight leg raising test in the lying position. If the patient experiences no pain in the sitting position, a previous positive straight leg raising test in the lying position probably suggests a nonorganic basis.

c. The patient may be asked to kneel on a chair; in this position the hamstrings are relaxed and the tension on the sciatic nerve is reduced; reluctance to bend forward while in this position is suggestive of a false-positive straight leg raising test.

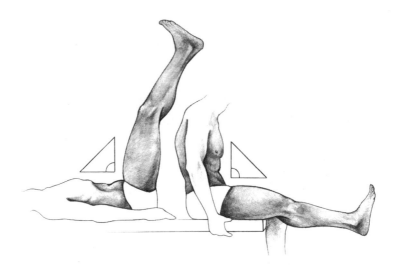

Figure 17-5. If the examiner suspects the straight leg raising test to be unreliable in the supine position, the examiner can surreptitiously raise the leg while the patient is in the sitting position. If the lesion is organic, radiating pain should be experienced in both positions.

While performing the straight leg raising test, hip joint mobility should also be evaluated. This is done by passive rotation of the leg at the hip (Figure 17.6). A patient with pathologic spinal changes will have no pain or restriction on rotary movements of the hip, but the patient with hip disease (who may present as a back pain problem) will show a marked aggravation of the pain when the hip is rotated internally or externally.

4. Concentrate on those aspects of the neurologic examination that may be helpful in confirming nerve root compression:

   a. Unilaterally absent or diminished patellar (L-4), internal hamstring (L-5), or Achilles (S-1) tendon reflexes localize an involved nerve root with reasonable accuracy. Be aware of the occasional patient who may show hyperactive reflexes in the presence of acute back pain due to keeping the lower extremity muscles tense; in such a patient the plantar response will remain flexor.

   b. Absent cremasteric reflexes suggest an upper lumbar root or conus medullaris lesion (see Figure 17.7).

   c. Unequal superficial abdominal reflexes may suggest a thoracic lesion from the T-9 to the T-12 level (see Figure 17.8).

   d. A dermatomal sensory loss, if typical, is useful in localizing the root involved.

   Caution: Never make a diagnosis on the basis of sensory loss alone.

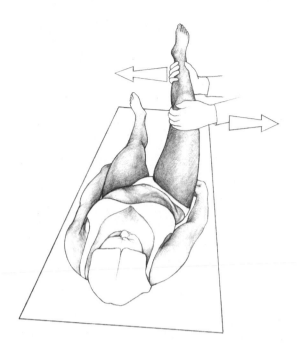

Figure 17-6. Hip rotation: With the hip and knee flexed, inward rotation of the lower leg with the knee flexed will cause pain if there is hip joint disease.

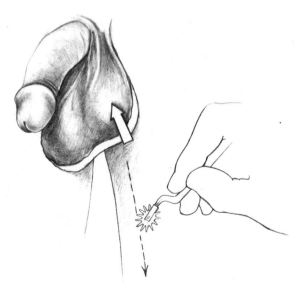

Figure 17-7. Cremasteric reflex: A light stroke downward on the inner surface of the thigh produces an upward movement of the testicle.

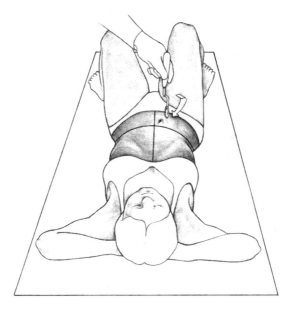

Figure 17-8. Abdominal reflex: A light stroke toward the umbilicus will normally cause muscle contraction with movement of the umbilicus toward the stimulus. The pinwheel is a more effective and reliable stimulus than a sharpstick.

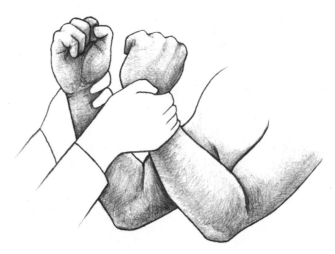

Figure 17-9. Test comparable muscle strength simultaneously if there is a suspicion of nonorganicity. It is very difficult to give way with one muscle while maintaining strength in another.

    e. Motor weakness demonstrated by specific muscle testing may confirm a motor root lesion. Muscle testing may also demonstrate involvement of multiple roots.

    f. Bilateral simultaneous muscle testing is a valuable method of detecting hysterical weakness. The patient is unable to coordinate hysterical "giving way" between both extremities (see Figure 17.9).

5. The physical examination should also include abdominal palpation, palpation of the lower extremity pulsations, and listening for a bruit over the aorta, the iliac arteries, and the femoral arteries.

6. A rectal examination is quite important in evaluating patients with persistent back pain or back and leg pain to detect pelvic pathologic changes and sphincter involvement. The anal reflex, which is often lost in conus medullaris and cauda equina lesions, should also be tested (Figure 17.10).

Clinical Investigations

The history and physical findings should narrow the differential diagnosis. The investigations are chosen on the basis of the most likely diagnoses. When evaluating the investigations keep in mind the false-positive and false-negative results for each:

1. Plain films of the lumbar and sacral spine: Anteroposterior (AP), lateral, and oblique views are done to look for abnormalities in the vertebral bodies, intervertebral disc spaces, and intervertebral foramina and for any abnormal shadows.

   Caution: Asymptomatic bony abnormalities are not uncommon and do not always correlate with neurologic deficit.

2. A CT scan of the lumbar spine is highly useful, particularly in disc lesions, to obtain good visualization of the vertebral body, intervertebral disc, neural arch, zygapophyseal joints, and intervertebral foramina.

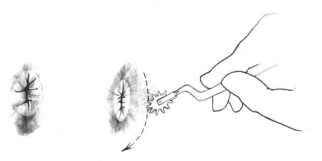

Figure 17-10. A light stroke with a pinwheel in the perianal area normally causes the anus to pucker.

Caution: The CT scan is useful only if on neurologic examination the physician can identify the level of the lesion.

3. MRI is particularly useful in visualizing lesions in the spinal cord or nerve roots (conus medullaris and cauda lesions).

4. Bone scanning is particularly useful when metastatic disease is suspected as a cause of low back pain. It is also often positive in inflammatory diseases of the spine and in fractures.

5. Electromyography: Function of the nerve root should be assessed by EMG and nerve conduction studies; myelography and CT scan show only the anatomy. In experienced hands it provides accurate localization of the root involved and serves as a complementary test to CT scan and myelography. It is useful in distinguishing between peripheral neuropathies and radiculopathies. It is particularly useful in patients who have had surgery before and are having recurrence of symptoms, where myelography and CT scans could be confusing.

6. Myelography: Myelography using metrizamide is the most useful test in differentiating a disc from a tumor. The test involves injection of a contrast material into the subarachnoid space. Pantopaque (lipid-soluble contrast) is known to produce arachnoiditis and hence water-soluble agents such as metrizamide are the contrast media of choice. If myelography is followed by CT scanning, additional information may be obtained.

   Remember: Myelography is an invasive test and should be considered seriously only when surgery is contemplated, or when the diagnosis is in doubt.

7. When metabolic bone disease or metastases are suspected, ESR, calcium, phosphate, and alkaline and acid phosphatase assays may be done. When disc space infections or inflammatory disease is suspected, ESR, antinuclear antibodies, and rheumatoid factor assays need to be done. When myeloma is suspected, x-ray studies of other parts of the skeleton, the urine for Bence Jones protein, serum protein electrophoresis, and a bone marrow examination are necessary.

Protruded Intervertebral Disc

1. The most important diagnostic feature is the onset of low back pain followed by radiation down one lower extremity.

   Caution: All such pain is not due to disc prolapse; any condition that afflicts the nerve root can present similarly.

2. The initial attack may be provoked by an identifiable precipitating event (often lifting a weight or a twisting movement). The pain may be described as severe enough to "take the breath away" and cause the patient to be completely immobilized.

3. The area of pain is usually well localized, and the extension can be traced with a finger. There is a feeling of associated tingling in the distal extension of the pain.

4. During subsequent episodes, which may again be precipitated by physical activity, the pain is often less severe and may disappear within a few days; less severe attacks are usually precipitated by movement and may be relieved by change of posture or rest.

5. The pain is improved by flexion of the thigh and the knees; individual patients may be worse at night or during the day; activity relieves pain in some patients but more often aggravates symptoms in others. The patient will often move about gingerly for fear of aggravating the pain.

6. The patient may complain of extremity weakness, numbness, and paresthesias in localized areas of the leg or foot. Infrequently, there may be interference of bowel, bladder, or sexual function; these symptoms are more common in midline disc herniation, involving the sacral nerve roots of both sides.

7. The physical examination reveals one or more of the following:
    a. The patient often stands in a listed position and tends to walk with the affected leg slightly flexed at the knee and at the thigh. There may be difficulty standing in an upright position with the leg fully extended.
    b. There may be difficulty supporting weight on the toes or heels. Walking on the heels often acutely aggravates the pain.
    c. Hopping is often difficult to perform, but if performed, a tendency for the knee to buckle suggests quadriceps weakness and the possibility of an L-3 or L-4 root lesion.
    d. Examination of the back shows paravertebral muscle spasm with limitation of bending forward or backward. Bending forward is more often limited in ruptured disc at the L-5 - S-1 interspace; bending backward is often limited in ruptured disc at the L-3 - L-4 or L-4 - L-5 interspaces. Frequently a scoliosis with convexity toward the symptomatic side may be seen.
    e. Percussion over the spine may produce radiation of the pain into the affected leg.
    f. The straight leg raising test is positive on the symptomatic side. Occasionally there is a positive crossed straight leg raising test with pain extending into the leg opposite the one being raised (this is suggestive of an extruded fragment).
    g. The patient will flex the knees and thighs and roll with legs flexed in the process of turning over or getting out of bed.

h. Over 90% of ruptured lumbar discs with nerve root compression affect either L-5 or S-1 roots producing the neurologic alterations described in Table 17.1.

Caution: Sensory deficits must be interpreted very carefully, taking into account an intuitive assessment of patient reliability and examiner's experience.

8. Investigations

a. The routine laboratory and plain x-ray studies in protruded lumbar intervertebral discs seldom show diagnostic abnormalities. Electromyography may provide objective evidence of denervation due to damage to ventral (motor) root. The dorsal (sensory) root function can be evaluated by doing H reflex and dermatomal somatosensory-evoked potential studies.

b. A CT scan of the lumbar spine has been found to be quite useful in evaluating patients with lumbar disc prolapse.

c. Myelography (often combined with CT scanning) is considered when there is progressive neurologic deficit or when surgery is contemplated.

9. Management

a. In acute disc prolapse, ten days of conservative treatment should

Table 17.1.
Symptoms of Lumbosacral Root Lesions

A. **S-1** root lesion (see Figure 17.11)
  1. Diminished or absent Achilles tendon reflex (ankle reflex)
  2. Sensory deficit in the lateral aspect of the heel and the lateral aspect of the sole of the affected foot
  3. Difficulty standing on tiptoe on the affected extremity (suggests calf weakness)

B. **L-5** root lesion (see Figure 17.12)
  1. Trouble supporting weight on heel or presence of foot drop; the patient may complain that his toes get caught on carpet
  2. Sensory deficits over the anterolateral aspect of the affected leg below the knee and extending to the dorsum of the foot and the big toe
  3. Diminished or absent internal hamstring tendon reflex

C. **L-4** root lesion
  1. Diminished or absent patellar tendon reflex
  2. Weakness in the quadriceps muscle of the affected leg
  3. Sensory deficit extending from the knee down the medial aspect of the lower portion of the affected leg as well as the medial malleolus.

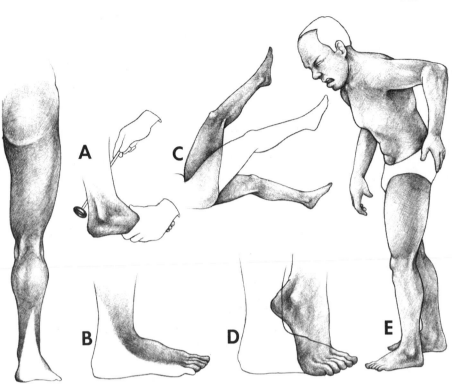

Figure 17-11. Summary of an S-1 root lesion: Diminished Achilles reflex (A), sensory disturbance over the lateral aspect of the heel and toe (B), positive straight leg raising (C), difficulty standing on tiptoe (D), pain worse bending forward (E).

be tried unless there is rapidly progressive neurologic deficit. This includes:

i. Strict bed rest (except for bathroom privileges); the bed should be firm (firm mattress or bed board) and flat. Slight flexion of the leg using a pillow under the knee is found to be comforting by most patients.

ii. Pelvic traction with 5 to 7 kg of weight may be useful in overcoming lumbar spasm and decreasing scoliosis.

iii. Analgesics and muscle relaxants should be used to control the pain and spasm. Aspirin 600 mg q4h plus diazepam 5 to 10 mg bid is one suggested regimen. Superficial heat using hydrocollator packs or infrared heating may be useful. Some patients find better relief with ice packs or ice massage. Transcutaneous electrical nerve stimulation (TENS) may be useful in pa-

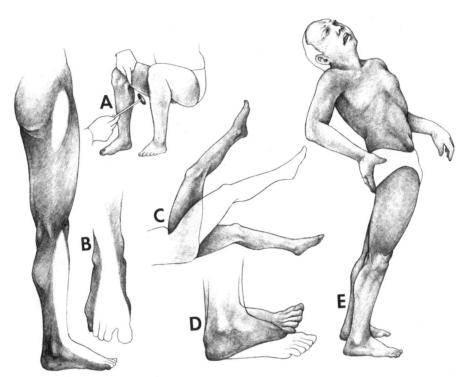

Figure 17-12. Summary of an L-5 root lesion. Diminished internal hamstring reflex (A), sensory disturbance over dorsum of foot and great toe (B), positive straight leg raising (C), foot drop (D), pain worse bending backward (E).

tients either with acute low back pain or those with low back pain and radicular pain.

   iv. After recovery from the acute attack a concerted program of back exercises (see Appendix E) should be undertaken for at least 6 weeks.

  b. Failure to respond to conservative treatment: may result from noncompliance with strict bed rest, incorrect diagnosis, persistent or worsening nerve root compression, unstable spine, secondary gain, litigation, or other psychosocial factors. A comprehensive evaluation is needed at this stage to determine the reason for nonimprovement. If the patient has progressive or persistent neurologic deficit, surgical treatment needs to be considered.

  c. Chemonucleolysis: During recent years, chemonucleolysis has emerged as an alternative form of treatment to surgery in selected patients with herniated nucleus pulposus. This involves intradiscal injection of chymopapain for enzymatic dissolution of the nucleus pulposus. The technique is useful only in those patients in whom there is nerve root compression resulting from prolapsed intervertebral disc. It is not useful in those with bony instability or root compression from bony encroachment of the foramen. It should only be performed by a physician experienced in the technique.

d. Surgical treatment consists of discectomy which involves usually a week's stay in the hospital, a 10% complication rate in the best of hands, and a 10% recurrence rate. In patients with unstable bony structure, lumbar fusion may be necessary.

Sprain or Fracture

1. Paravertebral muscle spasm is one of the commonest causes of acute low back pain. The most important clue to the diagnosis is pain specifically related to an injury that reaches a crescendo (quickly or over a period of days) and gradually tapers to a plateau that may persist for weeks to months.

2. The pain is described as diffuse backache with associated stiffness, spasm, and limitation of motion. Stiffness may extend up to the neck and down to the pelvis and legs.

3. Extension of the pain is vague unless a fracture has produced nerve root compression. In the facet syndrome (due to tearing of the capsule of the facet joint) the pain may extend to the buttock and posterior thigh of the involved side.

4. The pain is relieved somewhat by reclining, changing position, analgesics, and heat. Massage or manipulation often gives temporary relief, but may be dangerous in an unsuspected fracture. There is no relationship of the pain to the time of day or night.

5. Temporary ileus or difficulty in initiating urination may occur in the acute phase of pain.

6. Damage or compression of the spinal cord or nerve root by fracture may produce deficits in motor, sensory, bowel, bladder, and/or sexual function.

7. On examination:

    a. The gait *should not* be tested during the acute phase until x-ray examination has excluded the presence of an unstable vertebral fracture.

    b. Initially there may be palpable swelling or hematoma. Palpation of the back usually reveals an area of focal tenderness over the spinous processes in the region of the injury. Reversal of the spinal curve may be palpable at the level of the compression fracture.

    c. Because a common site of fracture is the T-12 vertebra, examination of sensation in the perianal area is mandatory to exclude injury to the conus medullaris without simultaneous nerve root injury. There may be loss of bowel and bladder function, sexual dysfunction in the male, and loss of anal reflex or a patulous anal sphincter.

d. In all patients careful documentation of reflex, motor, and sensory function is important in the acute phase so that comparison can be made with follow-up examinations.

8. In the case of low back sprain, spine x-ray films reveal few changes other than obliteration of normal spinal curvature resulting from paravertebral muscle spasm.

9. In the case of spinal fracture, spine x-rays are the diagnostic tool for identifying the lesion.

   Caution: Unsatisfactory x-ray films or films taken too low or too high in the spine result in many fractures being missed.

10. Management

    a. Back sprain

       i. In the acute phase, this includes bed rest, limitation of activity, local heat, muscle relaxants, and mild analgesics.

       ii. In the chronic phase, this consists of heat (diathermy or ultrasonic therapy), range of motion exercises, and progressive back stretching to restore the full range of motion.

    b. Spinal fracture requires absolute bed rest on a flat, firm surface (bed board) and consideration of surgical treatment by decompression laminectomy and/or surgical stabilization.

Structural Bony Lesions

1. The conditions that may lead to low back pain due to structural bony abnormalities include osteoporosis, old fracture, congenital bony abnormalities such as partially sacralized lumbar vertebrae, unilateral pedicle defect, spondylolisthesis, facet asymmetry, and spinal stenosis.

2. Most of these conditions present with chronic low back pain of long duration; the patient may trace the onset to injury.

3. The major feature is chronic, nagging, and centrally located back pain without radiation to the lower extremities; the notable exceptions are spondylolisthesis and spinal stenosis in which radicular pain spreading to the lower extremities may occur.

4. Pain is precipitated or aggravated by lifting, standing, or prolonged forward bending, and is aggravated by work, sexual, physical, and recreational activity; the pain is often relieved by sitting or lying down; it is seldom troubling at night.

5. An important clue to the diagnosis is that the pain is least troublesome on arising from bed, but increases with activity during the day.

6. No complaints of motor, sensory, bladder, bowel, or sexual dysfunction occur except in cases of spinal stenosis or spondylolisthesis with nerve root involvement.

7. Physical examination shows normal gait, with ability to walk on heels and toes, a negative straight leg raising test, and normal reflexes, muscle strength, and sensory perception. The abnormality is easily identified by x-ray films. The CT scan can be of immense help in locating and characterizing the defect.

8. Acute back pain resulting from structural bony abnormality should be treated with bed rest, analgesics, and muscle relaxants followed by progressive ambulation and a program of back exercises. Excessive weight in the abdominal area (potbelly) should be eliminated by a weight reduction program (Figure 17.13).

Lumbar Stenosis

1. Although this is also a structural abnormality, it is mentioned separately since the clinical presentation is somewhat typical. There is narrowing of the nerve root foramina and spinal canal resulting in compression of the lumbosacral nerve roots. A congenitally narrow canal with acquired factors like hypertrophy of vertebral bone and interspinal ligamentous

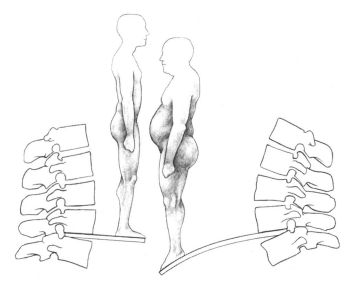

Figure 17-13. A potbelly increases stress on the lumbar spine. The length of the springboard is proportional to the distance between the navel and the spine.

tissue as well as displacement of the intervertebral discs may result in lumbar stenosis.

2. The most important clue to diagnosis is the occurrence of symptoms suggestive of bilateral lumbosacral radiculopathy, either acutely following minor trauma or insidiously.

3. Typical features include claudication (pain usually involves the lower extremities, is provoked by exertion, and relieved by sitting), postural aggravation of symptoms (exacerbation of radiating leg pain, paresthesia, numbness or weakness when standing erect or bending backward; patient may complain of sudden onset of severe pain in the legs on reaching for objects overhead, which is quickly relieved by bending forward). A typical patient will be one with bilateral sciatica who enters the examining room hunched over and walking with a short cane.

4. The diagnosis is confirmed by x-ray examination of the lumbar spine and CT scan. The treatment is surgical and consists of wide laminectomy with bilateral foraminotomy.

Inflammatory Disease Affecting the Spine

A. *Ankylosing Spondylitis:* Persistent low back pain may be caused by inflammatory disease of the spine, such as ankylosing spondylitis. This condition is estimated to occur in about 1% of the population. The characteristic features include:

1. Onset between ages 20 and 40 years, often in a male.
2. Insidious onset of chronic low back pain without sciatica.
3. Feeling of stiffness and pain aggravated by maintaining one position for a long time and improved by mild activity.
4. Absence of motor or sensory abnormalities; the straight leg raising test is negative.
5. Discomfort may be present on hip rotation with general reduction in movements of the lumbar spine in all directions.
6. The diagnosis is confirmed by typical x-ray appearances (involvement of sacroiliac joints, and calcification of anterior and posterior spinal ligaments) and elevated ESR.

B. *Rheumatoid arthritis* may lead to persistent low back pain. The most useful diagnostic features include involvement of other joints and laboratory data supporting the diagnosis.

C. *Infection*

1. Both acute and chronic infection of the spine may present with back pain.
2. Disc space infection, which may occur following surgery or as a complication of systemic infection, presents with severe back pain,

local spinal tenderness, and paraspinal spasm. X-rays, bone scan, CT scan, and blood studies are often diagnostic.

3. Involvement of the spine may also occur in conditions such as tuberculosis, brucellosis, and typhoid. Spinal tuberculosis may present with pain and spinal deformity (gibbus) in the lower thoracic area; cold abscess may form and compress the spinal cord and produce acute or subacute onset of paraplegia. The radiologic appearance is characteristic, showing rarefaction and often collapse of the adjacent vertebrae with paraspinal mass.

Intraspinal or Spinal Neoplasm

1. Intraspinal or spinal neoplasms occur with metastatic prostatic or breast carcinoma and primary tumors such as meningioma, neurofibroma, or ependymoma.

2. The most important clue to the diagnosis is steady relentless progression of symptoms (as opposed to static or intermittent pain noted with most other causes).

3. With a progressive increase in the severity and constancy of the pain the patient may describe radicular extension of the pain (often with motor and sensory deficits).

4. Pain is aggravated by activity and unrelieved by any therapeutic measures; there is slight improvement on reclining with the knees flexed; prolonged lying aggravates the pain and may wake the patient at night; with arousal and ambulation pain may lessen; pain may be increased by the Valsalva maneuver (but does not necessarily differentiate this cause of pain from other causes of back pain).

5. Progression of the lesion often results in impairment of bowel and bladder control and sexual dysfunction in the male.

6. The examination shows:

   a. Evidence of a spinal lesion manifested by:
      i. Muscle spasm
      ii. Area of focal tenderness
      iii. Reflex alterations
      iv. Sensory deficits
      v. Motor group weakness

   b. Examination of the breast or prostate may lead to diagnosis of the underlying metastatic neoplasm in a high percentage of cases.

7. Primary intraspinal neoplasms have no characteristic laboratory abnormalities.

8. Metastatic spinal neoplasms may exhibit laboratory findings of malignancy such as anemia, elevated ESR, and elevation of the alkaline phos-

phatase and/or acid phosphatase levels.

9. Spinal x-ray films may be negative or may show widening of the spinal canal, erosion of the pedicles, or even scalloping of the vertebral bodies. Metastatic neoplasms may show erosion of elements of the vertebral body or osteoblastic changes.

10. A bone scan may show evidence of metastatic lesions when the plain films are negative. Pain usually precedes x-ray changes by several weeks.

11. A CT scan is particularly useful in showing the extent of the lesion. An MRI may provide even clearer images.

12. A myelogram is usually necessary to identify and localize primary intraspinal neoplasms but should only be performed where adequate facilities for immediate neurosurgical treatment are available.

Treatment:

1. Early diagnosis may obviate the need for neurosurgical treatment and may avoid serious neurologic sequelae in cases of metastatic lesions.

2. Late diagnosis usually necessitates immediate neurosurgical decompression.

3. In almost all cases of malignant neoplasms intensive anticancer chemotherapy and radiotherapy is necessary. Short-term corticosteroid therapy is useful when there is cord compression.

4. Early surgical treatment of benign intraspinal tumors such as neurofibroma and meningioma leads to excellent results.

Retroperitoneal Lesions

1. The most important diagnostic clue is the pain, which is described as deep and burning and radiates from the abdomen through to the back. When the nerve plexus is involved, there is usually acute neuralgic pain, or burning paresthesia, which may radiate from the abdomen to the back, groin, or the lower extremities.

2. The pain may be related to ingestion of food and may be aggravated by lying flat, by emptying the bladder or by moving the bowels; pain may occur related to menstrual flow.

3. Activity has little or no effect on the pain.

4. Examination

   a. The back examination and neurologic examination are normal, unless the lumbosacral plexus has been affected.

   b. Percussion of the costovertebral angle may produce pain (this maneuver does not produce pain in other causes of back pain).

   c. Hyperextension of the leg at the thigh may produce pain if there is psoas muscle irritation.

    d. Rectal examination may reveal a presacral or pelvic mass.

    e. Evidence of lumbosacral plexus involvement may be present.

5. Laboratory studies may show evidence suggesting inflammatory or neoplastic disease.

6. Routine x-ray films are seldom helpful; a CT scan of the abdomen is often highly useful in identifying the lesion.

7. Special studies, such as a GI series or intravenous pyelography IVP may be of value in the diagnosis.

8. EMG studies may be useful in determining the extent and severity of lumbosacral plexus involvement.

9. Treatment must be directed toward the primary disease process.

Emotional Disorder

1. The most important diagnostic clue is that the patient is inconsistent with regard to the chronological history, description of pain, factors affecting the pain, and relationship of the pain to the time of day or night; if the pain is injury-related, the circumstances of the injury are usually presented in explicit detail in contrast to the vague description of the nature of the pain problem.

2. The history may be misleading if the patient has had previous exposure to leading questions by other examiners.

3. Sometimes the patient may purposely mislead the examiner.

4. Examination

    a. The patient exhibits overreaction to the examiner's physical contact.

    b. The patient reacts to palpation in a manner disproportionate to the lack of objective findings in the examination.

    c. The patient frequently exhibits an oscillatory giveaway weakness on muscle testing and exhibits vague, indefinite, and unphysiologic sensory alterations.

    d. The appearance and attitudes of the patient may vary from inappropriate cheerfulness to indifference and apathy, inappropriate distress, or hostility.

    e. Simultaneous muscle testing (see Figure 17.9) or an inappropriate straight leg raising test (Figure 17.5) may be clues to an underlying emotional disorder.

5. Do not be misled by nonspecific laboratory and x-ray findings.

    Treatment:

    Appropriate management of the underlying emotional problem is often indicated without denying the distress the patient is experiencing from the problem.

BIBLIOGRAPHY

Blumer D: Psychiatric and psychological aspects of chronic pain. *Clin Neurosurg* 1978; 25:276-283.

Condon RH: Modalities in the treatment of acute and chronic low back pain, in Finneson BE (ed): *Low Back Pain*, Philadelphia, JB Lippincott Co, 1981, pp 204-232.

Goldsmith MF: Chymopapain injection-an often fruitless endeavor? *JAMA* 1984; 251:13-14.

Hall S, Bartleson JD, Onofrio BM, et al: Lumbar spinal stenosis. *Ann Intern Med* 1985; 103:271-276.

Hardy RW, Plank NW: Clinical diagnosis of herniated lumbar disc, in Hardy RW Jr (ed): *Lumbar Disc Disease*, New York, Raven Press, 1982, pp 17-28.

Kelsey JL, White HH, Pastides H, et al: The impact of musculo-skeletal disorders on the population of the United States. *J Bone Joint Surg* 1979; 61A:959-964.

McCulloch JA, Macnab I: Selection of patients for chemonucleolysis, in McCulloch JA, Macnab I (eds): *Sciatica and Chymopapain*, Baltimore, William & Wilkins Co, 1983, pp 103-127.

Nakano K: *Neurology of Musculoskeletal and Rheumatic Disorders*. Boston, Houghton Mifflin, 1979.

Shields CB, Williams PE Jr: Low back pain. *Am Fam Physician* 1986; 33:173-182

XVIII

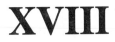

CERVICAL SPINE DISEASE

The grave implications of quadriparesis from spinal cord involvement or the severe disability of an arm from nerve root damage make it imperative that symptoms relating to the neck be thoroughly investigated. Otherwise, management of cervical spine disease usually consists of treating a "pain in the neck." This chapter is labelled Cervical Spine Disease rather than "neck pain" because a number of conditions affecting the cervical spine may occur without any symptomatic neck pain. Cervical spine disease may be classified as follows:

1. With neurologic involvement
    a. Acute spinal cord trauma
    b. Tumor
    c. Protruded disc
    d. Spinal canal stenosis
    e. Infection
2. Without neurologic involvement
    a. Meningeal irritation
    b. Sprain, strain, or fracture
    c. Degenerative or inflammatory disease
    d. Lesions of the vertebrae
    e. "Tension" or emotional disturbances

History

Patients with neck pain should be interviewed with particular attention to neurologic dysfunction. In most respects the same types of questions should be used to assess the patient with cervical spine disease as in the patient with low back pain (see Chapter 17). In addition, the following information may be specifically important in disease of the cervical spine:

1. As in other pain syndromes, information should be gathered through non-leading questions. For example, ''Does bending your head forward produce funny feelings?'' If the patient has shock-like feelings in the legs and/or arms on flexion or extension of the neck, Lhermitte's sign is present.

2. If the patient volunteers sensory or motor symptoms, obtain specifics as in low back pain (see Chapter 17).

3. Part of the examination must include careful observation of the patient during the history taking. Such observation often gives clues as to the extent of the disability. Particular attention should be paid to a patient's facial expression during head movements (a patient who freely moves the head without evidence of pain during the history taking but complains of pain during examination is suspect). Pay attention to the manner in which the patient changes position (for example, the neck will be held stiffly during head movements in the patient with painful organic spine disease).

Examination

1. Hyperactive tendon reflexes in the lower extremities (patellar and Achilles reflex) combined with upgoing plantar responses suggests spinal cord involvement.

2. Hyperactive tendon reflexes in the lower extremities and upgoing plantar responses associated with hypoactive or absent reflexes in the upper extremities (biceps, triceps, or brachioradialis) localizes the lesion to the cervical spinal cord. This could occur with an extrinsic lesion involving the nerve roots as well as the cord (extramedullary lesions as in meningioma or bony tumors) or in lesions involving the central portion of the cord (intramedullary lesion as in syringomyelia).

3. Presence of a sensory level is highly suggestive of spinal cord involvement. This may best be demonstrated by having the patient run his own fingers up the trunk until sensation changes (see Figure 18.1). In lesions of the central portion of the spinal cord there is selective loss of pain and temperature sensations in the arms and trunk with sparing of the sacral region (see Figure 18.2).

4. Weakness, hyperreflexia, a Babinski reflex, and loss of position and vibration sensation in the lower extremity on one side, associated with a deficit in pinprick and temperature sensation in the other leg (Brown-Séquard syndrome), suggests pathologic changes in the lateral half of the spinal cord.

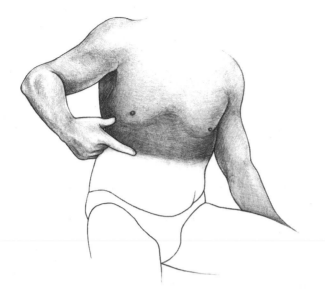

Figure 18.1. The cooperative patient may be able to outline a sensory change with his own finger more accurately than an examiner with multiple pinpricks.

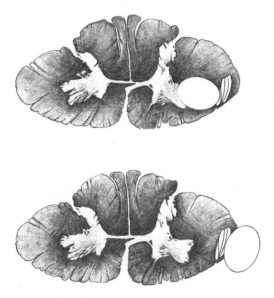

Figure 18.2. In the spinothalamic tract, the sacral pain fibers are more lateral than cervical pain fibers; destructive lesions in the center of the cord may spare the sacral fibers and sacral sensation. An extrinsic lesion may damage the sacral fibers first and produce a sensory disturbance in the sacral area as well as a bladder disturbance.

5. A diminished deep tendon reflex in one arm associated with a normal reflex in the other suggests unilateral nerve root involvement and is usually accompanied by other motor and sensory deficits in the distribution of that nerve root (Table 18.1).

6. Examination of the neck should be carried out with the patient in the sitting position and with the patient's hands folded in a relaxed position on the lap.

   a. Palpate the cervical and occipital muscles for spasms or masses.

   b. Palpate the posterior cervical triangle for masses or tenderness (see Figure 18.3).

   c. Assess the bulk and strength of the sternocleidomastoid muscles.

   d. Palpate and percuss the spinous processes for abnormalities or tenderness.

   e. The examiner should determine the passive range of motion in flexion, extension, side bending, and rotation of the neck.

   f. Radicular pain caused by nerve root compression may be reproduced by the following maneuvers:

      i. Hyperextend and tilt the neck to the affected side and apply downward pressure over the vertex (Spurling's maneuver). This

TABLE 18.1
LOCALIZING FINDINGS IN CERVICAL RADICULOPATHY

Nerve Root	Muscle Involved	Motor Weakness	Sensory Loss	Reflex Abnormality
C5	Deltoid Supraspinatus	Shoulder abduction	Lateral upper arm	Biceps
C6	Biceps	Elbow flexion	Thumb and index fingers	Biceps
	Extensor carpi radialis	Wrist extension		Brachio-radialis
C7	Triceps	Elbow extension	Middle and index fingers	Triceps
	Flexor carpi radialis	Wrist flexion		
C8	Flexor digitorum	Finger flexion	Little and ring fingers	Finger flexor
T1	Interossei	Abduction and adduction of fingers	Medial forearm and medial upper arm	

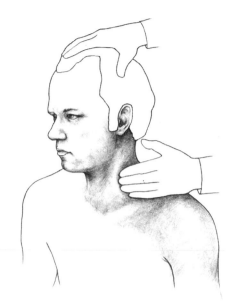

Figure 18.3. Palpation posterior to the sternocleidomastoid muscle may reveal masses and/or tenderness of the roots and/or upper brachial plexus.

may cause pain in the affected root.

ii. A light blow to the patient's forehead in the previous position (see Figure 18.4) will often cause pain when hyperextension and tilting do not.

iii. A light blow to the top of the head with the neck in the normal position may also cause pain in the distribution of the affected root.

Caution: Do not perform these tests in suspected cervical spine trauma or instability.

g. If flexion of the neck produces shocklike sensations down the back or arms, cervical cord abnormalities are suggested (Lhermitte's sign).

7. A Horner's syndrome (ptosis, miosis, decreased sweating) may occur in diseases that affect the cervical cord or the T-1 root.

8. Examination of sensation over the posterior part of the head can reveal sensory impairment from a lesion involving the second and third cervical roots (see Figure 18.5).

9. Hyperabduction and external rotation of the shoulder will obliterate the pulse in a thoracic outlet syndrome (also see Chapter 15) or will cause severe pain in periarthritis of the shoulder (see Figure 18.6).

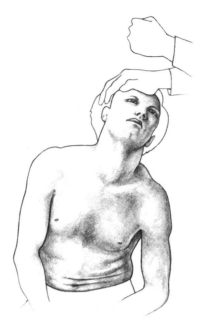

Figure 18.4. Spurling maneuver: Extension and tilting of the neck toward the affected arm may reproduce the pain by further compressing a nerve root in its exit from the foramen. Light percussion on the head as illustrated may accentuate this phenomenon.

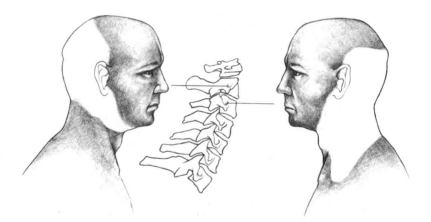

Figure 18.5. A fracture of the upper cervical vertebrae may result in a sensory loss in the distribution of C-2 or C-3. Failure to detect this sensory loss in upper cervical spine fractures may lead to dislocation of upper cervical vertebrae and severe quadriparesis or death. *Remember*: C-1 root innervates the meninges and has no cutaneous representation, and the root of C-2 exits above the vertebral body of C-2.

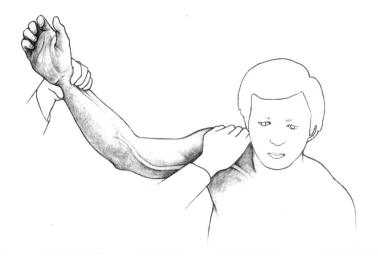

Figure 18.6. Rotation of the shoulder posteriorly when the arm is held in the illustrated position may obliterate the radial pulse at the wrist and be a clue to the thoracic outlet syndrome. As the shoulder is rotated posteriorly, the pulse should be obliterated in the affected arm sooner than the normal arm.

Acute Spinal Cord Trauma

1. In a patient with acute cervical trauma, evaluation and management must be carried out simultaneously.

   Caution: Until a complete evaluation has been carried out, the neck must be immobilized as completely as possible with sandbags, wrap around collar, or head-halter traction and with the head and shoulders supported on a board.

2. Adequate suctioning, administration of oxygen, and the maintenance of a good airway are important if the patient presents with paralysis.

   Caution: Under no circumstances should the head be hyperextended for insertion of an endotracheal tube. It is safer to do a tracheostomy if no other way of maintaining a good airway is possible.

3. Circulatory stability must be maintained since acute cervical cord injury often results in peripheral vasodilation and shock; volume expanders are usually not necessary; vasopressors are usually indicated (see Chapter 13).

4. An indwelling urinary catheter should be inserted to prevent overdistention of the bladder.

5. The level of cord injury can be best evaluated by determining the sensory level utilizing pinprick, beginning in an anesthetic area and extending upward to the area in which sensation is perceived. Do not forget

to examine sensation in the arm and hand beginning with the lower dermatome in the axilla (T-2) and ending with the higher dermatome over the deltoid (C-5).

6. If paralysis or cervical fracture is not present, muscle function should be tested by the ability of the patient to perform antigravity movements in the legs and by testing the strength of the elbow flexion and extension, wrist extension, and grip and finger extension.

7. Deep tendon reflexes should be tested; in the acute phase these reflexes may be diminished or absent (spinal shock).

8. An accurate history of the details surrounding the injury should be obtained as soon as possible. The history is most reliable immediately after the injury.

9. The patient should be examined carefully for associated injuries, especially fractures of the long bones, rupture of abdominal organs, and injury to the chest or lungs.

   Remember: The patient with paralysis and sensory loss may not be able to feel the pain of a broken bone or ruptured viscus below the level of the lesion.

10. X-ray examination should be performed after the patient's vital functions have been stabilized.

    a. If the patient has paralysis from a cervical spine injury, a single good lateral x-ray film will usually reveal the pathologic changes. In order to visualize adequately *all cervical vertebrae and the top of the first thoracic vertebra*, the shoulders must be depressed by pulling the arms toward the feet during the process of taking the x-ray film. If the film is normal but a neurologic deficit is present, a CT scan and/or myelogram is indicated.

    b. If the patient does not have paralysis or neurologic dysfunction, lateral views as described previously and AP cervical spine films should be obtained. Views of the odontoid (through the mouth) are important to rule out a fracture through the base of the odontoid. If no fracture is demonstrated, then oblique views, flexion-extension views, and occasionally tomograms should be done to evaluate suspicious areas.

Treatment:

1. For the patient with paralysis or severe spinal fracture, referral to an appropriate specialist is indicated.

   Caution: The patient should always be transported with the neck immobilized, preferably in head-halter traction.

2. The patient having cervical pain with no fractures or neurologic deficit probably has neck strain or sprain. Such a patient should be treated with:
   a. Bed rest with the patient lying flat with the neck flexed 30 degrees; the neck should be stretched using head-halter traction with no more than 1.5 kg of weight.
   b. Treat the pain with medication on demand and a muscle relaxant around the clock. (A combination of diazepam 2 to 5 mg with aspirin 650 mg tid may be effective.)
   c. During the ambulatory phase, the patient's neck can be supported with a soft, wrap around cervical collar.
   d. Remove the collar after 1 to 2 weeks and begin an intensive program of physical therapy consisting of heat, massage, and range of motion exercises to restore mobility to the cervical spine.

Tumor

Tumors of the cervical spine may be primary bone tumors, primary intraspinal tumors, or secondary tumors such as multiple myeloma, lymphoma, and metastatic carcinoma (common primary sources include breast, prostate, lungs, and kidneys). Spinal cord damage may occur either from compression by metastatic tumor in the epidural space (more commonly) or by direct invasion of spinal cord parenchyma.

1. *The most important clue to the diagnosis* is a relentless progression of pain and/or neurologic deficit (as opposed to static or intermittent pain noted with other causes).
2. Initial symptoms may vary with the location of the tumor:
   a. A bone tumor (tumor of the vertebrae) usually presents with pain often begins as a pain in the neck, and later progresses to radicular pain (pain in the arm).
   b. A neoplasm in the spinal canal may present with pain or a painless progressive neurologic deficit; the pain is radicular (extending into the arm) and may be associated with a Lhermitte's sign.
3. The examination may show:
   a. A stiffly held neck.
   b. Palpable masses, commonly in the posterior triangle or over the paraspinal areas.
   c. Areas of focal tenderness over the cervical spine.
   d. Fasciculations and atrophy of muscles of the upper extremities with hyperactive tendon reflexes in the lower extremities and Babinski

reflexes suggest compression of the spinal cord by an extrinsic or intrinsic tumor (see Table 18.2).

4. Cervical spine films may be negative (with tumors growing within the spinal cord itself) or may show destruction (as a result of bony or metastatic tumors) or erosion (from pressure effects by intraspinal tumors).

5. The CT scan and myelogram are the most valuable investigations in a patient with suspected spinal tumor. If an intramedullary tumor is suspected and the CT scan is negative, an MRI scan should be performed.

6. When symptoms strongly suggest a cervical spine neoplasm but the x-ray film is negative, a bone scan should be performed, especially when multiple metastatic lesions are suspected.

TABLE 18.2
DIFFERENTIAL DIAGNOSIS OF COMBINATION OF
ATROPHY OF ARM MUSCLES AND SPASTICITY OF LEGS

Disorder	Age of Onset	Diagnostic Features	
		Clinical	Investigative
Spondylitic myelopathy	<50 yr	Progressive spasticity and sensory ataxia with fasciculations restricted to one or two myotomes in the upper extremities	Spondylitic changes often with narrowing of foramina and/or spinal canal on plain x-ray films, CT scan, and myelography
Amyotrophic lateral sclerosis (ALS)	<40 yr	Generalized fasciculations (including bulbar muscles) with hyperactive tendon reflexes even in atrophic muscles and lack of sensory symptoms or signs	Normal x-rays films and myelogram; EMG findings diagnostic
Cervical syringomyelia	<40 yr	Dissociated sensory loss (absent pain and thermal sensation with intact touch) in the upper extremities and trunk with sacral sparing; fasciculations limited to a few myotomes of upper extremities	Widening of cord on myelogram and CT scan; best seen on MRI
Extramedullary tumor	Any age	Radicular pain and paresthesia with loss of touch and pain below the level of compression	Typical appearance on myelogram; CT scan and MRI valuable

7. Primary neoplasms of the cervical spine have no characteristic laboratory abnormalities, but secondary neoplasms may exhibit laboratory findings of malignancy such as anemia, elevated ESR, and elevation of serum alkaline and/or acid phosphatase.

Treatment:

1. Acute or subacute signs of spinal cord compression constitute a neurologic emergency. Immediate referral to an appropriate specialist is necessary if the diagnosis is suspected. CSF should be obtained during myelography.

   Caution: If bone erosion is present, support the neck in a collar (preferably a Philadelphia hard collar).

2. Acute management of cord compression from metastatic lesion includes dexamethasone 100 mg IV immediately followed by 24 mg qid for three days, then 20 mg qid for three days, and taper.

Protruded Cervical Disc

1. *The most important clue to the diagnosis* is the patient frequently awakening with a pain in the neck and within hours or days developing radiation of the pain in the distribution of the affected nerve root. (This is in contrast to tumor in which there is a longer duration of cervical pain prior to radicular involvement.)

2. A protruded cervical disc may present with or without a history of trauma.

3. The pain is usually aggravated by the patient's assuming an upright position and is often relieved by lying supine with the arm abducted at the shoulder.

4. The Valsalva maneuver often exacerbates the pain.

5. Examination may show:

   a. Limitation of range of neck motion.

   b. A positive Spurling's maneuver.

   c. Neurologic deficits in the distribution of the affected nerve root. About 80% of all ruptured discs compress either the C-6 or C-7 nerve roots. The salient features are given in Table 18.1 and in Figures 18.7 and 18.8.

6. Cervical spine films may show narrowing of the intervertebral disc space at the site of the disc protrusion. The oblique views (which should be done in all patients) may show encroachment on the intervertebral foramen.

7. The CT scan is a highly useful noninvasive method for demonstrating narrowing of intervertebral foramen and disc protrusions. It is particularly valuable when used in conjunction with water-soluble contrast media in the subarachnoid space (following the myelogram).

A   B

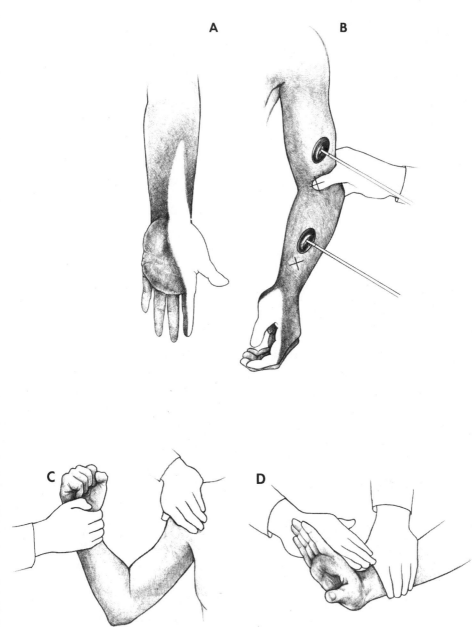

C   D

Figure 18.7. C-6 root lesion: The sensory disturbance is primarily over the thumb and the lateral aspect of the index finger (A); this sensory disturbance is most easily appreciated on the palmar surface of the hand. Decreased biceps and brachioradialis reflexes (B), weak flexion of the elbow (C), and weak extension of the wrist (D) may also be present.

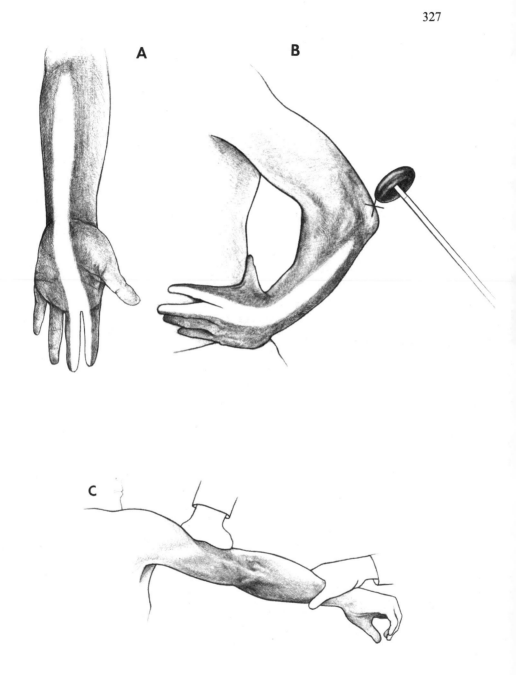

Figure 18.8. C-7 root lesion: The sensory disturbance occurs in the index and middle fingers (A) and this is also most easily appreciated on the palmar surface of the hand. A decreased triceps reflex (B) and weak extension of the elbow (C) may also be present.

8. The EMG provides objective evidence of denervation and identifies the ventral roots or roots that are affected.
9. A myelogram will identify the lesion but is indicated only if the patient has not responded to conservative treatment or is showing a rapidly progressing neurologic deficit. It should be done in an institution where neurosurgical facilities exist.
10. The clinical laboratory studies may show no consistent abnormalities.

Treatment:
1. Cervical traction is an effective treatment for a protruded cervical disc with or without mild neurologic deficits:
   a. The patient should be at strict bed rest (except for bathroom privileges).
   b. Traction should be applied continually. More than 1.5 kg of weight may cause irritation to the jaw.
   c. The head should be in a head halter; the neck should be in slight (30 degrees) flexion (see Figure 18.9).
   d. Traction should be continued for 1 week.
2. If the patient has improved, upright traction may be used intermittently to complete the therapeutic regimen. Use an over-the-door head-halter traction apparatus with 5 to 7 kg of weight for a period of 20 minutes 2 or 3 times daily (see Figure 18.10). The patient should face the door. An alternate method is to seat the patient in a recliner and place a pulley in the ceiling.
3. For mild recurring attacks, upright traction may be used effectively.
4. If the patient's pain does not respond to traction or if the neurologic deficit persists or becomes progressive, neurosurgical evaluation is indicated.

Inflammation and Infection

Inflammation and infection typically occur with rheumatoid arthritis or spondylitis, hypertrophic osteoarthritis, gouty arthritis, disc space infection, tuberculosis, or Paget's disease.

1. *The most important clue to the diagnosis* is an insidious onset with exacerbations and remissions. Acute disc space infection may have a rapid onset with no remissions. The history of exacerbations and remissions helps to differentiate chronic inflammation from tumor.
2. The patient experiences a feeling of general stiffness aggravated by movement and by maintaining one position for a long period ("jelling effect"), such as after spending the night in bed, and pain that may be worse in the late afternoon or evening, especially after an active day.

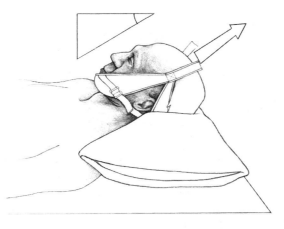

Figure 18.9. Cervical traction in the supine position: The direction of pull is 30 degrees upward from the horizontal.

3. Radicular symptoms are rare, but the pain may extend into the trapezius muscles.
4. There may be a history of related pain in other joints.

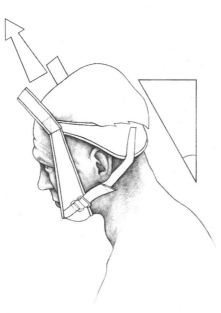

Figure 18.10. Cervical traction in the sitting position: Note the head is flexed 30 degrees, and the direction of pull is 30 degrees from the vertical.

5. Examination shows:

    a. A stiffly held neck and evidence of pain on extremes of motion in all directions.

    b. Tightness but not spasm in the cervical, occipital, and trapezius muscles.

    c. Normal reflexes, muscle strength, and sensation.

6. In the early phases, cervical spine films may be normal. In the late stages, degeneration of the discs and facet joints becomes apparent. In tuberculosis of the spine there is often collapse of adjacent vertebrae.

7. The ESR may be an important diagnostic clue, but an elevated ESR is not diagnostic, and a normal ESR does not exclude certain inflammatory processes such as gouty arthritis or Paget's disease.

8. Other valuable studies for inflammatory disease include a CBC, the presence of rheumatoid factor, antinuclear antibody studies, serum uric acid, and serum calcium, serum alkaline phosphatase determinations, *Brucella* agglutination tests, and tuberculosis skin tests.

Treatment:

1. Specific treatment for the underlying inflammatory process is necessary.

2. In acute disc space infection, immobilization of the cervical spine is mandatory. The patient should be in bed with head-halter traction until infection has subsided, then placed in a halo brace or Philadelphia hard collar. In tuberculosis of the spine, apart from immobilization, appropriate antibiotic treatment is instituted. Surgical treatment is needed if there is spinal cord compression.

3. In inflammatory arthritis, physical therapy such as diathermy and ultrasound, anti-inflammatory drugs, and temporary immobilization with a soft cervical collar may relieve the pain.

Structural Bony Abnormalities

Structural bony abnormalities typically include degenerative arthritis, osteoporosis, facet asymmetry, nonunion of the odontoid, absence of bony structure, Klippel-Feil disease, and spinal canal stenosis (cervical spondylosis or cervical bars).

Cervical Spondylosis

Cervical spondylosis is a degenerative process involving the cervical spine and constitutes a common cause for cervical pain. The degenerative changes begin in the intervertebral space leading to narrowing of the disc space, and protrusion of the disc with calcification and bar formation at multiple levels, most prominently at the C4 - C5, C5 - C6, and C6 - C7 levels. The clinical features are as follows:

1. *The most important clue to the diagnosis* is the occurrence of chronic, nagging, centrally located cervical pain, which may radiate to the occipital areas, arms, or chest; the pain is least troublesome on arising from bed, but increases with activity during the day. Recurrent episodes of neck pain with limitation of neck movement and bouts of upper extremity, intrascapular, or shoulder pain are characteristic.

2. Onset is usually after age 50 years.

3. The symptoms are of relatively long duration (there may be a history of injury preceding the symptoms).

4. With spinal canal stenosis, the patient describes progressive weakness and wasting of muscles of the arms with a feeling of stiffness and difficulty in controlling movements of the legs.

5. Dizzy spells related to neck rotation may occur in those patients in whom the degenerative changes encroach on the vertebral artery foramen.

6. Dysphagia may occur with anterior bars compressing the esophagus.

7. Minor neck trauma may precipitate major neurologic deficit in patients with cervical spondylosis, particularly when there is significant narrowing of the spinal canal.

8. Physical findings:
   a. Cervical muscle spasm and limitation of neck movement.
   b. When radiculopathy is the main feature, signs of nerve root compression are seen.
   c. When there is an accompanying spinal cord involvement (spondylitic myelopathy) due to compression by bony bars or ischemia the patient may show atrophy, fasciculation, and decreased tendon reflexes in the upper extremities with hyperreflexia, spasticity, and Babinski reflexes in the lower extremities. Myelopathy occurs more often when there is a spinal canal stenosis. The differential diagnoses of spondylitic myelopathy include ALS, syringomyelia, and extramedullary compression (see Table 18.2).

9. EMG studies are often necessary to distinguish between spondylolisthetic myelopathy and ALS.

10. Investigations:
    a. X-ray films of the cervical spin will reveal bars, narrowing of foramina, and the extent of narrowing of the spinal canal.
    b. The CT scan is an excellent technique to demonstrate osteophytes and spinal stenosis. When combined with a metrizamide myelogram the visualization is much better.
    c. MRI is the best method to visualize the changes in the spinal cord.

    d. Myelography is particularly useful in documenting the extent of cord and root compression.

Treatment:

1. The treatment must at first be conservative except when progressive neurologic deficit occurs. During the acute phase analgesics and muscle relaxants are given. A combination of aspirin (650 mg) and diazepam (5 mg) may be useful.

2. A soft cervical collar to limit neck movements may be helpful in the acute phase.

3. Surgical management (decompression of roots and spinal cord) is indicated in patients with persistent radicular pain and/or increasing neurologic deficit.

Meningeal Irritation

Meningeal irritation typically occurs with hemorrhage or infection in the subarachnoid space.

1. The symptoms of cervical pain begin acutely or subacutely.

2. The pain is associated with nonthrobbing occipital headache.

3. The patient complains of stiffness of the neck and a pulling sensation in the lower back with forward flexion of the neck.

4. Examination shows:

    a. An ill-appearing patient.

    b. Hyperextension of the neck.

    c. Guarding of the neck against forward flexion. Flexion increases the cervical pain and may produce pain between the scapulae.

    d. No aggravation of pain with rotatory neck movements.

    e. An elevated temperature.

    f. Kernig's and Brudzinski's signs (see Chapter 14).

5. Patients with either hemorrhage or infection in the subarachnoid space may show elevation of the peripheral white blood count with a shift to the left.

6. Abnormal CSF often confirms the diagnosis (be sure to culture the CSF).

Treatment:

1. Appropriate antibiotic therapy in the case of meningitis (see Chapter 14).

2. Treat subarachnoid hemorrhage with analgesics, and sedation if necessary, limiting visitors, and absolute bed rest with no bathroom privileges. Neurosurgical consultation is indicated.

Cervical Muscle Spasm from Tension

Cervical muscle spasm from tension typically occurs from emotional stress or a work-related circumstance (such as a secretary sitting over a typewriter all day).

1. Pain radiates down both shoulders, up the occiput, and often over the top of the head into the forehead.
2. The pain frequently disturbs the patient at night.
3. The patient may be anxious, despondent, angry, or hostile.
4. Examination shows:
   a. A straight neck with tense and tender cervical muscles. This is best appreciated in the supine position.
   b. Resistance to passive movement of the neck in all directions.
   c. No neurologic abnormalities.
5. Do not be misled by nonspecific laboratory and x-ray findings.

   Remember: The cervical spine films in most patients over age 40 years will show some degenerative changes.

Treatment:

1. For symptomatic job-related stress, a change of work activities may be indicated.
2. Appropriate treatment of any underlying emotional disturbance is indicated.

   Remember: Even though the underlying problem is emotional, the patient still experiences pain from the muscle spasm

BIBLIOGRAPHY

Brain WR, Baron J, Wilkinson M: *Cervical Spondylosis and Other Disorders of the Cervical Spine*. Philadelphia, WB Saunders Co, 1976.

Hoppenfeld S: *Orthopedic Neurology: A Diagnostic Guide to Neurologic Levels*. Philadelphia, JB Lippincott Co, 1977.

Jenkins DG: Differential diagnosis and management of neck pain. *Physiotherapy* 1982; 68:252-255.

Patchell RA, Posner JB: Neurologic complications of systemic cancer. *Neurol Clin* 1985; 3:729-750.

Schmidek HH: Cervical spondylosis. *Am Fam Physician* 1986; 33(5):89-99

XIX

THE PATIENT WITH A HEAD INJURY

Head trauma is perhaps the most common cause of brain damage in the young adult. Some of this damage is avoidable if prompt management is undertaken soon after the injury. However, many physicians feel apprehensive and insecure in managing the unconscious head-injured patient. This chapter outlines the initial evaluation and treatment, which should be carried out before transfer to a tertiary care center.

Remember: Evaluation and management of the patient must be carried out simultaneously.

Acute Management of the Head-Injured Patient

Following a head injury, the patient may present to the emergency room in an alert state or be brought in in a state of coma. While the alert patient will need only a CT scan and careful observation the comatose patient needs urgent measures.

1. Initial Management
   a. Stabilizing vital functions
      i. A good airway and adequate blood oxygenation must be maintained.
         (a) Insert an oropharyngeal airway; suction adequately to remove secretions. Insert an endotracheal tube if the patient is comatose. It is important to do this procedure rapidly and without causing any distress since even short periods of hypoxia and hypercarbia may increase the brain volume and initiate herniation. A tracheostomy is needed ur-

334

gently only in cases of severe maxillofacial and neck injuries.

(b) In the patient with respiratory distress, for whatever reason, oxygen in high concentration must be administered.

Note: Prompt endotracheal intubation and hyperventilation sufficient to drop P_aCO_2 to 30 torr may have contributed to the recently noticed decrease in morbidity and mortality following head injury.

ii. Circulatory stability must be maintained.

    (a) IV fluids should be held to a minimum in patients with possible brain herniation.

    (b) The patient with a low blood pressure and rapid pulse may have reduced circulating blood volume (blood loss). The source of hemorrhage may not be apparent since the comatose patient cannot complain of pain or exhibit typical signs of bleeding (eg, rigidity of abdominal wall in intraperitoneal hemorrhage). An IV line must be established and treatment aimed at maintaining adequate cerebral circulation by replacing blood loss and administering vasoconstrictors. A hemogram and type and cross-match should be obtained as soon as possible. P_aO_2 and P_aCO_2 should be monitored.

2. Immediate Management

  a. Once the vital functions are stabilized, there must be an ongoing determination of the level of consciousness and neurologic function (refer to Chapter 13) by determining:

    i. The level of consciousness: The most important criterion in the initial evaluation and follow-up of patients with head injury is the level of consciousness. The Glasgow Coma Scale (based on eye opening, best motor response, and verbal response; see Chapter 13) is simple enough for repeated recording by nurses, paramedical personnel, or physicians and has been shown to provide a reliable indication of prognosis. In one study 87% of patients with a score of more than 11 in the first 24 hours had good recovery, while 87% of those with scores of less than 5 remained in a vegetative state or were dead.

    ii. Pupillary size and reaction to light are highly useful in detecting impending herniation. With uncal herniation through the tentorial notch, the ipsilateral pupil dilates, and becomes poorly reactive to light, followed by similar changes in the contralateral pupil. In a large study, 50% of patients with intact pupillary reaction made good recovery while 91% with nonreactive pupils (in the first 24 hours after coma) either died or remained in a vegetative state.

   iii. Any focal deficit as evidenced by asymmetry of tendon reflexes or plantar response or movements in response to painful stimulation.

b. An indwelling urinary catheter should be inserted to obtain a urine specimen for analysis, to evaluate urinary output, and to avoid over-distention of the bladder.

c. Insert a nasogastric tube attached to suction to prevent abdominal distention and vomiting.

d. Hyperthermia should be treated by placing the patient on a cooling blanket or by applying ice water and alcohol to the skin.

e. Seizures should be controlled with IV anticonvulsants (see Chapter 11).

f. Extreme restlessness may be treated with barbiturates and codeine (phenobarbital 60 mg q4h IM and codeine 60 mg q4h IM given on an alternating q2h schedule).

Caution: The most important clinical criterion in a comatose patient is the level of consciousness; it is not possible to assess this properly if sedatives are administered to the patient. Hence, never use morphine,and give sedatives only sparingly to a patient with head injury.

g. Rapidly appraise associated injuries to identify intrathoracic or intra-abdominal hemorrhage, fractures, or lacerations with excessive blood loss. Appropriate management of such problems must be instituted immediately.

h. It is not sufficient to assume that the unconsciousness has resulted solely from the head injury. It may be the result of shock, alcohol or drug intoxication, adrenal insufficiency, stroke, diabetic acidosis, insulin shock, or other metabolic disturbances (see Chapter 13). Do the relevant blood studies.

i. As soon as the vital signs are stable all patients with head injury should undergo CT scan study. X-ray films of skull, spine, chest, abdomen, or other areas should be done depending on the clinical presentation. In a comatose patient fractures of the extremities or pelvis can be easily missed since the patient will not complain of pain.

Caution: Always suspect a cervical spine injury until excluded by lateral cervical spine x-ray (see Chapter 18).

j. A description of the nature and mechanism of injury from any available sources of information should be obtained. Appropriate consultations with neurosurgery, general surgery, cardiopulmonary surgery, or orthopedic surgery staff should be requested as the need for specialized care is identified. Transfer to a specialized center may be necessary.

3. When the patient's condition has been stabilized, a more complete neurologic examination should be performed (see Chapter 13). This examination should include the following:

   a. State of consciousness.

   b. Respirations: Slow, deep, or irregular respirations suggest serious intracranial abnormalities, while shallow rapid respirations are more commonly associated with pathologic changes extrinsic to the nervous system, such as shock related to blood loss.

   c. The degree of paresis of extremities: Early complete flaccid paralysis occurring unilaterally suggests marked damage to the opposite cerebral hemisphere, while spasticity of all four extremities suggests severe brainstem or cervical spinal cord injury.

   d. The presence of peripheral cranial nerve palsies is suggestive of a basilar skull fracture.

   e. Spinal fluid draining from the ear or nose is diagnostic of a basilar skull fracture.

   Caution: Basilar skull fractures usually cannot be seen on routine skull films.

Classification and Management of Cranial Injury

Injuries to the Scalp

1. Abrasions should be treated by careful cleansing with soap and sterile water; hair need not be removed; particles embedded in the scalp should be removed with a surgical brush to avoid the tattoo effect of retained particles. The area may be left either exposed to the air or covered with a sterile nonadherent dressing.

2. Contusions (bruises) may be treated by cold compresses.

3. Lacerations should be closed by suturing after the hair has been shaved from around the area and the area has been carefully cleansed. If a laceration extends through the galea, it is desirable to close the galea with absorbable suture *separately* from the closure of the skin.

4. Avulsions constitute a serious problem and in all cases the avulsed scalp should be preserved in normal saline. Microvascular surgical anastomoses of the vessels to restore circulation to the avulsed tissue is necessary.

Injuries to the Skull

1. Linear skull fractures are often difficult to identify on routine skull x-ray films and may be confused with vascular markings or suture lines.

Linear fractures may be particularly difficult to see if they occur in the base of the skull. Often basilar skull fractures can only be identified by:

    a. Blood behind the eardrum and/or Battle's sign (black-and-blue discoloration over the mastoid).

    b. Raccoon eyes (ecchymoses around the eyelids) suggest a frontal fracture.

2. Stereoscopic x-ray films of the skull are the most helpful study for evaluating linear skull fractures. Obtaining skull films in minor head trauma may not be necessary, but remember that skull fractures may occur without loss of consciousness. A patient with a skull fracture that crosses a venous sinus or a branch of a meningeal artery should be hospitalized and observed with hourly cranial checks for 24 hours (see Chapter 12).

3. A patient with a compound comminuted skull fracture should be treated with debridement and neurosurgical reconstruction.

4. Depressed skull fractures should be surgically elevated.

Injuries to the Dura and Leptomeninges

1. Injuries to the dura and leptomeninges are usually associated with a skull fracture.

2. An injury to the dura and leptomeninges over the paranasal sinuses or mastoid allows admission of air and/or infection to the intracranial contents and escape of CSF. Unless contraindicated for other reasons, patients with CSF leakage should be placed in a position with the head elevated to a 45 degree angle. This minimizes retrograde infection into the cranial cavity and encourages tamponade of the brain into the fistula tract. Prophylactic use of a broad-spectrum antibiotic in a therapeutic dose should be considered. Watch for signs of meningitis (see Chapter 14). The patient should be instructed to avoid blowing the nose. If CSF drainage persists beyond 2 weeks, neurosurgical consultation is indicated.

3. Intracranial hemorrhage may occur in skull fractures with meningeal involvement from injury to the blood vessels:

    a. *Extradural (epidural) hematoma* (bleeding from damage to a dural artery, most commonly the middle meningeal artery):

        i. Progressive drowsiness may follow a lucid interval, or the patient may remain unconscious from the time of the initial trauma.

        ii. Progressive headache may be a presenting symptom.

        iii. A dilating pupil on the side of the hemorrhage is highly suggestive of extradural hemorrhage (due to herniation).

        iv. A hemiparesis opposite to the side of the hemorrhage may be present.

        v. A focal motor seizure in the extremities opposite the side of the hemorrhage may occur.

vi. A slowing of the pulse and respirations and an increase in blood pressure are late and ominous signs. Progressive hemiparesis occurring on the same side as the dilated pupils suggests brain-stem involvement and indicates a grave prognosis.

Caution: This condition represents one of the most acute of all emergencies. Prompt neurosurgical evacuation of the clot usually results in complete functional recovery; delayed intervention results in permanent brain damage or death. If a diagnosis is suspected, immediate neurosurgical consultation is indicated. The diagnosis can be confirmed by CT scan.

b. *Acute subdural hematoma* usually results from damage to the venous sinuses or to the veins communicating between the cortex and the venous sinuses. Patients may show a variety of neurologic findings such as seizures, progressive deepening coma, progressive headache, progressive hemiparesis, confusional state, and signs of increased intracranial pressure.

Caution: Although the progressive deterioration in the patient with acute subdural hematoma is not usually as rapid as that in extradural hematoma, prompt neurosurgical treatment is still necessary. As with extradural hematoma, the diagnosis can be confirmed by CT scan.

Injuries to the Brain

A. *Cerebral concussion* may be defined as a temporary impairment of cerebral neuronal function due to a blow to the head and may be divided into the following categories:
1. Mild concussion - impaired neurologic function lasting less than five minutes.
2. Moderate concussion - impaired neurologic function lasting more than five minutes but less than three hours.
3. Severe concussion - impaired neurologic function lasting more than three hours. There are no demonstrable structural abnormalities in cerebral concussion. Patients with concussion recover completely, although sometimes a postconcussional syndrome consisting of headache, dizziness, and personality changes may occur.

Treatment:
1. The patient with either mild or moderate cerebral concussion can be managed at home if someone is ready to observe the patient's responsiveness, pupillary size, and ability to move the extremities on an hourly basis for 24 hours.

2. If the patient is hospitalized, hourly evaluation of the level of consciousness and the pupillary reactions should be performed (see Chapter 12).

B. *Cerebral contusion* is an impairment of neuronal function resulting from structural damage ("bruised brain"). Focal contusions occur under the site of impact or more often in the undersurface of the frontal or the anterior part of the temporal lobes from impact against the lesser wing of the sphenoid (the lesser wing of the sphenoid has been called the "dashboard" of the cranial cavity). Clinical findings include focal neurologic abnormalities and loss of consciousness.

Treatment:

The patient should be hospitalized with at least hourly neurologic evaluations (see Chapter 12) during the acute phase. Supportive care should be provided based on the degree of neurologic impairment.

Note: For medical, legal, and prognostic purposes, concussion and contusion may be differentiated by CT scans and serial EEGs. In the case of cerebral concussion, the EEGs show only temporary changes, whereas in the case of cerebral contusion, they show persistent abnormalities. CT scans usually show blood at the site of a cerebral contusion and are normal with a concussion.

C. *Cerebral lacerations* are secondary to depressed skull fractures or penetrating wounds.

Treatment:

Lacerations require immediate (within six hours) neurosurgical treatment. Emergency management should include control of hemorrhage from the scalp at the site of the injury and application of a sterile dressing. Accompanying scalp lacerations should not be sutured until after neurosurgical reconstruction has been performed.

D. *Traumatic subarachnoid hemorrhage* should be suspected when the patient presents with headache and stiff neck with or without other neurologic signs. Subarachnoid hemorrhage may also be present in the patient with coma and stiff neck. The diagnosis can be confirmed by CT scan.

Treatment:

Support of vital functions, elevation of the head to approximately 30 degrees, and careful observation with at least hourly neurologic evaluations (see Chapter 12) are required. Lumbar puncture should be deferred for 72 hours or longer if the patient is unstable. Symptomatic improvement may be obtained by removal of bloody CSF with repeated lumbar punctures. CSF will be xanthochromic and under elevated pressure. The amount of fluid removed should only be the volume necessary to reduce the spinal fluid pressure to one-half of the initial reading.

E. *Traumatic intracerebral hematoma* is suggested by increased intracranial pressure, progressive focal neurologic deficits, and a deteriorating state of consciousness. The presence of blood can be readily demonstrated by CT scan. Neurosurgical consultation is indicated.

Common Complications

A. *Increased Intracranial Pressure*

Increased intracranial pressure following head trauma is common. It may be due to simple causes such as airway obstruction with accompanying hypoxia and hypercarbia, or the presence of an intracranial hematoma, or sometimes no specific cause is demonstrable on the CT scan. It is possible that edema of the brain can develop following injury and may account for the increased pressure.

Treatment:

Increased intracranial pressure has a deleterious effect on the outcome, and prompt treatment should be undertaken depending on the cause. It is common practice now to monitor the intracranial pressure using an epidural, subdural, or intraventricular pressure monitor. Such procedures can be done only in a neurosurgical unit. The measures used in such centers include:

a. Hyperventilation: Hyperventilation is an effective way of reducing intracranial pressure rapidly. The rate of respiration should be adjusted such that the P_aCO_2 is around 30 torr. The effect achieved on intracranial pressure is by reduced intracranial blood volume and perhaps by decreased CSF formation.

b. Infusion of hyperosmolar agents like 20% mannitol: Use only after neurosurgical consultation unless the patient happens to be in a state of impending herniation.

c. Corticosteroids: There is no uniformity of opinion as to the efficacy of corticosteroids in posttraumatic cerebral edema.

d. In children with posttraumatic cerebral edema (with no surgically treatable cause) induction of barbiturate coma is undertaken in some centers.

B. *Posttraumatic Epilepsy*

While seizures may occur early in the course of a head injury, late posttraumatic epilepsy is one of the most frequent delayed complications. It occurs in about 5% of all patients admitted to hospitals after nonmissile head injury. The risk of epilepsy is higher when there has been intracranial hematoma or a compound depressed skull fracture or when there has been an early seizure (in the first week after injury). The onset is most common during the first 2 years although it has been reported even after 10 years.

Treatment: See Chapter 11.

C. *Postconcussional Syndrome*

    1. Following head trauma, 30% to 80% of patients have been reported to develop one or more of the following symptoms:

        a. Chronic posttraumatic headache: a constant, dull, nonthrobbing headache often described as a tight band around the head; sometimes associated with local area of tenderness or pain especially if a scar is present; rarely intermittent throbbing headaches may also occur. May last for several weeks to months or sometimes years.

        b. Dizziness, either intermittent or chronic, may be a major symptom (see Chapter 4).

        c. Amnesia, poor concentration, and learning difficulties in children.

        d. Emotional lability: irritability, aggressiveness, and hyperkinesis.

    2. The syndrome may occur following open and closed head trauma. There is no consistent correlation with duration of unconsciousness, posttraumatic amnesia, skull fracture, or blood in the CSF.

    3. Pre-existing psychiatric problems (eg, depression) and pending litigation are believed to be predisposing factors.

Treatment:

Amitriptyline hydrochloride 50 to 100 mg daily over a period of several weeks to months has been found to be effective, especially for the chronic posttraumatic headache. Reassure the patient and, if necessary, institute psychotherapy.

BIBLIOGRAPHY

Diamond S, Friedman AP: Management of post-traumatic headache, in Diamond S, Friedman AP (eds): *Headache. Contemporary Patient Management Series.* New York, Medical Examination Publishing Co, 1983, pp 65-70.

Jennett B, Teasdale G: *Management of Head Injuries.* Philadelphia, FA Davis Co, 1981.

Vogel HB: Trauma of the head, spine and peripheral nerves, in Earnest MP (ed): *Neurologic Emergencies,* New York, Churchill Livingstone, 1983, pp 177-217.

XX

NEUROLOGIC EMERGENCIES

By the word "emergency," we mean those conditions which, if not treated immediately, may result in death or permanent nervous system damage. There are conditions, such as the excruciating pain of trigeminal neuralgia, that may require immediate treatment but which are not included here because lack of treatment will not result in permanent damage. What is "neurologic" is also open to discussion; delirium tremens, threat of suicide, and acute glaucoma are ordinarily not considered neurologic problems, although clearly they are emergencies and if untreated may lead to permanent nervous system damage. Table 20.1 lists neurologic conditions that we consider emergencies with a brief statement of just why we consider them so. The remainder of the chapter is devoted to evaluation of symptoms we consider emergencies.

Coma

See Chapter 13 for examination, differential diagnosis, and management.

Immediate measures for all comatose patients include the following:

1. Determine the need for cardiopulmonary resuscitation (CPR).
2. Stabilize the patient.
   a. Establish and maintain a clear airway; provide ventilatory assistance, if necessary.
   b. Establish access to the circulation with an IV line, drawing blood at the same time for hematology and biochemistry tests.
   c. Maintain blood pressure with elevation of legs and/or volume expanders (blood or plasma, normal saline, lactated Ringer's solution).

Table 20.1
NEUROLOGIC CONDITIONS CONSIDERED TO BE EMERGENCIES

PROCESS	REASON FOR EMERGENCY
Coma	Many causes of coma such as drug overdose, hypoglycemia, or expanding cerebral mass may cause irreversible brain damage if not treated immediately
Transient ischemic attacks	Cause of attacks may be treatable (eg, embolus); untreated, permanent brain damage may occur
Stroke	Cause of paralysis could be reversible, such as a subdural hematoma, instead of the over-used diagnosis of intracerebral atherosclerosis
Bacterial meningitis	Delayed treatment results in irreversible brain damage or death
Spinal cord compression	Unless pressure on the cord is relieved within a few hours, permanent paralysis will result
Status epilepticus	Prolonged seizures may result in brain damage or death
Fracture of the spinal column	Inappropriate movement of the patient may permanently sever the spinal cord
Thiamine deficiency	Delayed treatment results in an irreversible organic brain syndrome
Temporal arteritis	The process may spread to intracranial arteries and cause cerebral infarction or blindness
Severe muscle spasms	These are usually caused by severe hypocal-cemia or tetanus, both of which are treatable
Myasthenia gravis	Respiratory failure in a crisis may occur suddenly and without warning
Guillain-Barré syndrome	Respiratory failure may occur suddenly without warning in a patient who is not severely weak

    d. Administer glucose (after a blood sugar has been drawn) in the form of 25g in a 50% glucose solution.

  3. Determine the cause of the coma.

Status Epilepticus

Convulsive status epilepticus is a medical emergency because of the respiratory compromise and subsequent hypoxic brain damage that may occur. Nonconvulsive status is not a medical emergency because no respiratory compromise occurs. See Chapter 11 for management.

Head Trauma

See Chapter 19 for management of head trauma.

Fracture of the Spinal Column and Spinal Cord Compression

Cervical spine fracture must be suspected following any neck trauma from falls, being thrown from a car, or blows to the neck. If a patient is also comatose, cervical spine fracture must be ruled out by lateral cervical spine films *before* undue manipulation of the neck. If there is a neurologic deficit and the plain x-ray films are normal, a CT scan of the spinal column and cord and/or a myelogram is indicated. For management, see Chapter 18.

Spinal cord emergencies present with acute paralysis of the legs, and with varying involvement of the trunk and upper extremities depending on the level of the compression. There is a sudden and rapidly progressive onset of sensory and/or motor loss of function in the trunk and extremities below the level of the lesion.

> *Remember*: If decompression laminectomy can be performed or radiation therapy initiated (for malignancy) before all neurologic function (below the level of the lesion) has been lost, complete recovery of function is possible. Steroids may provide temporary relief.

If pain occurs, it is often radicular from involvement of the sensory spinal nerves at the level of the spinal cord lesion; pain seldom involves the trunk or extremities below the level of the lesion.

The etiologies of spinal cord emergencies include the following:

1. Sudden compression of the spinal cord during trauma, usually secondary to a compression fracture or fracture-dislocation of the spine
2. Collapse of a vertebra from involvement by infection (tuberculosis, osteomyelitis) or neoplasm (metastatic carcinoma, multiple myeloma)
3. A ruptured intervertebral disc
4. Ischemia of the spinal cord from aortic occlusive disease or progressive compression by a neoplasm, primary or metastatic, intra-axial or extra-axial; or thrombosis of anterior spinal artery
5. Spontaneous hemorrhage into the spinal cord from a vascular malformation

6. Acute or subacute infection (subdural empyema) or inflammation of the spinal cord (transverse myelitis)

Findings

1. Motor deficits resulting from lesions of the spinal cord may be identified by hyperactive reflexes in the lower extremities combined with Babinski reflexes. In acute spinal cord damage there is often a temporary flaccid paralysis with absent deep tendon reflexes in the lower extremities from "spinal shock."

2. A sensory level is an important clue to spinal cord involvement.
   a. Begin sensory testing in an anesthetic area and work toward an area of normal sensation (usually a pin is used).
   b. Test for sensory level on the back, as well as on the chest and abdomen.
   c. With a high thoracic or cervical lesion, examine sensation in the arms and hands beginning with the lower dermatome in the axilla (T-2) and ending with the higher dermatome over the deltoid (C-5).

3. Beevor's sign can help determine a motor level over the trunk, particularly the abdomen. The examiner places his index finger at the level of the umbilicus and asks the patient, who is lying flat, to look at the finger. If the umbilicus moves up, the level of the lesion is at T-10 or below. The normally strong upper abdominal muscles will contract, while the lower abdominal muscles (below the umbilicus, or T-10) will not, pulling the umbilicus up toward the head.

4. Spinal cord involvement localized to one half of the spinal cord will result in a Brown-Séquard syndrome.
   a. The leg on the same side will show weakness, hyperreflexia, a Babinski reflex, and loss of sensation to position and vibration.
   b. The opposite leg will show a deficit to pinprick.

5. A central cord injury of the cervical spinal cord may result in a flaccid paralysis of the muscles of the arms with absent deep tendon reflexes in the arms (due to damage involving the anterior horn cells), and hyperactive reflexes with Babinski reflexes in the lower extremities (due to damage involving the corticospinal tract).

   Management:
   1. In the patient with acute spinal column trauma associated with spinal cord injury, the spinal column must be kept immobile (see Chapter 17). These same principles should also be followed in cases showing acute involvement of the spinal cord from other lesions.
   2. Adequate blood pressure must be maintained, since acute spinal cord

damage often results in peripheral vasodilatation and shock.

   a. Elevate the legs.

   b. Administer peripheral vasoconstrictive agents (see Chapter 13).

3. An indwelling catheter should be placed as soon as practical to prevent overdistention of the bladder.

4. If respiratory insufficiency is present consider the following:

   a. Suctioning and the administration of oxygen

   b. Intubation with a soft cuff endotracheal tube or tracheostomy

5. Patients with acute spinal cord compression must be referred for urgent neurosurgical management.

Caution: Myelography should be avoided unless facilities are available for immediate neurosurgical decompression. If the patient has some residual neurologic function below the level of the lesion, decompression laminectomy may result in dramatic improvement in more than 50% of cases.

Transient Ischemic Attacks

TIAs (see Chapter 12) are episodes of temporary CNS dysfunction, usually lasting minutes, but always lasting less than 24 hours. Approximately one third of patients with TIAs go on to develop stroke.

Caveat: Transient dysfunction today could be a permanent dysfunction tomorrow. Many of the causes are treatable.

1. Thromboemboli from the heart (atrial fibrillation, valvular heart disease, or postmyocardial infarction)

2. Platelet emboli from an ulcerated carotid plaque

3. Carotid or vertebral stenosis

4. Hypoglycemia

Treatment:

Adequate treatment depends on adequate diagnosis and this almost invariably includes the following:

1. CT scan of the brain, mainly to rule out hemorrhage

2. Digital intravenous subtraction angiography, or four-vessel cerebral angiogram

Caution: All TIAs are not "ischemic" and anticoagulation of the patient whose transient dysfunction was caused by bleeding could be dangerous to the patient's health!

Stroke in Progression

The only way to be certain of the diagnosis of stroke in progression is to actually observe the patient deteriorating over time. Since deterioration may be stuttering in temporal profile, this is a difficult judgment to make. If the neurologic deficit is progressive, it is imperative to determine first whether bleeding is occurring, such as in hypertensive hemorrhage, subarachnoid hemorrhage secondary to aneurysm or arteriovenous malformation, or hemorrhage into a tumor. An emergency CT scan of the brain is the procedure of choice. Barring that, if there are no contraindications (such as increased intracranial pressure or evidence of supra- or subtentorial mass), lumbar puncture may reveal bleeding.

If there is no evidence of subarachnoid, parenchymal or intraventricular hemorrhage, occlusive disease (ie, thrombosis or embolus) is the most likely cause. Within the first 24 hours or so, the CT scan may not show any decreased densities or evidence of infarct. Short-term anticoagulation may be considered (see Chapter 12).

1. There is universal agreement that anticoagulation with heparin first, and then oral anticoagulants later, is indicated for cardiogenic emboli. If the deficit is massive and the infarct is hemorrhagic, one may need to wait a week or more to initiate anticoagulation.

2. If there is evidence of progressive stroke and no evidence of either cardiogenic emboli or hemorrhage, use short-term anticoagulation beginning with heparin sodium, 10,000 units IV by infusion pump, followed by 1000 to 1200 units/hour through a pump in order to maintain the partial thromboplastin time (PTT) 1.5 to 2 times normal.

3. Subsequently, decisions can be made as to whether to institute long-term anticoagulation using warfarin compounds or aspirin (or aspirin plus dipyridamole). There are no good controlled studies yet published that show that surgical treatment (ie, endarterectomy) has any better results, in the long run, than medical therapy, although it may be helpful in selected patients; however, recent studies do show that extracranial-intracranial arterial bypass surgery definitely has no better results than medical therapy.

Stroke

For evaluation, see Chapter 12.

A stroke is the sudden occurrence of a neurologic deficit, usually due to vascular disease, but some of the other causes of stroke are curable. The preceding remarks under TIAs are appropriate for stroke. *DO NOT* assume that all strokes are caused by intracerebral atherosclerosis.

Fever and Central Nervous System Symptoms

See Chapter 14.

Meningitis

1. Consider the possibility of bacterial meningitis in any patient with fever

and even minimal mental or neurologic symptoms.

2. Whenever the diagnosis is suspected, a lumbar puncture must be performed and bacterial cultures obtained. When the CSF is abnormal, tuberculous and fungal cultures should also be obtained.

3. Prognosis depends on the interval between the onset of the illness and institution of therapy.

Treatment:

1. If the CSF examination is suggestive of bacterial meningitis (increased nucleated cells, particularly neutrophils, and low sugar) and after cultures have been sent, the patient must be started on IV antibiotics. The choice of antibiotics depends on the patient's age and medical history (see Chapter 14), and the results of the Gram stain of the CSF. The antibiotic regimen can be modified later when culture and sensitivity results are known.

2. Management of complications may be necessary (see Chapters 11, 13, and 14).

Encephalitis

If severe headache, stiff neck, and Brudzinski's and Kernig's signs are absent, mental symptoms are prominent, and the CSF shows normal sugar, a low number of cells, or predominantly a mononuclear pleocytosis (lymphocytosis), encephalitis must be suspected. It is important early in the course of the illness to recognize or suspect *Herpes simplex* encephalitis since it has now been shown that acyclovir instituted early, and even without brain biopsy confirmation, has decreased the morbidity remarkably. Patients with *Herpes simplex* encephalitis classically present with an acute onset of mental and behavioral symptoms, often with an amnestic syndrome, and may have lateralized findings, such as mild hemiparesis or aphasia. They have an EEG with focal slowing over the temporal lobe and (at some point during the course) periodic lateralizing epileptiform discharges (PLEDS). The CT scan shows decreased density and swelling of the involved temporal lobe.

Treatment:

For *Herpes simplex* encephalitis begin acyclovir immediately at 10 mg/kg/day IV q8h for at least ten days; in some cases, brain biopsy may have to be performed for confirmation.

Guillain-Barré Syndrome

See Chapter 15.

Treatment:

1. Respiratory function initially must be closely monitored with frequent (at least hourly) bedside forced vital capacity (FVC) and inspiratory force

measurements. Respiratory function must be closely monitored even in patients with no apparent respiratory involvement, since rapid progression over several hours may lead to respiratory failure. If FVC falls below 1400 mL in the 70-kg individual, tracheostomy or insertion of a soft-cuff endotracheal tube must be very seriously considered. An inspiratory force (a direct reflection of respiratory muscular strength) of less than 25 cm also indicates the probable need for tracheostomy. The frequency of monitoring of respiratory function may be reduced as the patient shows signs of clinical improvement.

2. Respiratory insufficiency may have causes other than muscle weakness:
   a. Aspiration pneumonia from inability to swallow properly
   b. Pulmonary embolism from venous stasis of immobilized legs
   c. Pneumonia from decreased cough and hypoventilation
3. Early institution of plasmapheresis has been reported to hasten recovery and reduce morbidity.

Myasthenia Gravis (Myasthenic or Cholinergic Crisis)

See Chapter 15.

The patient with myasthenia gravis may present as a neurologic emergency or crisis in which there is rapidly progressive respiratory insufficiency. Crisis usually occurs in a patient with known myasthenia during added stress such as infection, anesthesia, surgery, or medication changes; occasionally a patient with undiagnosed myasthenia gravis will present primarily with respiratory failure. Crises are of two types:

1. *Myasthenic crisis* - an increase in severity of the disease relative to the treatment (ie, undertreatment).
2. *Cholinergic crisis* - an excess of anticholinergic activity (usually from anticholinesterase drugs) relative to the severity of the disease (ie, overtreatment).

It is difficult or impossible to differentiate these two types of crises at the time of presentation with imminent respiratory failure. Sometimes the evidence of excessive acetylcholine effect, such as abdominal cramps, sweating, lacrimation, bradycardia, miosis, muscle cramps, and fasciculations may suggest that the patient is in a cholinergic crisis; however, caution is necessary, since such signs may be absent in definite cholinergic crisis or present in a myasthenic crisis.

Treatment:

1. Maintain ventilation initially with an AMBU bag and later with a soft-cuff endotracheal tube or a tracheostomy. The soft-cuffed endotracheal tube may be left in place for up to a week without serious risk or distress to the patient.

2. Withdraw all medications used to treat myasthenia and all drugs with a curarelike action (such as antibiotics that end in "-mycin").
3. After 24 hours, gradually reintroduce antimyasthenic medication.
4. Some centers with appropriate equipment and trained personnel use plasmapheresis. The place of immunosuppressant drugs is still controversial.

Remember:
1. Myasthenia is a disease characterized by muscle fatigability; artificial ventilatory support will temporarily restore respiratory strength, which will then gradually decline.
2. Respiratory failure may occur in the presence of normal arm and leg strength.
3. Myasthenia kills only by respiratory failure.

Wernicke's Encephalopathy-Thiamine Deficiency

See Chapter 8.

The presentation is of a patient with an acute confusional state (characterized by disorientation and an amnestic syndrome) accompanied by extraocular muscle paralysis and evidence of polyneuropathy. Although it occurs primarily in nutritionally deficient alcoholics, it may occur in other settings, such as the hospitalized patient receiving IV feedings without thiamine supplements or individuals who are on diets deficient in thiamine.

Treatment:
Thiamine 100 mg IV (preferable) or orally immediately, followed by 50 mg bid maintenance dose.

Differential Diagnosis of Acute Paralysis of Extraocular Movement That May Have Emergency Implications

1. *Botulism* presents as paralysis of extraocular muscles rapidly progressing to involvement of swallowing, generalized weakness, and respiratory failure. It is most commonly associated with eating improperly home-canned acidic foods (such as green beans), and the diagnosis should be strongly suspected when several members of a family acquire symptoms.

   Treatment: Antitoxin should be administered immediately. Contact the local poison control center for a supply of antitoxin. Respiratory failure should be treated with mechanical ventilatory support.
2. *Myasthenia gravis* (see Chapter 15): Paralysis of extraocular movement in ocular myasthenia may occur acutely but presents no immediate danger, and there is no long-term danger if weakness is confined to those muscles. However, if generalized myasthenia develops, respiratory failure may result.

3. *Cavernous sinus thrombosis* presents with paralysis of extraocular muscles and a painful bulging red eye; it is often associated with sinus infection; four-vessel cerebral angiography may be necessary to establish the diagnosis.

   Treatment: Blood and CSF cultures must be obtained; skull films with sinus films or CT scan may reveal the source of infection. Massive doses of IV antibiotics, as if treating meningitis, should be given (see Chapter 14).

4. *Carotid-cavernous fistula*: The patient usually has suffered a recent head injury and presents with extraocular palsies and a painful bulging red eye, which pulsates synchronously with carotid pulsation. A bruit may be heard over the eye. Cerebral angiography will establish the diagnosis.

   Treatment: Neurosurgical intervention is usually necessary.

5. *Posterior communicating artery aneurysm*: The patient often presents with third cranial (oculomotor) nerve palsy (the affected eye is turned down and out and the pupil is dilated). The ocular palsy occurs most often when the aneurysm ruptures and the patient develops severe headache and stiff neck. Unlike the acute third nerve palsy of diabetes in which pupillary reactivity is intact, in the case of an aneurysm the pupil is dilated and poorly reactive to light on the the side of palsy. The diagnosis is established by four-vessel cerebral angiography.

   Treatment: Neurosurgical consultation is mandatory, and surgical intervention is necessary if the aneurysm has a neck that can be clipped.

Temporal Arteritis - Sudden Loss of Vision

1. A firm, tender temporal artery associated with an elevated ESR suggests a diagnosis of temporal arteritis.
2. Temporal arteritis presents as monocular visual loss accompanied by diffuse arthralgias and myalgias, and a stringlike, nonpulsatile temporal artery in a patient usually over 55 years of age.
3. An edematous retina with optic disc pallor may be visualized by ophthalmoscopy.

   Treatment:

   1. With headache as the only symptom, immediate treatment with prednisone 60 mg/day PO is recommended (see Chapter 3).
   2. If monocular visual loss has occurred, in order to prevent visual loss in the other eye, immediate IV corticosteroids, either methylprednisolone 120 to 500 mg IV followed by 120 mg/day, or dexamethasone 30 to 125 mg IV followed by 30 mg/day. This should be continued until ESR is normal, when the patient can then be switched to oral prednisone.

3. Temporal artery biopsy should be performed within two to three days to confirm the diagnosis.

Differential Diagnosis of Sudden Visual Loss

The sudden loss of all or part of visual function is a potential neuro-ophthalmological emergency.

1. The type of visual loss suggests the location of the disease.
   a. Monocular visual loss suggests disease of the optic nerve or globe.
   b. Partial loss in both eyes suggests CNS disease behind the optic chiasm.
2. Eye pain is associated with glaucoma, infection, or optic neuritis.
3. Transient visual loss in one eye associated with paralysis on the opposite side suggests emboli from an ulcerating plaque in the carotid artery (see Chapter 12).
4. Prodromal phenomena (zig-zag lights, stars, etc.) are seen both in CNS infarction and migraine.
5. A firm globe to palpation (tonometry is much more accurate) suggests a diagnosis of glaucoma.
6. An unreactive pupil or a Marcus-Gunn pupil (see Figure 10.1) suggests disease anterior to the optic chiasm.
7. With unilateral blindness, the cause can often be diagnosed with the ophthalmoscope:
   a. Intraocular hemorrhage
   b. Retinal detachment
   c. Emboli
   d. Retinal infarction
   e. Infection
8. A bruit over the neck raises the possibility of the carotid artery being a source of embolus to the ophthalmic artery.

Conditions Requiring Immediate Treatment

1. *Retinal artery or branch occlusion*
   A monocular defect is found in the visual field corresponding to an ischemic retina with reduced or absent arterial blood flow evident on ophthalmoscopy. Occasionally, an embolus can be visualized on ophthalmoscopy; small retinal hemorrhages and retinal edema may also be seen.

   If the blindness is transient and associated with a contralateral hemiparesis, the diagnosis of carotid artery stenosis or ulceration is strongly suggested.

   Treatment: Anticoagulants (heparin) to prevent further embolization while looking for site of origin of emboli.

2. *Optic or retrobulbar neuritis*

Subacute (over hours) unilateral or bilateral visual loss with patient complaining of eye pain with eye motion; the ophthalmologic examination may be normal; Marcus-Gunn pupil (see Figure 10.1) may be demonstrated. Unilateral optic neuritis is almost always associated with multiple sclerosis, while bilateral optic neuritis is most often associated with a toxic disturbance, such as methyl alcohol poisoning.

Treatment: If related to MS use prednisone 60 to 80 mg/day for the first ten days, then decrease by 10 mg/day every three days over 3 weeks.

Conditions Requiring Referral to an Ophthalmologist

1. *Acute glaucoma*: Usually the globe is hard (increased tension) with an unreactive dilated pupil and enlarged optic cup. Assess intraocular tension by palpation or preferably by tonometry. Sudden blindness may occur secondary to vascular occlusion due to the raised intraocular pressure.

   Treatment: Instillation of cholinergics (pilocarpine in sufficient dose to constrict the pupil); referral to an ophthalmologist to consider paracentesis of the eye.

2. *Retinal detachment*: Monocular visual loss in field corresponds to the area of retinal detachment; detachment is visible on ophthalmoscopic examination.

   Treatment: Avoid excessive head or eye movement. Refer to ophthalmologist for photocoagulation and/or surgery to prevent progression of the detachment to completion.

3. *Intraocular hemorrhage*: Monocular visual loss with blood is visible on ophthalmoscopic examination.

   Treatment: Ophthalmologic evaluation to determine cause of the bleeding and consideration of ocular paracentesis to reduce pressure.

4. *Intraocular infection*: Monocular visual loss with purulent material is evident on ophthalmoscopic examination; eye pain is common.

   Treatment: Ophthalmologic evaluation with paracentesis for culture, and immediate antibiotic treatment similar to that used for meningitis (see Chapter 14).

Neurologic Conditions That May Not Require Treatment

1. *Migraine*: A transient hemianopic field defect may occur, as well as transient monocular blindness. Headache is not invariably present, especially if this is the first presentation of migraine. The ophthalmologic examination is normal. The diagnosis is suggested by the

presence of a strong family history of migraine, use of birth control pills, or subsequent development of a unilateral throbbing headache.

Treatment: Acute treatment may not be necessary (see Chapter 3).

2. *Occipital lobe damage* presents as a binocular visual field defect, most commonly a hemianopsia from occlusion of the posterior cerebral artery; the remainder of neurologic examination may be normal. Bilateral occipital lobe damage presents as cortical blindness.

Treatment: See Chapter 12.

Severe Incapacitating Muscle Spasms

A. *Tetanus*

1. Patient has a fixed smile with teeth clenched (trismus). Remainder of muscles are in constant contraction.

2. Appears one to 54 days (in more than half of cases within 14 days) after a puncture or lacerating wound (but may appear without a demonstrable wound); especially common in older adults who have not been reimmunized for many years.

3. Autonomic disturbances may occur, resulting in cardiac arrhythmias and wide fluctuations in blood pressure.

Treatment:

1. Penicillin G should be given IV at a dose of 10 to 20 million units/day.

2. Tracheostomy should be performed in all but very mild cases. Continuous artificial ventilation is needed.

3. Analgesics should be used to relieve the pain from muscle contractions.

4. Toxin should be neutralized with human tetanus immune globulin (TIG-H) 3000 to 10,000 units IM at several sites, including the area of the presumed injury (infection).

5. Diazepam 80 to 230 mg/day is often effective in reducing spasms.

B. *Hypocalcemic Tetany*

1. Hypocalcemic tetany may be distinguished from tetanus by a milder degree of muscle spasm and by the presence of carpopedal spasm, Chvostek's sign (unilateral facial muscle spasm precipitated by tapping the facial nerve near the ear), and Trousseau's sign (carpal spasm precipitated by brief inflation above systolic pressure of a blood pressure cuff on the arm).

2. Most commonly seen in infants on cow's milk. It is important to recognize this disorder in infants because of the possible respiratory compromise and associated seizures.

3. Tetany in adults may be associated with hyperventilation syndrome (see Chapter 4).

4. Diagnosis is established by low serum calcium and high serum phosphate.

Treatment:

Slow IV administration of calcium gluconate (10% solution) should be given in severe cases (up to 10 mL in children and 30 mL in adults). Oral calcium gluconate and/or a change to commercially prepared formula feeding in the infant may be adequate treatment in milder cases.

BIBLIOGRAPHY

Cole (ed): *Harriet Lane Handbook*. Chicago, Yearbook Medical Publishers, 1984.

Orland MJ, Saltman RJ (eds): *Manual of Medical Therapeutics*. ed. 25. Boston, Little, Brown & Co, 1987.

Graef JW, Cone TE Jr: *Manual of Pediatric Therapeutics*. Boston, Little, Brown & Co, 1984.

Hyman SE: *Manual of Psychiatric Emergencies*. Boston, Little, Brown & Co, 1984.

O'Doherty DS, Fermaglich JL: *Handbook of Neurologic Emergencies*. Flushing, NY, Medical Examining Publishing Co, 1977.

Samuels MA: *Manual of Neurologic Therapeutics*. ed.2. Boston, Little, Brown & Co, 1982.

XXI

CONSIDERATIONS IN THE CARE OF PATIENTS WITH SEVERE AND IRREVERSIBLE NERVOUS SYSTEM DAMAGE

Advances in medical technology have provided clinicians with the means of preserving life at the expense of a great deal of unnecessary pain and suffering by patients. The decisions with regard to neurologic patients should be governed by the same general principles as those used in other disciplines of medicine. Usually, these problems have a way of providing their own solutions without the aid of complicated rules, regulations, and fancy machines. For example, cardiac resuscitation in patients with severe brain damage is rarely successful.

GENERAL PRINCIPLES

The following are a few principles that we feel are important in handling patients with severe and irreversible nervous system disease:

1. Always keep the family and loved ones fully informed about the patient's condition. Avoid technical jargon such as, "The cerebral angiogram showed bilateral cerebral hemisphere infarction"; preferable would be a statement such as, "When we injected dye into the arteries of the brain, we found that no blood is reaching those parts of the brain which control movement and thought. Without blood, brain tissue dies and does not have the capability of recovering."
2. Families relate better to one physician than to a team, which may seem to the family to be giving conflicting information.

357

3. Families and patients must be involved in the decision-making process. The physician has the responsibility to provide clearly and simply the facts that are necessary to make a decision. Often it is appropriate to give the family advice as to what action to take in a particular situation. The wishes of the patient and the family take precedence over the physician's preference.

4. Consider the quality of life before the current neurologic disability; for example, the patient with a clearly documented severe dementia who develops a sudden left hemiparesis may not need more than fluid and nutritional support.

5. Consider the quality of life after the neurologic disability; for example, most physicians do not provide respiratory support to patients with end-stage ALS or muscular dystrophy. A patient with ALS on a respirator faces the prospect of consciously watching the body wither away until the individual becomes little more than a "living uncommunicative brain in a fishbowl."

6. All discussions and decisions should be carefully documented in the hospital record.

7. The physician should promote the use of traditional patient and family support systems such as clergy, close friends, and fraternal organizations during times of severe stress.

8. Cases of suspected homicide, assault, child abuse, and the like require that the physician use special care in the decision-making process, and it is always wise to seek additional (including legal) opinions.

BRAIN DEATH

Once artificial life support systems have been instituted and irreversible coma or brain death is suspected, state and/or local hospital criteria for discontinuing respiratory support should be followed. These criteria often include recommendations from multiple consultants (medical and sometimes clergy and legal).

Human death is the irreversible loss of the capacity for consciousness and the capacity to breathe. Guidelines have evolved since the late 1960s for the determination of brain death:

1. Brain death is defined as the *irreversible cessation* of all clinically ascertainable functions of the entire brain, including the brainstem (but not necessarily including the spinal cord).

2. Cessation of brain function is interpreted as both:

   a. Cerebral unreceptivity and unresponsivity

   b. Absent brainstem reflexes

   Note: Spinal cord activity (reflexes) and peripheral nervous system activity may persist after brain death.

3. Minimal accepted clinical neurologic findings are:

   a. No spontaneous movement and no movement elicited by painful stimuli to the face or trunk (see Chapter 13).

   b. Pupils fully dilated or midposition and totally unreactive to light (examine under magnification with a bright light in a darkened room).

   c. Absence of oculocephalic (doll's eye) and oculovestibular (caloric) responses (see Chapter 13), absent corneal reflex, absent pharyngeal reflex (insertion and removal of a nasopharyngeal suction tube should not produce a cough or gag), and absent cough reflex (after suctioning and/or irrigation of the endotracheal tube). There should be no spontaneous blinking (eye opening) or swallowing.

   d. No spontaneous respirations (apnea) after the arterial carbon dioxide partial pressure (P_aCO_2) has reached a level that provides maximal respiratory stimulus (about 60 torr). Apnea testing should be performed with a protocol that permits pretest hyperoxygenation, exposure of the tracheobronchial tree to oxygen during the test, and monitoring of arterial P_aCO_2 levels (average rise of 4 torr/min during apnea).

4. Irreversibility is interpreted to mean:

   a. The *cause* of the coma is established, is sufficient to account for the coma, and is not a reversible condition.

   Caution: The frequent reversible conditions of metabolic and/or drug (sedative) intoxication, hypothermia, neuromuscular blockade, and shock must be excluded.

   b. The possibility of recovery of any brain function is excluded. Demonstration of a lack of blood flow to the brain is confirmation of irreversibility.

   Caution: Conventional cerebral angiography may falsely demonstrate flow in a brain-dead patient due to excessive injection pressure forcing dye into the intracranial vessels or injection with the head in a dependent position allowing contrast material to leak into vessels.

   c. The cessation of all brain function persists for an adequate observation period (six hours with confirmatory tests, 12 to 24 hours in the absence of confirmatory tests).

5. Confirmation of electrocerebral silence by EEG performed at least six hours after loss of clinically ascertainable brain function is desirable when confirmatory documentation is needed to substantiate the clinical findings.

   Caution: EEG tracings must be carried out utilizing the technical guidelines established by the American Electroencephalographic Society. These guidelines have been established to ensure that tracings for electrocerebral silence are not marred by artifacts and that all measures to maximize recording of minimal cerebral electrical activity have been performed.

Usually, if everything has been done by a registered EEG technologist (REEGT), and interpreted by an experienced electroencephalographer, this is assurance enough that the guidelines have been followed.

Note:
  a. Electrocerebral silence tracings may be seen in the potentially reversible situations:
     i. Barbiturate intoxication
     ii. Hypothermia
     iii. Such tracings may also be noted in the premature and full-term infant who is not brain dead.
  b. Brainstem auditory-evoked responses may also be used in the diagnosis of brain death. It is known that brainstem auditory-evoked responses can be present while an EEG shows electrocerebral silence, but may finally disappear when medullary function ceases.

6. Before respiratory support is discontinued, the family must be carefully informed of the situation.

7. Guidelines for the determination of brain death in children under the age of 5 years are still in the process of development. Clinical criteria similar to those in use for patients over age five years have been found to be applicable to infants and term newborns (38 weeks gestational age) older than 7 days of age. It has been recommended that two EEG tracings be performed in children under 1 year of age with these EEG tracings separated by an interval of 48 hours in those 7 days to 2 months of age and by an interval of 24 hours in those 2 months to 1 year of age. Beyond 1 year of age, laboratory tests are not necessary if an irreversible cause exists and clinical criteria for brain death are met.

BIBLIOGRAPHY

A definition of irreversible coma: Report of Ad Hoc Committee of the Harvard Medical School to Examine the Definition of Brain Death. *JAMA* 1968; 205:337-340.

American EEG Society: Minimum technical standards for EEG recording in suspected cerebral death, in Klass DW, Daly DD (eds): *Current Practice of Clinical Electroencephalography*. New York, Raven Press, 1979, pp 492-496.

Black PMcL: Brain death. *N Engl J Med* 1978;299:338-344, 393-401.

Goldie WD, Chiappa KH, Young RR, et al: Brainstem auditory and short-latency somatosensory evoked responses in brain death. *Neurology* 1981; 31:248-256.

Guidelines for the determination of death: Report of the Medical Consultants on the Diagnosis of Death to the President's Commission for the Study of Ethical Problems in Medicine and Biomedical and Behavioral Research. *JAMA* 1981; 246:2184-2186.

Kaufman HH, Beresford R, Bernat JL, et al: Brain death. *Neurol Neurosurg Update Ser* 1986;6:1-8.

Mosh SL, Alvarez LA: Diagnosis of brain death in children. *J Clin Neurophysiol* 1986;3:239-249.

Rowland TW, Donnelly JH, Jackson AH: Apnea documentation for determination of brain death in children. *Pediatrics* 1984;74:505-508.

Schwartz JA, Baxter J, Brill DR: Diagnosis of brain death in children by radionuclide cerebral imaging. *Pediatrics* 1984;73:14-18.

Task Force for the Determination of Brain Death in Children: Guidelines for the determination of brain death in children. *Ann Neurol* 1987;22:616-617.

Youngner SJ, Bartlett ET: Human death and high technology: the failure of the whole-brain formulations. *Ann Intern Med* 1983;99:252-258.

APPENDIX A
AUDIOLOGIC TEST BATTERY

Speech discrimination. Measures the patient's ability to repeat monosyllabic words spoken to the patient at a comfortable listening level. Considered abnormal if reduced scores are obtained in the absence of significant hearing loss. More sensitive if a competing noise is presented in conjunction with the words. An abnormal test suggests a lesion proximal to the cochlea.

Tone decay. Determines whether abnormal adaptation occurs over a one-minute period to a continuous tone. The signal is increased in 5-dB intervals each time the tone becomes inaudible. If the signal must be increased more than 25 dB at one particular frequency, then a lesion is suggested proximal to the cochlea.

SISI (short increment sensitivity index). Determines the ability to detect 1 dB increments of sounds in the presence of a continuous tone that is 20 dB above threshold. Patient with lesions proximal to the cochlea will have difficulty detecting these sound increments.

ABLB (alternate binaural loudness balance). A pure tone is presented alternately to the patient's ears. The intensity is held constant in the affected ear, and the patient is asked to balance the intensity in the normal ear. An increase in intensity is perceived louder in the abnormal ear and is known as recruitment. This is seen in cochlear lesions.

Békésy audiometry. Measures perceived differences in a continuous versus a pulsed tone. Tracings are usually categorized into five types:

Type I
No differences are perceived (seen in normal individual or patients with conductive hearing loss)

Type II
Continual and pulsed tones are heard equally at low frequency; at high frequencies (> 1000 to 5000 Hz) the continual tone is heard with greater difficulty (threshold higher) than the pulsed tone by 10 to 20 dB; this suggests a cochlear lesion

Type III
Continual and pulsed tones are heard equally at low frequencies but at high frequencies the continual tone is heard with extreme difficulty (threshold rapidly rises); this suggests a lesion proximal to the cochlea

Type IV
The continual tone is heard with greater difficulty at both high and low frequencies (by 10 to 20 dB); the tracings for the two tones are parallel; this tracing suggests a cochlear lesion

362

Type V

The patient always hears the continual tone better than the pulsed tone; this is physiologically impossible and suggests malingering.

Impedance tympanometry. The ability of the tympanic membrane to move is measured by varying air pressures: Little movement suggests otosclerosis or middle ear infection and a flaccid drum suggests that the middle ear bones are not properly connected.

Stapedial reflexes. A loud noise in one ear should normally cause the stapedius muscles in both ears to contract. If this does not happen, there is likely to be a problem (such as an acoustic neuroma) in the internal auditory canal.

Stapedial reflex decay. Normally, the stapedius muscle should be able to contract for 10 seconds in the presence of a loud sound; if it does not, a problem in the internal auditory canal (such as an acoustic neuroma) is suggested.

Appendix B

"Routine" Mental Status Examination

1. *Memory*

    a. *Immediate recall*: Have the patient repeat after the examiner, a series of numbers starting with a series of three numbers and continuing until the patient fails twice. For example, if the patient fails to repeat six digits forward 2 times, the score would be 5.

    b. *Recent memory*: The patient should be able to remember three unrelated words for three minutes (for example, "fox," "car," "blue"). When these words are initially given, the patient should be told that he will be asked to recall them. Additionally, in obtaining the patient's history, questions regarding the last few hours (if the examiner can confirm the facts) are also indicative of recent memory ability.

    c. *Remote memory*: Testing of remote memory can be incorporated with obtaining family and social histories. Information such as the patient's age, date of birth, number and order of siblings, marriage date, and number and names of children is appropriate. The examiner may also use readily available historical facts.

2. *Ability to follow instructions* can usually be assessed during physical and neurologic examination.

3. *General information*: Rather than asking questions that are indicative of education and reminiscent of school examinations, it is as meaningful and less threatening to ask about the patient's occupation or hobbies. The patient should discuss either with interest and reasonable knowledge. Another useful line of questioning may concern a favorite television show and the plot from a recent episode. This combines recent memory with the ability to tell a story and may give insight into the patient's character as well.

4. *Calculation*: Simple, everyday problems of calculation should be used such as, "If a man buys 6 cents worth of stamps and gives the clerk 10 cents, how much change should he get back?" or "A newsman collected 25 cents from each of six customers. What is the total amount he collected?"

    Note: Serial-sevens (subtracting seven from 100 and continuing to subtract seven from each number obtained) is *not* a simple calculation problem. It involves calculation as well as recent memory and ability to concentrate. Even normal patients may have difficulty with serial-sevens under stress. Also, poorly educated normal individuals may be unable to perform this task.

5. *Judgment and abstract thinking* are difficult to assess but may be the earliest functions to be impaired. Evidence of poor judgment often can be

obtained by a history of occupational performance and daily activities. The following questions also may be useful:

a. "If you traveled to an unfamiliar city to visit a friend, how would you go about finding him?"

b. "If you got into your car one morning to go to work and it didn't start, what would you do?"

Another useful test involves similarities and differences. Ask the patient how two items are alike, such as an orange and a banana, a dog and a lion, or a coat and a dress; the best answers would be conceptual ones such as fruit, animals, or clothing, while concrete answers may be given such as both are edible, have four legs, or have sleeves. Patients with dementia often can give differences, but not similarities.

> *Note*: Interpretation of proverbs such as "People who live in glass houses shouldn't throw stones" or "A golden hammer breaks an iron door" is often used by physicians as a test of judgment, but may be difficult even for normal individuals, especially if they are from a different cultural background.

Six Item Orientation-Memory-Concentration Test
(Mini Mental Status Test)

This simple test, easily administered by a nonphysician, discriminates between mild, moderate, and severe cognitive defects. The results correlate with Alzheimer neuritic plaque counts at autopsy and accurately predict scores on a more comprehensive mental status questionnaire. Normal subjects have a weighted score of 6 or less; scores greater than 10 are consistent with a dementing process and a completely demented patient would have a score of 28.

Item	Instruction	Maximum Error	Raw Error Score	Weighting Factor	Weighted Error Score
1	What year is it now?	1	_____	X 4	= _____
2	What month is it now?	1	_____	X 3	= _____
3	Repeat this phrase after me: John Brown, 42 Market Street, Chicago (memory phrase)	1	_____	X 3	= _____
4	Count backward 20 to 1	2	_____	X 2	= _____
5	Say the months in reverse order	2	_____	X 2	= _____
6	Repeat the memory phrase	5	_____	X 2	= _____

Score 1 for each incorrect response; maximum weighted error score = 28

APPENDIX C

International Classification of Seizures (Modified)

I. Generalized seizures

Primary - absences, tonic-clonic convulsions, akinetic, myoclonic, clonic, tonic

Secondary - partial onset, secondarily generalized

II. Partial (focal) seizures

Simple - motor, sensory

Complex (psychomotor, temporal lobe)

International Classification of Epilepsy (Modified)

Primary (idiopathic) generalized epilepsy

  Petit mal epilepsy

  Grand mal epilepsy

Primary (idiopathic) partial epilepsy

  Benign centrotemporal epilepsy

Secondary (symptomatic) generalized epilepsy

  Infantile spasms syndrome

  Lennox-Gastaut syndrome

Secondary (symptomatic) partial epilepsy

  Simple partial epilepsy (focal motor, jacksonian)

  Complex partial epilepsy (psychomotor, temporal lobe)

APPENDIX D
Head Circumference Charts

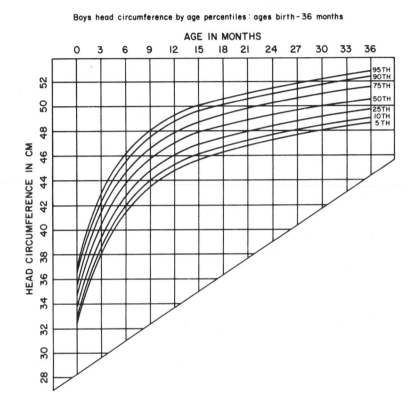

Boys head circumference by age percentiles: ages birth-36 months

Growth charts courtesy of National Center for Health Statistics: NSCH Growth Charts, 1976. Monthly Vital Statistics Report, Volume 3, Supplement (HRA) 76-1120 Health Resources Administration, Rockville, Maryland.

GROWTH CHARTS*

Girls head circumference by age percentiles : ages birth - 36 months

Denver Developmental Test

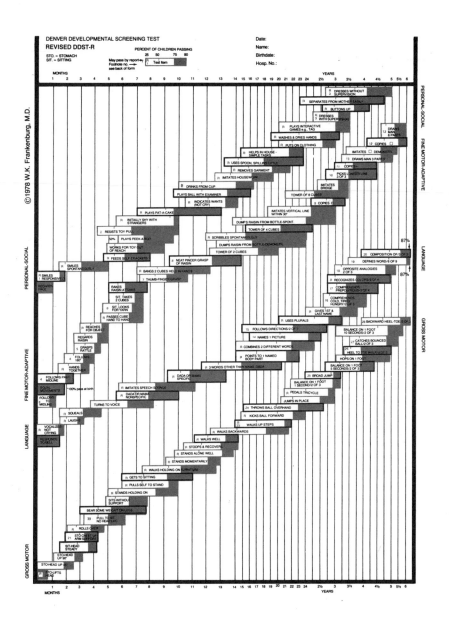

By William K. Frankenburg, MD, and Josiah B. Dodds, PhD, University of Colorado Medical Center.

1. Try to get child to smile by smiling, talking or waving to him. Do not touch him.
2. When child is playing with toy, pull it away from him. Pass if he resists.
3. Child does not have to be able to tie shoes or button in the back.
4. Move yarn slowly in an arc from one side to the other, about 6" above child's face. Pass if eyes follow 90° to midline. (Past midline; 180°)
5. Pass if child grasps rattle when it is touched to the backs or tips of fingers.
6. Pass if child continues to look where yarn disappeared or tries to see where it went. Yarn should be dropped quickly from sight from tester's hand without arm movement.
7. Pass if child picks up raisin with any part of thumb and a finger.
8. Pass if child picks up raisin with the ends of thumb and index finger using an over hand approach.

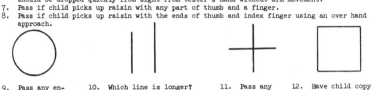

9. Pass any enclosed form. Fail continuous round motions.
10. Which line is longer? (Not bigger.) Turn paper upside down and repeat. (3/3 or 5/6)
11. Pass any crossing lines.
12. Have child copy first. If failed, demonstrate

When giving items 9, 11 and 12, do not name the forms. Do not demonstrate 9 and 11.

13. When scoring, each pair (2 arms, 2 legs, etc.) counts as one part.
14. Point to picture and have child name it. (No credit is given for sounds only.)

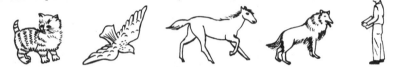

15. Tell child to: Give block to Mommie; put block on table; put block on floor. Pass 2 of 3. (Do not help child by pointing, moving head or eyes.)
16. Ask child: What do you do when you are cold? ..hungry? ..tired? Pass 2 of 3.
17. Tell child to: Put block on table; under table; in front of chair, behind chair. Pass 3 of 4. (Do not help child by pointing, moving head or eyes.)
18. Ask child: If fire is hot, ice is ?; Mother is a woman, Dad is a ?; a horse is big, a mouse is ?. Pass 2 of 3.
19. Ask child: What is a ball? ..lake? ..desk? ..house? ..banana? ..curtain? ..ceiling? ..hedge? ..pavement? Pass if defined in terms of use, shape, what it is made of or general category (such as banana is fruit, not just yellow). Pass 6 of 9.
20. Ask child: What is a spoon made of? ..a shoe made of? ..a door made of? (No other objects may be substituted.) Pass 3 of 3.
21. When placed on stomach, child lifts chest off table with support of forearms and/or hands.
22. When child is on back, grasp his hands and pull him to sitting. Pass if head does not hang back.
23. Child may use wall or rail only, not person. May not crawl.
24. Child must throw ball overhand 3 feet to within arm's reach of tester.
25. Child must perform standing broad jump over width of test sheet. (8-1/2 inches)
26. Tell child to walk forward, ⇐⇒⇐⇒⇐⇒→ heel within 1 inch of toe. Tester may demonstrate. Child must walk 4 consecutive steps, 2 out of 3 trials.
27. Bounce ball to child who should stand 3 feet away from tester. Child must catch ball with hands, not arms, 2 out of 3 trials.
28. Tell child to walk backward, ←⇐⇒⇐⇒⇐⇒ toe within 1 inch of heel. Tester may demonstrate. Child must walk 4 consecutive steps, 2 out of 3 trials.

DATE AND BEHAVIORAL OBSERVATIONS (how child feels at time of test, relation to tester, attention span, verbal behavior, self-confidence, etc,):

SUGGESTED READINGS FOR PARENTS

Down's Syndrome

Horrobin JM, Rynders JE: *To Give an Edge: A Guide for New Parents of Down's Syndrome Children.* Minneapolis, The Colwell Press, Inc, 1978.

Hunt N: *The World of Nigel Hunt. The Diary of a Mongoloid Youth.* New York, Garrett Publications, 1967.

Roberts N: *David.* Richmond, Va, John Knox Press, 1968.

Hearing-Impaired and Speech-Handicapped Child

Semple JE: *The Hearing-Impaired Preschool Child.* Springfield, Ill, Charles C Thomas, 1970.

Van Riper C: *Your Child's Speech Problems: A Guide for Parents.* New York, Harper & Row, 1961.

Autism

Greenfeld J: *A Child Called Noah.* New York, Pocket Books, 1970.

Morgan SB: Helping parents understand the diagnosis of autism. *Dev Behav Pediatrics* 1984;5:68-85.

Retarded Child

Blodgett HE: *Mentally Retarded Children: What Parents and Others Should Know.* Minneapolis, University of Minnesota Press, 1971.

Buckler B: *Living with a Mentally Retarded Child: A Primer for Parents.* New York, Hawthorn Books, 1971.

Carlson BW, Ginglend D: *Play Activities for the Retarded Child.* Nashville, Abingdon Press, 1961.

Dittman LL: *The Mentally Retarded Child at Home, A Manual for Parents.* Children's Bureau Publications. No. 374-1959. Superintendent of Documents, U.S. Government Printing Office.

What Everyone Should Know About Mental Retardation. A Scriptographic Booklet. South Deerfield, Mass, Channing L. Bete Co, 1978.

Hyperactivity (Attentional Deficit Disorder with Hyperactivity)

Silver L: *Attention Deficit Disorders.* Summit, NY, CIBA Pharmaceutical Co, 1980.

Stewart MA, Olds SW: *Raising a Hyperactive Child.* New York, Harper & Row, 1974.

Tonner L: *The Difficult Child.* Des Plaines, Ill, Bantam Books, 1985.

Learning Disabilities

Clarke L: *Can't Read, Can't Write, Can't Talk Too Good Either*. Baltimore, Md, Penguin Books, 1974.

The Journal of Learning Disabilities, 101 East Ontario St, Chicago, IL 60611

McCarthy JJ, McCarthy JF: *Learning Disabilities*. Boston, Allyn & Bacon, 1969.

Ross AO: *Learning Disability: The Unrealized Potential*. New York, McGraw-Hill Book Co, 1977.

Cerebral Palsy (Static Congenital Encephalopathy)

Cruickshank W (ed): *Cerebral Palsy, A Developmental Disability*, ed 3. Syracuse, Syracuse University Press, 1976.

Behavior Management

Becker WC: *Parents Are Teachers*. Champaign, IL, Research Press, 1971.

Carter R: *Help! These Kids Are Driving Me Crazy*. Champaign, IL, Research Press, 1972.

Deibert AN, Harmon AJ: *New Tools for Changing Behavior*. Champaign, IL, Research Press, 1970.

Smith JM, Smith DEP: *Child Management: A Program for Parents and Teachers*. Champaign, IL, Research Press, 1976.

APPENDIX E

Exercises for the Lower Part of the Back

At the beginning do each exercise 5 times, twice each day. As strength is gained, increase the number of times and intensity of each exercise. Do the first four exercises for 2 weeks, then do the next four for 2 weeks, then the last four for 2 weeks. Then after 1 month off (no exercises), repeat the cycle.

Exercises

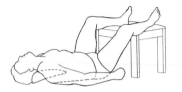

1. Lying on back, place legs up on a stool, with a folded towel between the shoulders and arms at the sides; hold this position for five minutes.

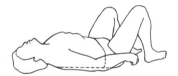

2. Lying on back with knees bent and feet flat on floor; (a) inhale and draw in entire abdomen, (b) exhale and force lower back to the ground. Keep abdomen in and chest up.

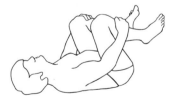

3. Lying on back: Draw both knees toward the chest and then grasp knees with hands and pull them toward chest.

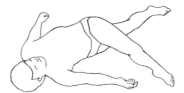

4. Lying on the back, legs extended and wide apart: Roll hips completely over and touch right foot to floor across left; repeat using left foot.

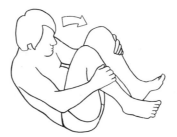

5. Lying on the back: Draw both knees to chest, and then roll forward and up to the sitting position.

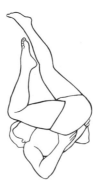

6. Lying on the back: Raise the knees high and well up over the chest and head (may prop hips with hands), then move legs slowly in large circles as in bicycle riding.

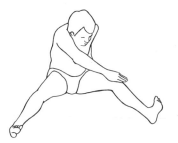

7. Sitting on the floor with legs spread and toes turned in, arms raised at the sides to shoulder height: (a) Swing right hand to left foot, left arm behind; (b) return and swing left hand to the right foot.

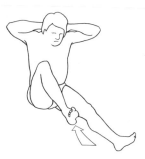

8. Sitting on the floor with legs straight, hands folded behind the neck: Bring one knee at a time (alternately) up to chest without changing the position of the trunk.

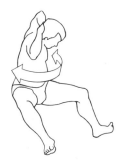

9. Sitting on the floor with hands folded behind the neck keeping the head erect, chest held high and elbows well back: Slowly twist the trunk as far as possible to the right; then return and twist the trunk to the left.

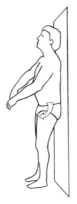

10. Stand against a wall, with heels 4 in. from the wall and with head, shoulder, and hips touching the wall; pull in abdomen and push lower back against the wall.

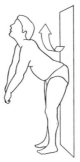

11. Stand 4 in. away from the wall. Bend the body forward at the hips with the back arched, then slowly straighten up until the lower back, shoulders, and head touch the wall.

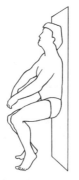

12. Standing with the back against the wall, raise up on the toes and bend knees (knees together and back straight) to perform a deep knee bend; then straighten legs to resume standing position.

INDEX

Abdominal reflex, figure, 300
Acetest tablets, 28
Acetoacetic acid, 27
Achilles reflex, figure, 199
Acoustic neuroma, 59
Acquired immunodeficiency syndrome (AIDS), 217, 222–223, 234
Active jaw reflex, 82
Acycloguanosine, 221
Acyclovir, 221, 225
Advanced sleep–phase syndrome, 76
Affective disorders, 71, 119
AIDS. *See* Acquired immunodeficiency syndrome
Akathisia, 108, 136
Al-Anon, 119
Al-Ateen, 119
Alcohol abuse, 70, 79
  blackouts, 113–114
  clinical clues to, 112, 113
  in dementia, 86
  diagnosis of, 110–114
  nutritional diseases with, 117–118
  peripheral neuropathy associated with, 117–118
  questions to ask patient, 111–112
  withdrawal syndrome, 114–117
Alcoholic cerebellar degeneration, 118
Alcoholic dementia, 118
Alcoholic hallucinosis, 115
Alcoholic myopathy, 118
Alcoholics Anonymous (AA), 119
Allergies, 63
Alzheimer's disease, 88, 89, 96, 276
Alzheimer's Disease and Related Disorders Association, 89
Amantadine hydrochloride, 98, 143
Amaurosis fugax, 175
Aminoglycosides, 60
Amitriptyline, 40
Amitriptyline hydrochloride, 36, 124, 143, 285
A-mode echoencephalography, 25
Amphetamines, 134
Ampicillin, 40, 61
Amyotropic lateral sclerosis (ALS), 24, 235–236, 324
Anemia, 63
Aneurysm, posterior communication artery, 352
Ankylosing spondylitis, 310

Anterior horn cell disease, 227
Anticholinergic psychosis, 124
Anticoagulation, in treatment of stroke, 182
Anticonvulsants, 157–163
  weaning from, 163–164
Antigen-antibody studies, 206
Antihistamines, 39, 61
Antipyrine, 27
Antisocial personality, 137
Antispasticity agents, 143
Antivert, 55
Anxiety, 126–128
Aphasia, 134, 185–188
  anomic, 186, 188
  Broca's, 186–187
  global, 187
  summary of language problems, table, 186
  Wernicke's, 187
Argyll Robertson pupil, 87
Arsenic, 233
Arthritis, inflammation of, 328
Association for Children with Learning Disability, 291
Astereognosis, 140
Asterixis, figure, 102
Atenolol, 35, 114
Athetosis, 92
Atrophy, of arms with spasticity of legs, table, 324
Attentional/activity disorder with hyperactivity, 285–287
Attention deficit disorder (ADD), 281, 289
Audiograms, pure tone, 59
Audiologic tests, 362–363
Aura, 32, 56
  uncinate, 156
Autism, infantile, 284–285

Babinski reflex, 6–7, 9, 88, 140
Back pain
  clinical investigations of, 301–302
  emotional disorders causing, 313
  examination of patient, 294–301
  exercises for, 373–376
  forming a hypothesis for, 294
  history of patient, 293
  inflammatory disease affecting spine, 310–311
  intraspinal or spinal neoplasm, 311–312